Peter A. Reichart/Hans P. Philipsen
Odontogenic Tumors and Allied Lesions

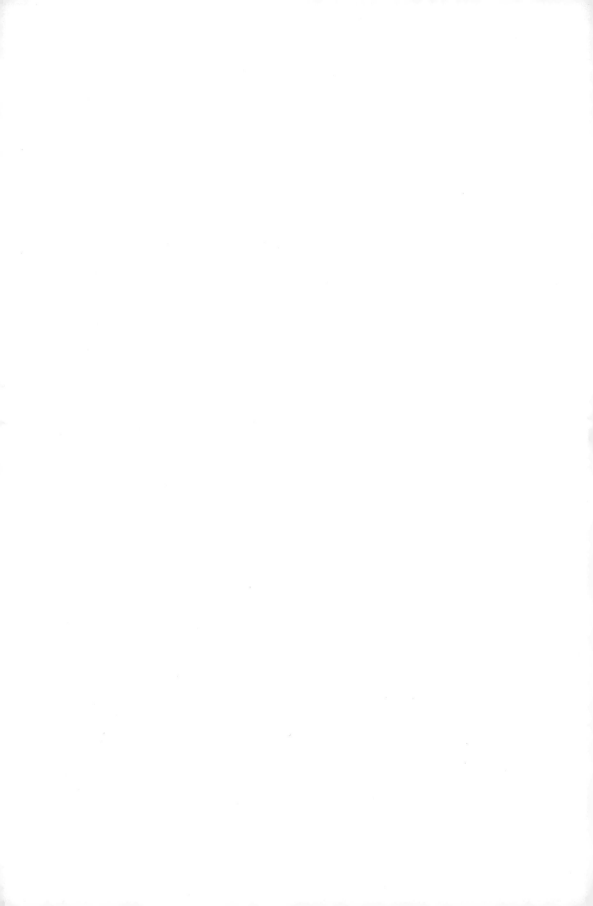

DATE OF RETURN
UNLESS RECALLED BY LIBRARY

PLEASE TAKE GOOD CARE OF THIS BOOK

Odontogenic Tumors and Allied Lesions

Prof Dr Peter A. Reichart
Humboldt-University of Berlin
Berlin, Germany

Prof Dr odont Hans P. Philipsen
Guadalmina Alta, Spain

Quintessence Publishing Co Ltd

London, Berlin, Chicago, Copenhagen, Paris, Milan, Barcelona,
Istanbul, São Paulo, Tokyo, New Delhi, Moscow, Prague, Warsaw

British Library Cataloguing in Publication Data

Reichart, P. (Peter)
   Odontogenic tumors and allied lesions
    1. Odontogenic tumors 2. Odontogenic cysts 3. Jaws – Cancer
    I. Title II. Philipsen, H. P. (Hans P.)
    616.9'92314

ISBN 1850970599

Quintessence Publishing Co, Ltd
Grafton Road
New Malden, Surrey KT3 3AB
United Kingdom
www.quintpub.co.uk

ISBN 1-85097-059-9

Contents

Foreword

In the years since the Second World War, and particularly in the past three decades, there have been considerable advances in understanding of the natural history, structure and behaviour of the odontogenic tumors. Prior to this, there was of course interest in the subject and attempts were made to classify them in a logical manner. As early as 1887, Bland-Sutton had proposed subdividing the 'odontomes' into those arising from aberrations of the enamel organ, aberrations of the follicle, of the papilla, and aberrations of the whole tooth germ. He also included a fifth group of anomalous odontomes. The report of the British Dental Association, published in 1914 and authored by Gabell, James and Payne, included both radicular and dentigerous cysts as odontomes, and also grouped the lesions into three categories, those of epithelial, composite and connective tissue origin.

The 1946 classification published by Thoma and Goldman separated the odontogenic tumors into those of ectodermal, mesodermal and mixed origin. This was widely accepted in textbooks and formed the basis of the 1950 classification approved by the American Academy of Oral Pathology.

In 1958, Pindborg and Clausen (Finn Prætorius) proposed a classification that separated the epithelial odontogenic tumors into two groups according to whether or not there were inductive changes in the connective tissue. This concept was developed and modified by an international panel of oral and anatomical pathologists appointed by the World Health Organization and chaired by Jens Pindborg. Their recommendations were published in 1971 in the work *Histological Typing of Odontogenic Tumours, Jaw Cysts, and Allied Lesions.* These proposals were refined further in 1992 in the Second Edition of this WHO series under the simpler heading *Histological Typing of Odontogenic Tumours.* This 1992 classification classified both benign and malignant odontogenic tumors into those of odontogenic epithelium without odontogenic ectomesenchyme, those of odontogenic epithelium with odontogenic ectomesenchyme, and those of odontogenic ectomesenchyme.

Contemporaneously, large numbers of clinicopathological and laboratory studies of the range of odontogenic tumors have been published in peer-reviewed journals, contributing greatly to our understanding of these lesions. Peter Reichart and Hans Peter Philipsen, the authors of this book, have themselves made valuable contributions to scholarship in this field in a series of meticulously documented reviews and descriptions of topics such as the ameloblastoma, unicystic ameloblastoma, desmoplastic ameloblastoma, adenomatoid odontogenic tumor, and most recently a suggestion for revisions of the 1992 WHO classification. It is worth recording here that it was Philipsen who, with Birn, introduced the term adenomatoid odontogenic tumor in 1969. Philipsen also named and described the odontogenic keratocyst in 1956 while still a senior dental student working in Jens Pindborg's department in Copenhagen.

This productive academic partnership of Reichart and Philipsen has harnessed the talents of a skillful clinician-pathologist with those of an experienced and innovative oral pathologist. Both are meticulous in the accumulation and presentation of their published material. Their recently published book *Color Atlas of Dental Medicine - Oral Pathology*, Georg Thieme Verlag (publisher) Stuttgart, New York 1999, was an exquisite-ly produced authoritative work which promises to become a collector's item.

The present book has the same promise. It devotes a separate chapter to each of the odontogenic tumors, and includes descriptions and illustrations of clinical features, radiology, pathogenesis, pathology, with notes on treatment and prognosis. I have very much enjoyed reading the pre-publication proofs of a book that will be an invaluable teaching, diagnostic and research resource.

Prof. em. Mervyn Shear
Simonstown
Republic of South Africa

Preface

We have made an effort to present the chapters of this book in a uniform and easy-to-use format. In some instances, however, we have had to deviate from the "beaten track" and introduce an extra paragraph or section when appropriate. The terminology of the chapter titles may not immediately be familiar to you. We have a priori chosen the terms agreed on today by a majority of investigators, and those we, based on the most recent suggestions, find the most appropriate. The subtitle (in brackets) may, however, be met with a nod of recognition.

The reader will appreciate that the tumors and lesions covered in the text are rare in relation to the frequency of benign and malignant tumors in all locations; Baden[1] gave a conservative estimate of about 0.002% to 0.003% of all surgicals received in large centers. If only neoplasms were considered, the frequency would increase to about 0.006%. Bhaskar[2] found that odontogenic tumors comprise 2.4% of all lesions biopsied in a dental office. A more recent comparable figure from Mexico City[3] was 2.5%.

Odontogenic tumors, neoplasms, and other lesions related to the jawbones have for years been recognized as presenting clinical, radiologic, and histopathologic challenges. The first appearance of World Health Organization (WHO) Histologic Typing of Odontogenic Tumors in 1971[4] made a marked impact on the general interest in the study of this particular field of oral pathology,

as witnessed by a rather steep increase in publications on lesions covered by the classification. The purpose of the WHO classifications was clearly expressed by Kramer et al[5] when they wrote the following: "The publications in the series International Histological Classification of Tumours are not intended to serve as textbooks, but rather to facilitate the adoption of a uniform terminology that will facilitate and improve communication among cancer workers. For this reason literature references have been omitted and readers should refer to standard works for bibliographies."

There is no doubt that the publication of the WHO classifications intensified the zeal for doing research in the field of odontogenic tumors and publishing the results, because terminology and a diagnostic framework were now available. We have, however, generally been disappointed in trying to trace "standard works for bibliographies." A true standard work on odontogenic tumors does not exist, apart from Baden's, which is now 30 years old but was comprehensive at the time.

We undertook to write this book because we felt a need to fill this gap by compiling the increasing amount of data within this field. What initiated thoughts of embarking on this project were both the innumerable times we had to look up passages in the blue WHO books over the years and the fact that we did not always agree with the authors. Having devoted many years of research to this field and having coauthored and published a considerable number of related articles, we regarded ourselves as reasonably competent to do the job. Now, our readers—undergraduate and postgraduate students, surgeons, radiologists, oral as well as general pathologists, and anyone doing research in this field—have to judge whether we have, not accomplished, but at least approached the task.

The references in each chapter have been selected based on their merit of priority or their inclusion of a recent, thorough review of the condition in question. We hope that the mention of appropriate literature will stimulate further studies of the many types of lesions. The reader will realize that, in the vast majority of the lesions discussed, there is a strong need for more case reports and, for the more common lesions, a need for smaller or larger series of studies. It is our experience that for the latter category it is of great importance to present data in detail, including all relevant information for each and every patient.

The information presented in this book is taken from previously published cases. Such a retrospective approach suffers from several disadvantages, including the inconsistency of both the data provided in the different articles and the classifications used. We regret to say that this is the best we can do at present. Significant additional knowledge about the biologic profile of odontogenic tumors and other lesions of the jaws would be gained from a large prospective study in which such variables as clinical features, microscopic diagnosis, treatment, and follow-up can be accurately recorded. To establish a prospective study would, however, be difficult because the rarity of a considerable number of lesions would necessitate multi-institutional cooperation if sufficient examples are to be obtained. It may seem an insurmountable task to engage in such a project. However, we believe that it is very desirable to learn more about the lesions described in the present book. It surely can be done, provided that financial support can be obtained, but it must be appreciated that very few of these tumors and conditions constitute a public health problem.

We consider the preparation of this book to be a great academic challenge and the final result as a valuable, practical aid in the early diagnosis of odontogenic tumors and lesions. As readers will see, the number of new entities, additional subvariants of existing lesions, and modified concepts have increased substantially during the period (1971–1992) between the first and second editions of the WHO classifications. The amount of new knowledge accumulated in the field since 1992 is quite astonishing and, already at this stage, there seems to be a need for a revision of the definitions of odontogenic tumors and allied lesions as suggested in chapter 2.

This book includes an extensive number of illustrations, most of which have been collected by the authors over more than three decades. As is well known to all those who have dealt with the diagnosis and treatment of odontogenic neoplasms, some of these (such as odontomas) are relatively common, while others are exceedingly rare and one may see only one or two cases of them during a professional lifetime. While we were able to illustrate most of the common tumors quite well, our material on rare lesions was not always sufficient. So we asked our colleagues around the world to provide us with needed examples, including clinical radiographs, computed tomographs, and magnetic resonance images, as well as histologic slides and photomicrographs of particular lesions.

We would like to express our sincere gratitude and thanks to all who have helped us so generously. The following colleagues provided radiographic illustrations, histologic slides, or photomicrographs: Prof M. Altini, Johannesburg, Republic of South Africa; Prof E. Ariji, Japan; Prof A. Eckardt, Hannover, Germany; Prof G. Jundt, Basle, Switzerland; Prof C. Opitz, Berlin, Germany; Prof R.J. Radlanski, Berlin, Germany; Prof J. Reibel, Copenhagen, Denmark; Prof J.J. Sciubba, Baltimore, USA; Prof I. van der Waal, Amsterdam, The Netherlands; Prof W. Wagner, Mainz, Germany; Prof J. Wolf, Berlin, Germany.

The photographic documentation would not have been possible without the dedicated professionalism of photographers J. Eckert and R. Hoey. The graphic art was done by W. Lorenz. We express our sincere gratitude to these three individuals.

Our thanks also go to Ilona Trettin, our secretary, who never got tired of making yet another correction and addition to the text. We are also grateful for her skillful preparation of the bar graphs for the individual chapters. Also, we would like to thank Sylvia Kaatz for helping to retrieve references in the different libraries of Berlin.

In particular, we would like to express our gratitude to the publisher of Quintessence, Herrn Haase, and all his wonderful coworkers who made this project possible.

Finally, we are very grateful to our wives, Kirsten and Barbara, who supported us during the years it took to finish this book.

Hans P. Philipsen,
Guadalmina Alta, Spain

Peter A. Reichart,
Berlin, Germany

July 2003

References

1. Baden E. Odontogenic tumors. Pathol Annu 1971; 6:475–568.

2. Bhaskar SN. Synopsis of Oral Pathology. 3d ed. St. Louis: CV Mosby, 1969:225–226.

3. Mosqueda-Taylor A, Ledesma-Montes C, Caballero-Sandoval S, et al. Odontogenic tumors in Mexico. A collaborative retrospective study of 349 cases. Oral Surg Oral Med Oral Pathol Oral Radiol Endod 1997;84:672–675.

4. Pindborg JJ, Kramer IRH. Histological Typing of Odontogenic Tumours, Jaw Cysts, and Allied Lesions. Berlin: Springer-Verlag, 1971.

5. Kramer IRH, Pindborg JJ, Shear M. Histological Typing of Odontogenic Tumours. 2d ed. Berlin: Springer-Verlag, 1992.

Section One

**General Introduction: Classification,
Normal Odontogenesis, Radiography**

Chapter 1

Introduction:
Odontogenic Tumors and Allied Lesions

Odontogenic tumors (OTs) have been a topic of considerable interest to oral pathologists, who have studied and catalogued them for several decades. Odontogenic tumors, the term *tumor* being used throughout this book in its broadest sense, constitute a group of heterogenous lesions that range from hamartomatous or non-neoplastic tissue proliferations to malignant neoplasms with metastatic capabilities. These lesions are of varying rarity within odontogenic tissues, but very rare (and in some cases, extremely rare) when viewed in the context of the entire human tumor pathology.

Odontogenic tumors are lesions derived from epithelial, ectomesenchymal, and/or mesenchymal elements that are, or have been, part of the tooth-forming apparatus. These tumors, therefore, are found exclusively within the jawbones (intrabony or centrally located) or in the soft mucosal tissue overlying tooth-bearing areas (peripherally located). The tumors may be generated at any stage of an individual's life.

The reader is reminded that correlation of histologic features with complete historical, clinical, and radiographic information is not only helpful but also, in a considerable number of instances, essential to ensure an accurate diagnosis of tumor pathology. Diagnoses predicated on microscopic appearance alone may prove inconclusive or unreliable. Knowledge of the basic epidemiological features, such as age, gender, and location, can be extremely valuable in developing differential diagnoses. An understanding of the biologic behavior of OTs is of fundamental importance to the final diagnosis and to treatment planning. This book aims at giving the reader a thorough insight into the field of odontogenic tumor pathology; clinical and radiologic data, as well as histopathologic aspects, form an important part of each chapter.

The book covers a total of 27 neoplasms, hamartomatous or tumorlike lesions all arising from the odontogenic apparatus. In addition, it covers 11 distinctive jaw lesions that must be distinguished from odontogenic tumors. Some of the tumors included have been reported only in recent years. Thus, only preliminary clinical and histopathologic characteristics of such cases can be presented. However, it is hoped that the literature references cited will urge pathologists to report more cases in order to increase the detailed knowledge of these characteristics.

Over the years—in fact, since 1867 when the French physician Broca[1] proposed a classification of tumors originating from dental tissues—several histologic classifications have been devised to help comprehend this complex group of lesions. Most of the early attempts were rather complicated and the nomenclature used was inconsistent.

It should be appreciated that it takes considerable time for any center to accumulate representative cases in sufficient numbers, and with adequate follow-up information, for useful comparative data to emerge. Further, due to the complexity of the tissues involved, it is only recently that classification attempts have been successful and applicable.

Among the prerequisites for comparative studies of oncology is international agreement on histologic criteria for the definition and classification of tumors types and a standardized nomenclature. As a result of a 5 year collaborative effort organized by the World Health Organization (WHO) and carried out by the International Reference Centre at the Department of Oral Pathology, Royal Dental College, Copenhagen, Denmark, the first consensus on taxonomy of odontogenic tumors, cysts, and allied lesions was published in 1971.[2] The classification was based on the concept suggested by Pindborg and Clausen in 1958[3] that the characteristic interactions between epithelial and ectomesenchymal tissue elements occurring during normal tooth development also operate to a certain extent in the pathogenesis and histodifferentiation of odontogenic tumors. The WHO effort was the first authoritative and useful guide to the classification of odontogenic tumors; an updated second edition appeared in 1992.[4]

This classification, as well as other volumes of the WHO series *International Histological Classification of Tumours* (published since 1967), was not intended to serve as a textbook but rather as a guide facilitating the adoption of a uniform terminology that will ease communication among oncologists. Although the WHO classification focuses on histology, it also contains certain sporadic, short accounts on epidemiological information such as age and gender distribution, location, and radiologic features pertaining to the individual tumor entities.

The scope of the present book covers updated information on relevant epidemiological features, radiologic characteristics, and full accounts on the histopathology of individual tumours. In addition, recurrence rates and—where appropriate—notes on latest views on treatment also are presented. Whereas the WHO classifications do not contain references for each chapter, the present authors have chosen to include a number of relevant citations. A literature search covering all chapters was terminated in the first months of 2002.

Although it has been only 12 years since the second edition of *Histological Typing of Odontogenic Tumours* was published, the amount of new information and accumulated knowledge in this field has already grown considerably. Based on the most recent advances in the understanding of the origins and interactions of odontogenic tissues in tumor development, as well as on recent reports of hitherto unknown tumor entities and variants, the authors thought it appropriate to let these new advances make an impact by suggesting a revised version of the 1992 classification.[5]

In March 2003, the authors of this book were invited to participate in *Pathology and Genetics of Tumours of the Head and Neck*, the fifth volume of the new WHO Blue Book series *WHO Classification of Tumours*, started in the year 2000. *Tumours of the Head and Neck* includes a chapter on the odontogenic tumors (chapter 6). At the Editorial and Consensus Conference in Lyon, France (IARC) in July 2003, a final classification was developed based on the present authors' revised version of the 1992 WHO classification.[5] Thanks to the courtesy of our publisher, Quintessenz, at a late stage in the production of this book we were able to include the entire new tumor classification (see chapter 2 of this book) as it will appear in the new WHO volume, which is scheduled for publication in spring 2004.

The reader will note that reference is made to the 1992 WHO classification in the present book (see "Histologic definitions" from chapter 5 on), despite the fact that a new WHO classification is pending. This is mainly for historical purposes.

References

1. Broca PP. Recherches sur un nouveau groupe de tumeurs désignées sous le nom d'odontomes. Paris 1867.

2. Pindborg JJ, Kramer IRH. Histological Typing of Odontogenic Tumours, Jaw Cysts, and Allied Lesions. Berlin: Springer-Verlag, 1971.

3. Pindborg JJ, Clausen F. Classification of odontogenic tumors. A suggestion. Acta Odontol Scand 1958;16:293–301.

4. Kramer IRH, Pindborg JJ, Shear M. Histological Typing of Odontogenic Tumours. 2d ed. Berlin: Springer-Verlag, 1992.

5. Philipsen HP, Reichart PA. Revision of the 1992 edition of the WHO histological typing of odontogenic tumours. A suggestion. J Oral Pathol Med 2002; 31:253–258.

Chapter 2

Classification of Odontogenic Tumors and Allied Lesions

The following classification was approved at the Editorial and Consensus Conference held in Lyon, France (WHO/IARC) in July 2003 in conjunction with the preparation of the new WHO Blue Book volume *Pathology and Genetics of Tumours of the Head and Neck*. The pathology of odontogenic tumors is the subject of chapter 6 of that volume.

Neoplasms and tumor-like lesions arising from the odontogenic apparatus

Benign

Odontogenic epithelium with mature, fibrous stroma; odontogenic ectomesenchyme not present[1]

Ameloblastomas[2]
   Solid/multicystic
   Extraosseous/peripheral
   Desmoplastic
   Unicystic
Squamous odontogenic tumor
Calcifying epithelial odontogenic tumor
Adenomatoid odontogenic tumor
Keratinizing cystic odontogenic tumor[3]

Odontogenic epithelium with odontogenic ectomesenchyme with or without dental hard tissue formation

Ameloblastic fibroma
Ameloblastic fibrodentinoma
Ameloblastic fibro-odontoma
Complex odontoma
Compound odontoma
Odontoameloblastoma
Calcifying cystic odontogenic tumor
Dentinogenic ghost cell tumor

Mesenchyme and/or odontogenic ectomesenchyme with or without included odontogenic epithelium

Odontogenic fibroma[4] (epithelium-poor and
   epithelium-rich types)
Odontogenic myxoma or fibromyxoma
Cementoblastoma

Malignant tumors (odontogenic carcinomas)[5]

Metastasizing, malignant ameloblastoma
Ameloblastic carcinoma
   (a) primary
   (b) secondary (dedifferentiated), intraosseous
   (c) secondary (dedifferentiated), extraosseous
Primary intraosseous squamous cell carcinoma (PIOSCC)

21

(a) PIOSCC solid type
(b) PIOSCC derived from odontogenic cysts
(c) PIOSCC derived from keratinizing cystic odontogenic tumor
Clear cell odontogenic carcinoma
Ghost cell odontogenic carcinoma

Malignant tumors (odontogenic sarcomas)

Ameloblastic fibrosarcoma
Ameloblastic fibrodentino- and fibro-odontosarcoma

Neoplasms and other lesions occurring in the maxillofacial skeleton

Osseous neoplasms
    Ossifying fibroma

Non-neoplastic lesions
    Fibrous dysplasia
    Osseous dysplasia
    Central giant cell lesion
    Cherubism
    Aneurysmal bone cyst
    Simple bone cyst

Comments on tumor classification

The numbering ([1-5]) refers to the preceding classification.

[1] An important aspect associated with the definition of this group of tumors lies in the characteristics of the tumor stroma. The stroma is relatively acellular and fibrous (and thus presumably has no capability of demon-strating epithelial-ectomesenchymal interactions) in contrast to tumors described in Section three, chapters 12 to 16 (so-called mixed odontogenic tumors).

[2] The plural form ("ameloblastomas") underscores what recent advances have clearly shown, that today it is not sufficient to diagnose a tumor merely as an ameloblastoma. There are several variants of this neoplasm and of utmost significance is that they show distinct variations in their clinical and demographic aspects as well as in their biologic behavior. These variants are described in chapters 5 to 8.

[3] As stated in the Preface, odontogenic cysts are not addressed in the present book. Recently, a wealth of clinical and molecular (genetic) evidence has indicated that the odontogenic keratocyst (OKC) now has to be regarded as a *benign cystic neoplasm*.[1-3] At the earlier mentioned Editorial and Consensus Conference (in July of 2003) in association with the preparation of the forthcoming WHO volume *Pathology and Genetics of Tumours of the Head and Neck*, there was consensus that the OKC should be included in chapter 6 (odontogenic tumors) under the term *keratinizing cystic odontogenic tumor* (KCOT). Because the present book was in the final stage of proofreading at the time the conference was being held, it was unfortunately not possible to add a new chapter on the KCOT.

[4] The odontogenic fibroma represents a rare and controversial tumor. At present two variants can be distinguished: the epithelium-poor type and the epithelium-rich type, formerly known as the simple and complex (or WHO) types, respectively.

[5] The terminology used to describe malignant epithelial odontogenic tumors (in particular chapters 22 to 26 of this book) has var-

ied since the WHO published the initial consensus (first edition, 1971) on the taxonomy of odontogenic tumors. Minor changes were introduced in the second edition (1992). It is only in very recent years that additional knowledge has accumulated, prompting Eversole[4] to refine the classification of malignant odontogenic tumors. The WHO-classification shown here is a further modification that deviates considerably from that of the WHO 1992 classification.

The reader should be aware of the fact that the present book covers more entities than the ones included in the above new WHO classification.

References

1. Shear M. The aggressive nature of the odontogenic keratocyst: Is it a benign cystic neoplasm? Part 1. Clinical and early experimental evidence of aggressive behaviour. Oral Oncol 2002;38:219–226.

2. Shear M. The aggressive nature of the odontogenic keratocyst: Is it a benign cystic neoplasm? Part 2. Proliferation and genetic studies. Oral Oncol 2002;38:323–331.

3. Shear M. The aggressive nature of the odontogenic keratocyst: Is it a benign cystic neoplasm? Part 3. Immunocytochemistry of cytokeratin and other epithelial cell markers. Oral Oncol 2002;38:407-415.

4. Eversole LR. Malignant epithelial odontogenic tumors. Sem Diagn Pathol 1999;16:317–324.

Chapter 3

Early Normal Odontogenesis with Special Reference to the Development and Fate of the Dental Laminae

In order to understand and appreciate the origin and development of odontogenic tumors and hamartomatous lesions, a knowledge of certain early stages of normal odontogenesis is a basic requirement. This chapter presents the processes involved in the development of the dental lamina complex and the final disintegration and fate of this interesting epithelial structure. There is presently increasing evidence that residues of odontogenic epithelium play a role in the histogenesis of odontogenic tumors, hamartomas, and cysts. However, the present authors do not agree with McClatchey's[1] claim that the ameloblastic carcinoma, the maxillary ameloblastoma, and the squamous odontogenic tumor are directly linked to and derived from the dental lamina.

Tooth development involves regional and temporal patterning of the individual tooth primordium. Odontogenesis comprises initiation, morphogenesis, and cytodifferentiation, controlled by sequential and reciprocal epithelial-ectomesenchymal interactions. Only certain aspects of the initiation, that is, the earliest stages of the formation of the tooth primordium, will be dealt with here.

Odontogenesis

The dental lamina (dental plate)

The first signs of tooth development appear during the sixth week of gestation. Ooé[2] observed the first sign of the dental anlage in embryos with a crown-rump (CR) length of 8 to 9 mm. At this stage the primitive oral cavity, or stomodeum, is lined by ectoderm, which consists of a basal layer of cuboidal to low columnar cells and a surface layer of flattened squamous cells. The rich glycogen content of their cytoplasm gives them an empty ("clear cell") appearance. The epithelium is separated from the underlying neural crest–derived ectomesenchyme by a basement membrane. Certain cells in the basal cell layer of the oral epithelium begin to proliferate at a more rapid rate than do the adjacent cells. As a result, an epithelial thickening arises on the mandibular, maxillary, and medial nasal processes and is interrupted by the nasal pit of the maxilla. This epithelial thickening, or primary epithelial band, has often been called the dental lamina but should correctly be termed the dental plate, analogous to neural plate and nasal plate (Figs 3-1 and 3-2).

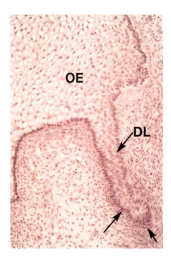

Fig 3-1 Photomicrograph showing the initial downgrowth from the primitive oral epithelium forming the dental plate. Notice the cell-rich ectomesenchyme (arrows); (hematoxylineosin [H&E] ×80). OE = oral epithelium; DL = dental lamina.

The dental and vestibular laminae

In embryos with 11 to 14 mm of CR length, the epithelial thickening begins to proliferate into the ectomesenchyme that shows a condensation of cells in the immediate vicinity of the dental plate. This leads to the formation of an epithelial sheet that forms a horseshoe-shaped structure in both developing jaws. Shortly thereafter, in embryos with 15-mm CR length, this sheet divides into two processes of which the inner (lingual or palatal) band develops into the primordium of the ectodermal portion of the teeth or the dental lamina (Fig 3-3). The free margin of the

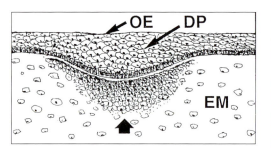

Fig 3-2 Schematic drawing of the events shown in Fig 3-1. OE = oral epithelium; DP = dental plate; EM = ectomesenchyme with condensation of its cells adjacent to the dental plate (*arrow*) (modified after Mjör and Fejerskov[3]).

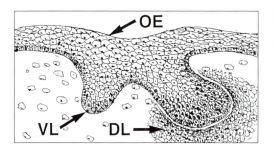

Fig 3-3 Schematic drawing showing the development of the dental lamina (DL) and the development of the vestibular lamina (VL) on the lingual side of the DL. OE = oral epithelium (modified after Mjör and Fejerskov[3]).

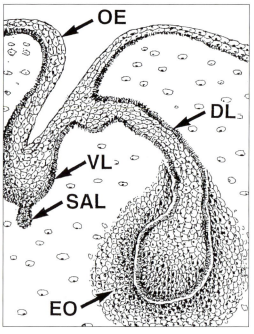

Fig 3-4 Formation of an epithelial bud (enamel organ, EO) at the end of the dental lamina (DL). Notice the cavitation of the vestibular lamina (VL), the first step toward formation of a vestibule. At the bottom of the VL there is an initial epithelial proliferation leading to the formation of accessory salivary glands (SAL) (modified after Mjör and Fejerskov[3]).

dental lamina is not linear but possesses a wavy contour. The outer (buccal or labial) band—often referred to as the lip-furrow band, the buccogingival lamina, or the vestibular lamina (see Fig 3-3)—develops somewhat later than the dental lamina. The vestibular lamina grows slowly into the mesenchyme, and at a certain stage the core cells disintegrate to produce cavitation. The slitlike cavity thus formed is the vestibule of the mouth (Fig 3-4). The epithelium that is retained contributes to the mucosal lining of the vestibule.

Later, further epithelial downgrowths into the connective tissue from the bottom of the vestibule result in the formation of the minor, accessory salivary glands. The ectoderm lining the labial and buccal wall of the vestibule demarcates the cheeks and the lips from the tooth-bearing regions. Thus, the vestibular lamina not only forms the oral vestibule but, in its developmental path, participates with the dental lamina in defining the maxillary and mandibular arches into which dental laminae will proceed in odontogenesis.

The enamel organ

At intervals along the length of the dental lamina, small rounded epithelial swellings or buds are formed shortly after establishment of the lamina. Each swelling is a result of the rapid proliferation of the epithelial cells and represents the enamel organ of the deciduous teeth (see Fig 3-4). The first tooth buds to appear are those of the anterior segment of the mandible (mandibular deciduous or primary incisors) and the initiation of the entire deciduous dentition occurs during the second month in utero. Ooé[2] found that the distance between the maxillary right and left deciduous central incisors was greater than the same distance in the mandible. He suggested that this difference could be responsible for the more frequent median diastema in the maxilla.

The lateral lamina and enamel niche

With the formation of the tooth germs for primary teeth on the labial (facial) aspect of the dental lamina, some of the dental lamina is extended labially as an epithelial bridge connecting the differentiating tooth organ with the dental lamina. This lateral extension is called the *lateral lamina* (Fig 3-5). Occasionally, growth forces of the mesenchyme adjacent to the lateral lamina produce a cavitation, called the *enamel niche*, between the lamina and the dental organ. Neither the lateral lamina nor the enamel niche is functionally important.

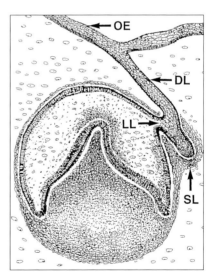

Fig 3-5 Formation of the deciduous tooth germs occurring on the labial aspect of the dental lamina (DL). An epithelial bridge (lateral lamina, LL) connects the DL with the bell-shaped tooth germ. The free tip of the DL proliferates into the ectomesenchyme as the successional lamina (SL), providing the anlage for a permanent tooth. OE = oral epithelium (modified after Mjör and Fejerskov[3]).

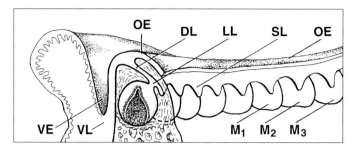

Fig 3-6 Schematic presentation of several important features in the (nonchronological) development of the dental laminae. The dental lamina (DL) provides tooth germs for deciduous teeth and through the successional lamina (SL) provides tooth germs for permanent incisors, canines, and premolars. Permanent molars (M_1, M_2, and M_3) develop from a distal extension of the DL, the accessional lamina, which is situated below the oral epithelium (OE). VE = vestibule; VL = vestibular lamina; LL = lateral lamina. Note that all three permanent molars exhibit a successional lamina that does not develop further.

The successional lamina

After the formation of the bell-shaped enamel organ, the free terminal or tip of the dental lamina begins to proliferate lingually (or palatally) into the ectomesenchyme to the enamel organ of each deciduous tooth; this occurs in the 4th month of fetal growth. This newly established growth center is known as the *successional* (succedaneous) *lamina* (see Fig 3-5) and is destined to provide the anlage for the permanent teeth replacing the primary predecessors, incisors for incisors, canines for canines, and premolars for primary molars. The process of producing the first 20 permanent teeth (incisors, canines, and premolars) occurs from the 5th fetal month (central incisor) to the 10th month of age (second premolar).

The accessional lamina

At $3\frac{1}{2}$ to 4 fetal months (160-mm CR length) the permanent molars that do not have deciduous predecessors begin to appear. They arise directly from a distal extension of the "original" dental lamina which grows backward underneath the oral epithelium (Fig 3-6). This part of the dental lamina complex is called the *accessional lamina* (the parent dental lamina, or lamina for permanent molars). These segments of the dental lamina elongate progressively, keeping pace with the lengthening of the arches and maturation of the maxilla and mandible. The earliest sign of the enamel organ of the first permanent molar is seen in the 4th fetal month. The second permanent molar appears shortly before birth and the third molar is initiated when the child is about 4 to 5 years of age. When the tooth germ of the third permanent molar is well defined, the dental lamina may extend farther distally and give rise to the epithelial primordium of a fourth molar—and even a fifth.

Proliferative activity may, however, terminate prematurely so the laminae and the associated tooth germs for the third molars are not produced. This accounts for the possible absence of the permanent third molars in some individuals. Meyer[4] and Ooé[5] among others have demonstrated that the first, second, and third permanent molar anlages all exhibit a successional lamina (see Fig 3-6) in the same manner as do the primary tooth primordia. However, this lamina does not develop into a successor (Ooé[5] called this lamina "an abortive successor") but rather shows fragmentation into epithelial remnants or disintegrates.

Disintegration of the dental lamina complex

The complex pattern of dental laminae begins to fragment or disintegrate due to ectomesenchymal invasion shortly after the establishment of the tooth germs. These processes occur initially in the lamina connecting the tooth bud to the overlying oral epithelium. From the area known as the orodental epithelial junction (the zone where the dental lamina joins with the oral epithelium), disorganization or fragmentation of the dental lamina progresses toward the developing enamel organ (Fig 3-7). Some cells of the lamina persist and tend to aggregate through proliferation into nests, known traditionally as epithelial pearls (Serres pearls).

The successional and accessional laminae also disintegrate and give rise to odontogenic epithelial remnants. It is widely held that the vast majority of these epithelial residues persist throughout life as vital, but mostly inactive ("resting"), cell clusters. However, some of these cell rests—or "waste products"—of normal human odontogenesis seem to be triggered by hitherto unknown mechanisms to proliferation and a resulting production later in life of well-known pathologic entities, like epithelium-lined cysts (dentigerous cysts, odontogenic keratocysts, gingival cysts of infancy, and lateral periodontal cysts) and epithelial odontogenic tumors such as ameloblastomas (see

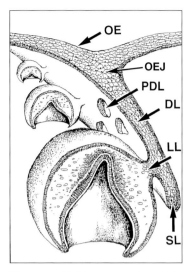

Fig 3-7 Initial fragmentation of the dental lamina (DL) starting at the orodental epithelial junction (OEJ). Several perforations (PDL) have occurred. LL = lateral lamina; SL = successional lamina; OE = oral epithelium.

chapter 5), adenomatoid odontogenic tumors (see chapter 11), and calcifying epithelial odontogenic tumors (see chapter 10).

Additional odontogenic epithelial cell residues

Remnants from the dental lamina complex are not the only epithelial residues persisting after the completion of the normal odontogenesis. When dentin formation has started, changes occur in the epithelial root sheath *(Hertwig root sheath),* which consists mainly of the inner and outer dental epithelium. It loses its continuity as ectomesenchymal cells from the surrounding dental follicle grow between the epithelial cells and the cementoblasts start to produce cementum matrix on the surface of the dentin. The fragmentation of the root sheath results in the creation of a network of epithelial cells around the root. Simpson,[6] who studied the fate of this epithelial network in the periodontium of 96 premolars from patients aged $8\frac{1}{2}$ to 64 years, found that the network in the youngest specimens resembled a perforated sheet rather than a net. With the passage of time the amount of epithelium diminished so that the network became a wide mesh and the strands of epithelium thinned. Later the network was seen to break up and many isolated strands and islands were observed. Finally, only scattered remnants of epithelium *(rests of Malassez)* were present. The author presented a graph indicating that the rests degenerate in a fairly regular manner over time. The rate is rapid at first but eventually becomes very slow, and the author concluded that it is unlikely that many adult periodontal membranes are completely free of epithelial residues.

Hodson[7] studied the epithelial residues in human jaws with special reference to edentulous jaw regions in 37 autopsies of subjects aged 23 to 87. In edentulous jaws, epithelial nests were found in 58% of the incisor and 14% of the third molar regions. They were located in the "eruption tract" (gubernacular canal), including its extension into the gum. Residues were found up to the age of 87 years. Often the odontogenic remnants were embedded intraneurally in the nerve fiber bundles of the gubernacular canal.

Interestingly, several years later, Eversole and Leider[8] reported the case of a 68-year-old edentulous man with an anterior maxillary defect which was considered to be a postextraction focus of bone deficiency. To rule out a pathologic process, a trephine bone biopsy was performed. Histology showed marrow spaces containing nerve fibers; within the nerve, surrounded by peripheral-oriented axis cylinders, were ovoid clusters of epithelial cells. The authors considered it highly unlikely that odontogenic epithelium would become intraneurally en-

cased even after tooth extraction. They concluded that these structures appeared to be identical to those found in the pterygomandibular space in a structure known as the organ of Chievitz. The reason for this problem may be explained by Hodson's findings.[7]

Valderhaug and Nylen[9] showed in their electron microscopic studies that the epithelial islands and strands were separated from the connective periodontal tissue by a typical basement lamina. Their study further revealed that the cells contained all the necessary components to meet whatever functional demands might be placed on them through environmental alterations. So, although the term *cell rest* must be considered an apt one, this does not preclude the possibility that the resting cell can return to a more active state if appropriately stimulated.

Whereas an inflammatory reaction does not seem to play a role in triggering dental laminae residues to proliferation resulting in odontogenic cyst and tumor development, inflammation is likely to be a main factor in the proliferative activity of the epithelial rests of Malassez that produces pathologic lesions. Some of the lesions believed to originate from the rests of Malassez are periapical (dental or radicular) cysts and paradental cysts.

Remnants arising from the outer enamel epithelium

Eriguchi[10] has produced evidence for the existence of yet another source of odontogenic epithelial remnants not previously recognized. During the bell stage of tooth development, the outer enamel epithelium consists of a layer of low cuboidal cells. In human embryos of 80-mm CR length, the author observed that some cells of the outer enamel epithelium tend to group together in small epithelial "pearl-like" structures, similar in morphology though smaller than those seen developing from the dental lamina. They do not persist as individual pearls but disappear fairly soon and are not traceable in the latter half of embryonic life. These remnants are not likely to play a role as nidi for development into pathologic lesions.

In embryos of 230- to 260-mm CR length, the author further demonstrated thin epithelial strands (in cross sections composed of 2 to 5 polyhedric cells) radiating from the outer enamel epithelium but corresponding only to the masticatory part of the presumptive crown. The strands tend to proliferate and may reach 1.5 to 1.8 mm in length; thus, they almost come in contact with the epithelial ridges of the overlying oral mucous membrane epithelium. The strands also show a tendency to join together, forming netlike configurations. They are often accompanied by or intermingled with small blood vessels, which should not be mistaken for the epithelial strands. The strands later show fragmentation, especially close to the oral epithelium, with the formation of several spherical epithelial pearls that blend with corresponding remnants from the dental laminae located in the connective tissue of the gingival lamina propria. These outer enamel epithelium–derived residues are, in contrast to the rests mentioned above, likely to act as a source for the development of pathologic lesions later in life.

Permanent molars

The permanent molars function throughout life without replacement so the question arises of whether they belong to the first dentition but have no successors, or to the second dentition but have lost their predecessors. Norberg[11] postulated that the second permanent molar belongs to the second dentition, since he believed it is derived from the successional lamina; in contrast, Meyer[4] and

Ooé[5] regarded the first, second, and possibly third permanent molars as belonging to the first dentition.

Although the overall activity of the various dental laminae thus covers a considerable period of time (from week 6 of embryonic development to the age of 4 years) any particular portion of it only functions for a very short period before differentiation, fragmentation into epithelial rests, or total disintegration.

The gubernaculum dentis

Although the successional teeth—that is, the permanent incisors, canines, and premolars—eventually become isolated in their own bony crypts, they maintain continuity with the connective tissue of the lamina propria of the overlying gingiva. This is achieved through the persistence of an intrabony canal or corridor called the *gubernaculum dentis*, or gubernacular canal, which connects the two.[12] This canal is occupied by the gubernacular cord which comprises mainly fibrous connective tissue that contains peripheral nerves, blood and lymphatic channels, and epithelial cells or cell clusters from the fragmented dental lamina. Thus, the gubernacular cord is the connective tissue link between the crypt (or perifollicular connective tissue) and the oral mucous membrane. It has been proposed that the gubernacular cord provides the directional path for eruption of the permanent teeth. The gubernacular canals, whose superficial orifices lie on the lingual (or palatal) aspect of the crowns of the deciduous teeth, can be recognized readily in dried jaws of children. The dental lamina remnants can thus be traced as "pearls on a string" from the gingival lamina propria down to the perifollicular tissue (tooth sac) surrounding the developing permanent tooth (Fig 3-8).

Based on these findings, Philipsen et al[13] suggested that the adenomatoid odontogenic tumor (AOT) (as well as several others) is derived from remnants of the dental lamina complex. The AOT (see chapter 11) occurs in both an intraosseous and an extraosseous (peripheral) variant, and these variants all show identical histology. To conceptualize a unified source of origin for the diverse locations of the AOT, one has to look to odontogenic epithelium with a widespread occurrence through the entire gubernacular canal. Only one candidate matches the requirements: the epithelial remnants of the dental lamina complex.

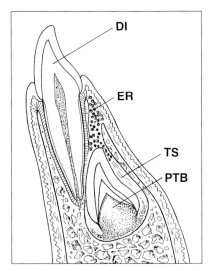

Fig 3-8 Epithelial remnants (ER, shown as tiny circles) from the dental lamina localized to the gubernacular canal that links the tooth sac (TS) around the developing permanent tooth bud (PTB) with the lingual gingiva. DI = deciduous incisor (drawing modified after Scott and Symons[14]).

References

1. McClatchey KD. Tumors of the dental lamina: A selective review. Semin Diagn Pathol 1987; 4:200–204.

2. Ooé T. On the early development of human dental lamina. Okajimas Folia Anat Jpn 1959:32: 97–108.

3. Mjör IA, Fejerskov O, eds. Histology of the Human Tooth. 2d ed. Copenhagen: Munksgaard, 1979, chapter 2.

4. Meyer W. Lehrbuch der normalen Histologie und Entwicklungsgeschichte der Zähne des Menschen. Munich, 1932:195–208.

5. Ooé T. Development of human first and second permanent molar, with special reference to the distal portion of the dental lamina. Anat Embryol (Berl) 1979;155:221–240.

6. Simpson HE. The degeneration of the rests of Malassez with age as observed by the apoxestic technique. J Periodontol 1965;36:288–291.

7. Hodson JJ. Epithelial residues of the jaw with special reference to the edentulous jaw. J Anat 1962;96:16–24.

8. Eversole LR, Leider AS. Maxillary intraosseous neuroepithelial structures resembling those seen in the organ of Chievitz. Oral Surg 1978; 46:555–558.

9. Valderhaug JP, Nylen MU. Function of epithelial rests as suggested by their ultrastructure. J Periodontal Res 1966;1:69–78.

10. Eriguchi K. Über die Entstehung und Involution der aus der Zahnleiste sowie aus dem Schmelzepithel herstammenden Epithelperlen. Yokohama Med Bull 1959:10:352–373.

11. Norberg O. Studies of the human jaws and teeth during the first years of life. Z Anat Entwicklungsgesch 1960;122:1–21.

12. Hodson JJ. The gubernaculum dentis. Dent Pract Dent Rec 1971;21:423–428.

13. Philipsen HP, Samman N, Ormiston IW, Wu PC, Reichart PA. Variants of the adenomatoid odontogenic tumor with a note on tumor origin. J Oral Pathol Med 1992;21:348–352.

14. Scott JH, Symons NBB. Introduction to Dental Anatomy. 9th ed. Edinburgh: Churchill Livingstone, 1982:107–108.

Chapter 4

Christian Scheifele

Radiography as an Important Tool in Diagnosing Odontogenic Tumors and Allied Lesions of the Maxillofacial Skeleton

1. Introduction

Radiography is often the first step in diagnosing an odontogenic tumor; a screening radiograph is made and evaluated. It can also be the final step before creating a working diagnosis, after a complete history has been taken and physical and laboratory examinations have been done. In both instances, a number of considerations have to be made relating to the application of imaging procedures that are presently available.

Odontogenic tumors are composed of a number of different soft and hard structures, including components derived from ectoderm, ectomesenchyme, and mesenchyme proper. Pulpal tissue and enamel represent the extremes in radiographic density and, in a number of lesions, may be closely associated. Therefore, their radiographic appearance may vary from complete radiolucency to mixed radiolucency/radiopacity to complete radiopacity (Table 4-1).

For lesions of the jaws, any suitable imaging procedure requires radiation exposure, except for magnetic resonance imaging (MRI) and sonography. While radiation dose values in dental radiography are comparatively low, radiation dose burdens may be considerable with computed tomography (CT), which has been applied extensively in dentomaxillofacial radiology during the last decade. This is particularly relevant when there are long-term postoperative follow-up examinations which are necessary for a considerable number of odontogenic tumors. To keep exposure to diagnostic radiation to a minimum, the background for all radiographic examinations should be based on the principle "as low (exposure) as reasonably achievable (ALARA)."[1]

2. Summation images

2.1 Intraoral radiographs

Intraoral dental radiographs are usually the first step in clarifying the nature of suspicious findings in panoramic images, provided the region of interest is attainable. It has been stressed that intraoral imaging is, where applicable, an indispensable part of the diagnostic procedure for odontogenic tumors. This has especially been shown in the early stages of both adenomatoid odontogenic tumors and odontomas in which it otherwise may be impossible to demonstrate discrete foci of calcified deposits.[2,3] Occlusal views of the jaws provide easy imaging of displaced teeth in a second plane. In all intraoral and extraoral projections, the radiographic evaluation may be disturbed by superimposing structures.

Table 4-1 Suggested imaging techniques according to odontogenic tumor type

	Intraoral radiography	Orthopantomography	Extraoral, lateral oblique projection	CT	MRI	Scintigraphy
Neoplasms and tumor-like lesions arising from the odontogenic apparatus						

Benign

Odontogenic epithelium with relatively acellular fibrous stroma, odontogenic ectomesenchyme not present

	Intraoral radiography	Orthopantomography	Extraoral, lateral oblique projection	CT	MRI	Scintigraphy
Ameloblastomas — Solid/multicystic	(+)	+		(+)		
Extraosseous (peripheral)	+	(+)				
Desmoplastic	(+)	+				
Unicystic		+	(+)	(+)		
Squamous odontogenic tumors	+	+				
Calcifying epithelial odontogenic tumor		+	(+)	(+)	(+)	
Adenomatoid odontogenic tumor	+	+		(+)		

Odontogenic epithelium with odontogenic ectomesenchyme with or without dental hard tissue formation

	Intraoral radiography	Orthopantomography	Extraoral, lateral oblique projection	CT	MRI	Scintigraphy
Ameloblastic fibroma and fibrodentinoma (neoplastic and non-neoplastic)	(+)	+				
Complex and compound odontoma	(+)	+				
Ameloblastic fibro-odontoma	(+)	+	(+)			
Odontoameloblastoma	(+)	+				
Ghost cell odontogenic tumor	(+)	+		(+)	(+)	

Odontogenic ectomesenchyme and/or mesenchyme with or without included odontogenic epithelium

	Intraoral radiography	Orthopantomography	Extraoral, lateral oblique projection	CT	MRI	Scintigraphy
Odontogenic fibroma	(+)	+		(+)		
Odontogenic myxoma or myxofibroma	(+)	+	(+)	(+)		
Cementoblastoma	(+)	+	(+)			

Malignant

	Intraoral radiography	Orthopantomography	Extraoral, lateral oblique projection	CT	MRI	Scintigraphy
Odontogenic carcinomas and sarcomas		+		+	+	(+)

CT = computed tomography; MRI = magnetic resonance imaging; + = first choice; (+) = supplementary.

2.2 Extraoral special projections

Special projections of the jaws and skull are of minor significance today. They are used for a survey of lesions not substantially exceeding the alveolar bone, including those in the jaws and facial structures. A second objective is often to demonstrate lesions in a second plane. Common special projections include the lateral oblique projection of one half of the mandible, the posterior-anterior projection (PA, or Clementschitsch view) of the mandible, and the lateral (cephalometric) and PA views of the skull. These techniques are advisable for the demonstration of lesions if other facilities are not available.

2.3 Digital imaging in intra- and extraoral projections

Intraoral imaging was one of the first areas within radiology where digital methods were effectively able to replace the conventional film-based image.[4,5] Due to the small file size of intraoral dental images, the storage and exchange of these radiographs have never been a problem. Today, there are two methods of image acquisition in intraoral dental radiography: sensors and the imaging plate system.[5,6]

At present, the spatial resolution of sensor systems exceeds that of the imaging plate systems, while the latter show a broader dynamic range in respect to radiation exposure. Clinically, both are accepted and proven to deliver equal or even better images than conventional radiography.[7-11] Projections and views in digital systems are identical to those of conventional radiography. Digital image processing and enhancement, however, allow operators to adjust brightness and contrast scales over a broad range. From that point of view, digital systems may be superior to conventional systems in describing early calcifications and small density differences, as described earlier.[7]

3. Dental panoramic radiographs and conventional tomograms

3.1 Dental panoramic radiographs

The first descriptions of odontogenic tumors in dental panoramic radiographs were published in the 1970s.[12] At present, dental panoramic radiographs provide the state-of-the-art view of the jaws and are mandatory for any screening protocol in oral radiology.[13,14]

Like all tomograms, dental panoramic images show a somewhat lower resolution (2 to 3 line pairs/mm) than comparable plain film radiographs, especially intraoral radiographs (> 30 line pairs/mm). However, the speed and ease that allow the clinician to obtain a complete survey at low exposure doses strongly counterbalance this disadvantage.

3.2 Cross-sectional views in dental panoramic units

In modern units, the position of the image layer itself and the x-ray tube are programmable within a wide range. This has made possible a variety of cross-sectional imaging methods, which include cross-sectional views of the jaws, the sinus, and the temporomandibular joints.[15]

4. Computed tomography

4.1 Axial and coronal views

Differentiation of a benign lesion from a malignant one may be difficult with only plain film radiographs. Therefore, it is easy to understand that CT was a crucial advance in imaging the highly differentiated anatomy of the skull.[16]

The main advantage of classic CT was that it could eliminate superimposition of skull structures. This provided a tremendous gain in information about the size and spatial orientation of any findings in (at that time) primary reconstructed axial tomograms. Years before general digital radiography, CT was able to identify tissues in respect to their attenuation in the radiograph. With the attenuation factor, expressed in Hounsfield units (HU), a physically calibrated characteristic was found that may, along with the structure observed, contribute to differential diagnosis. Thus, differences in density of less than 1% can be detected, but this does not necessarily apply to the imaging of soft tissues.

Metal dental restorations may cause massive superimpositions both in primarily axial or coronal reconstructed views. By and large, it is possible to partially eliminate these problems by using appropriate algorithms. Nevertheless, conventional CT is recommended in dentate patients for the demonstration of lesions outside the alveolar process. The evaluation of tumor extent into the paranasal sinuses, the nasopharynx, the base of the skull, or the cervical spine are typical applications.

4.2 Secondary reconstructed views

At present, state-of-the-art CT is characterized by a couple of improvements that have enhanced both image quality and simplicity of application and evaluation: The spatial res-

olution has gradually been improved, and spiral CT, multislice CT, and combinations of both have been introduced.[17] These allow for fast imaging and considerably improved image quality with a reduced number of artifacts.[16,18]

Imperative, however, is the secondary reconstruction—also called multiplanar reconstruction—of freely selectable or predefined layers of the primarily reconstructed axial views. Dental examination protocols are available for most CT units and especially the Denta-CT software[16,18,19] and offer reconstructed panoramic as well as reconstructed cross-sectional images, facilitating and improving the interpretation of findings seen on plane film radiographs. In addition, artefacts resulting from dental restorations have often interfered with evaluation of lesional structures, especially in primarily reconstructed coronal CT views, which were produced by reclining the patient's head. With reconstruction of the coronal view from the axial high-resolution images, the number and size of these artifacts have decreased considerably.[16]

For the diagnosis of diseases of the jaws, including odontogenic tumors, CT interpretation covers both topography and fine structure of the lesion.[20] The involvement of surrounding tissue, the cortical margins, and the extent and relationship to adjacent teeth or roots are easily seen on dental CT images. Slow-growing benign lesions often expand the cortex, while rapidly growing malignant tumors destroy adjacent structures. Thus, additional valuable information about the tumor type may be achieved when the findings from conventional radiography are exhausted.[16,21–23]

With the combination of adequate bone or soft tissue window algorithms and thin sections, the resolution of recent CT images allows one to demonstrate the fine structures of mixed lesions. Subtle calcifications, bone and marrow changes, and even desquamated keratin may be seen with appropriate settings either directly or as increased attenuation areas.[23,24] The presence and kind of intralesional calcifications, bony septa, and other solid masses may be crucial in the differential diagnosis of odontogenic tumors.[20,21,23,25]

5. Magnetic resonance imaging

Magnetic resonance imaging has for some time been considered inappropriate to resolve the alveolar regions, due to the weak signals from hard tissues. However, it has been shown that even for this anatomic area adequate imaging will be possible. By rendering MRI data sets to commercial dental CT software reconstructed panoramic and cross-sectional images from MRI may be available soon.[26]

The general use of MRI for the differential diagnosis of jaw lesions that exceed the alveolar process and contain soft tissues has been demonstrated for years.[27–29] This method produces superior imaging of the soft tissues, differentiates exactly between cysts and solid tumors, and can reveal the tumor-tissue margins in a singular manner.

MRI is also able to detect essential macropathologic details like mural nodules, fibrous or incomplete calcified septa, or solid contents of a cyst.[21,25] For example, it has been postulated that MRI might be the only way to demonstrate a mural ameloblastoma in a preexisting follicular cyst.[21] Martin-Duverneuil et al[25] recently reported on the use of CT and MRI in the diagnosis of calcifying epithelial odontogenic tumors and calcifying odontogenic cysts with odontoma. It must be emphasized that the value of CT and MRI in diagnosing odontogenic tumors is not solely the imaging of the tumor margins or the reaction of surrounding tissues, but rather the

demonstration of fine intralesional fibrous tissue and its mineralization. In addition, the spatial orientation of mineralization as central, mural, or flecked appearance may be of importance in the differential diagnosis.[25] With this detailed information available, MRI may considerably increase knowledge in the field about the pathology of odontogenic tumors.

Finally, MRI has been described as superior to CT when evaluating the mandible, due to the registration of both cortical and medullar involvement.[21,26] In summary, the main advantages of MRI in evaluating odontogenic tumors, compared to CT, are the absence of artifacts, the improved soft tissue contrast, and the capacity to image exact tumor borders and small intralesional masses.[30]

6. Radionuclide imaging

Scintigraphy requires the ingestion or injection of specific radionuclides with short half-lives. Appropriate choice of these agents means that radionuclides concentrate selectively in the region or tissues of interest. In classic scintigraphy, the γ-rays from isotopes are detected by a gamma camera that records the scintigram. Thus, radionuclide imaging methods delineate regions of increased or decreased metabolism. As already described, the true extent of bone resorption, such as around an odontogenic tumor, is in most instances larger than that depicted in conventional radiographs. Since radionuclide imaging is based on the biologic activity of a given lesion, it is able to demonstrate changes not only more precisely but also earlier than other techniques. In a case of intramural ameloblastoma, for example, the intramedullary extension of the tumor beyond the cystic wall could be demonstrated as an increased activity in scintigraphy.[31] The imaging field of radionuclide methods can cover the whole body, providing an excellent overview of conditions like bony metastases or unknown primaries.

Radionuclide imaging, however, does not reveal the cause of bone resorption or bone formation, such as tumors, inflammation, degenerative changes, or trauma.[32] However, scintigraphy has been postulated to be part of the standard diagnostic program for the evaluation of malignant tumors of the oral cavity, including odontogenic carcinomas and sarcomas.[30]

References

1. Pasler F, Visser H. Zahnmedizinische Radiologie: Bildgebende Verfahren. 2 ed. Stuttgart and New York: Thieme, 2000.

2. Dare A, Yamaguchi A, Yoshiki S, Okano T. Limitation of panoramic radiography in diagnosing adenomatoid odontogenic tumors. Oral Surg Oral Med Oral Pathol 1994;77:662–668.

3. Oliver RG, Hodges CG. Delayed eruption of a maxillary central incisor associated with an odontome: Report of case. ASDC J Dent Child 1988;55: 368–371.

4. Horner K, Shearer AC, Walker A, Wilson NH. Radiovisiography: An initial evaluation. Br Dent J 1990;168:244–248.

5. Mouyen F, Benz C. Sonnabend E, Lodter JP. Presentation and physical evaluation of RadioVisioGraphy. Oral Surg Oral Med Oral Pathol 1989;68:238–242.

6. Kashima I, Sakurai T, Matsuki T, et al. Intraoral computed radiography using the Fuji computed radiography imaging plate. Correlation between image quality and reading condition. Oral Surg Oral Med Oral Pathol 1994;78:239–246.

7. Yoshiura K, Kawazu T, Chikui T, et al. Assessment of image quality in dental radiography, part 2: Optimum exposure conditions for detection of small mass changes in 6 intraoral radiography systems. Oral Surg Oral Med Oral Pathol Oral Radiol Endod 1999;87:123–129.

8. Youssefzadeh S, Gahleitner A, Bernhart D, Bernhart T. Konventionelle Dentalradiologie und Zukunftsperspektiven. [Conventional dental radiography and future prospectives]. Radiologe 1999; 39:1018–1026.

9. Schulze R, Krummenauer F, Schalldach F, d'Hoedt B. Precision and accuracy of measurements in digital panoramic radiography. Dentomaxillofac Radiol 2000;29:52–56.

10. Stamatakis HC, Welander U, McDavid WD. Physical properties of a photostimulable phosphor system for intra-oral radiography. Dentomaxillofac Radiol 2000;29:28–34.

11. Borg E, Attaelmanan A, Grondahl HG. Subjective image quality of solid-state and photostimulable phosphor systems for digital intra-oral radiography. Dentomaxillofac Radiol 2000;29:70–75.

12. Oikarinen VJ, Calonius PE, Meretoja J. Calcifying epithelial odontogenic tumors (Pindborg tumor) case report. Int J Oral Surg 1976;5:187–191.

13. Floyd P, Palmer P, Palmer R. Radiographic techniques. Br Dent J 1999;187:359–365.

14. Farman AG, Farman TT. Extraoral and panoramic systems. Dent Clin North Am 2000;44:257–272.

15. Molander B. Panoramic radiography in dental diagnostics. Swed Dent J Suppl 1996;119:1–26.

16. Abrahams JJ. Dental CT imaging: A look at the jaw. Radiology 2001;219:334–345.

17. Vannier MW, Hildebolt CF, Conover G, Knapp RH, Yokoyama-Crothers N, Wang G. Three-dimensional dental imaging by spiral CT. A progress report. Oral Surg Oral Med Oral Pathol Oral Radiol Endod 1997;84:561–570.

18. Lenglinger FX, Muhr T, Krennmair G. Dental CT: Examination method, radiation dosage and anatomy. Radiologe 1999;39:1027–1034.

19. Spitzer WJ, Binger T. Roentgen diagnosis in oromaxillofacial surgery. Mund Kiefer Gesichtschir 2000;4(suppl 1):270–277.

20. Bodner L, Bar-Ziv J, Kaffe I. CT of cystic jaw lesions. J Comput Assist Tomogr 1994;18:22–26.

21. Erasmus JH, Thompson IO, van Rensburg LJ, van der Westhuijzen AJ. Central calcifying odontogenic cyst. A review of the literature and the role of advanced imaging techniques. Dentomaxillofac Radiol 1998;27:30–35.

22. Scholl RJ, Kellett HM, Neumann DP, Lurie AG. Cysts and cystic lesions of the mandible: Clinical and radiologic-histopathologic review. Radiographics 1999;19:1107–1124.

23. Han MH, Chang KH, Lee CH, Na DG, Yeon KM, Han MC. Cystic expansile masses of the maxilla: Differential diagnosis with CT and MR. AJNR Am J Neuroradiol 1995;16:333–338.

24. Yoshiura K, Tabata O, Miwa K, et al. Computed tomographic features of calcifying odontogenic cysts. Dentomaxillofac Radiol 1998;27:12–16.

25. Martin-Duverneuil N, Roisin-Chausson MH, Behin A, Favre-Dauvergne E, Chiras J. Combined benign odontogenic tumors: CT and MR findings and histomorphologic evaluation. AJNR Am J Neuroradiol 2001:22;867–872.

26. Gahleitner A, Solar P, Nasel C, et al. Magnetic resonance tomography in dental radiology (dental MRI). Radiologe 1999;39:1044–1050.

27. Heffez L, Mafee MF, Vaiana J. The role of magnetic resonance imaging in the diagnosis and management of ameloblastoma. Oral Surg Oral Med Oral Pathol 1988;65:2–12.

28. Lee YY, Van Tassel P, Nauert C, Raymond AK, Edeiken J. Craniofacial osteosarcomas: Plain film, CT, and MR findings in 46 cases. AJR Am J Roentgenol 1988:150:1397–1402.

29. Becker J, Schuster M, Reichart P, Semmler W, Felix R. Principles of the clinical application of magnetic resonance tomography (MRT) in oral medicine. II: Clinical application of MRT. Dtsch Z Mund Kiefer Gesichtschir 1986;10:46–59.

30. Wood NK, Goaz PW. Differential Diagnosis of Oral and Maxillofacial Lesions. 5th ed. St. Louis: Mosby, 1997.

31. Shibuya H, Hanafusa K, Shagdarsuren M, Okada N, Suzuki S. The use of CT and scintigraphy in diagnosing a cystic ameloblastoma of the jaw. Clin Nucl Med 1994;19:15–18.

32. Hardt N. Knochenerkrankungen und tumorähnliche Knochenerkrankungen. In: Sitzmann F, ed. Zahn-, Mund- und Kiefererkrankungen. Atlas der bildgebenden Diagnostik. Munich and Jena: Urban & Fischer, 2000:245–390.

Section Two

Benign Neoplasms and Tumor-like Lesions Arising from the Odontogenic Apparatus Showing Odontogenic Epithelium With Mature Fibrous Stroma, Without Ectomesenchyme

Introduction to Ameloblastomas

A recently published biologic profile based on 3,677 ameloblastoma cases,[1] has clearly demonstrated that it is no longer appropriate in any scientific study to use the diagnosis of ameloblastoma without specifying the type. Based on clinical and radiographic characteristics, histopathology, and behavioral and prognostic aspects, three or four subtypes or variants of ameloblastomas can presently be distinguished:

- The classic solid/multicystic ameloblastoma (SMA)
- The unicystic ameloblastoma (UA)
- The peripheral ameloblastoma (PA)
- The desmoplastic ameloblastoma (DA), including so-called hybrid lesions

The first two variants (SMA and UA) may be broken down further according to their histomorphologic characteristics (see chapters 5 and 8). The last variant (DA) is added to the list of the first three commonly accepted variants because recent studies[2-6] lend support to the contention that it may well qualify as a subtype of ameloblastoma. The atypical morphology of the epithelial component, the marked stromal desmoplasia, the unusual radiologic appearance, and the difference in anatomic location compared to other forms of ameloblastomas suggests that this tumor variant may be considered a clinicopathologic entity and not just a histologic variant of the SMA.

Chapters 5 to 8 deal with each of the four variants separately. Each subtype has its own clinical, radiographic, and histologic characteristics and thus is worthy of individual consideration. As previously mentioned, it is only within the last 10 years or so that it has become evident that a splitting up of the old ameloblastoma concept into several variants is appropriate. It is of paramount importance to pathologists and maxillofacial surgeons to understand the true nature and biologic behavior of the individual variants of the ameloblastoma tumor complex. If ignored, it may lead to unnecessary extensive and often mutilating surgical interventions.

The term *solid/multicystic ameloblastoma* deserves some discussion. This "classic" intraosseous ameloblastoma commences as a solid epithelial tumor. In some cases, the epithelial islands remain relatively small, and consequently there is little tendency toward cystic degeneration of the epithelial component. The tumors remain solid. In other cases, the neoplastic epithelial islands grow and become cystic; this degenerative process starts in the center of the islands where the cells cannot receive sufficient supplies of nutrients. This phenomenon may spread to several islands, where it is first recognized microscopically and later grossly. This has led to the use of the term *cystic ameloblastoma*, primarily by clinicians. Unfortunately, this term causes confusion with the *unicystic* ameloblastoma, which has a basically different behavior—and a much better prognosis—than the typical solid/multicystic ameloblastoma. Thus, it is imperative to understand the difference between a unicystic ameloblastoma and one that is merely cystic.

The tumors to be described in chapters 9, 10 and 11, respectively, have for years been considered entities, a viewpoint that has not been changed in recent years.

References

1. Reichart PA, Philipsen HP, Sonner S. Ameloblastoma: Biological profile of 3677 cases. Eur J Cancer B Oral Oncol 1995;31B:86–89.

2. Philipsen HP, Ormiston IW, Reichart PA. The desmo- and osteoplastic ameloblastoma. Histologic variant or clinicopathologic entity? Case reports. Int J Oral Maxillofac Surg 1992;21:352–357.

3. Ashman SG, Corio RL, Eisele DW, Murphy MT. Desmoplastic ameloblastoma. A case report and literature review. Oral Surg Oral Med Oral Pathol 1993;75:479–482.

4. Kaffe I, Buchner A, Taicher S. Radiologic features of desmoplastic variant of ameloblastoma. Oral Surg Oral Med Oral Pathol 1993;76:525–529.

5. Thompson IOC, van Rensburg JL, Phillips VMJ. Desmoplastic ameloblastoma: Correlative histopathology, radiology and CT-MR imaging. J Oral Pathol Med 1996;25:405–410.

6. Sakashita H, Miyata M, Okabe K, Kuramaya H. Desmoplastic ameloblastoma in the maxilla: A case report. J Oral Maxillofac Surg 1998;56:783–786.

Chapter 5

Solid/Multicystic Ameloblastoma

1. Terminology

The tumor that meets today's diagnostic criteria for solid/multicystic ameloblastoma (SMA) has been known for about 180 years. In 1827 Cusack[1] published a report describing what obviously was an ameloblastoma. Broca[2] gave the first detailed description of an SMA in 1868. During 1884 and 1885 Malassez[3,4] studied odontogenic tumors and proposed the name "epithelioma adamantin" for the SMA; he also showed it could arise from odontogenic epithelial remnants ("debris epitheliaux"). The term *adamantinoma* was changed in 1930,[5] especially in the English-speaking countries, to the more appropriate term *ameloblastoma,* which is still in current use. The term *adamantinoma* may be considered a misnomer in as much as adamantin (enamel) is not a product of this tumor. The characteristic peripheral cylindrical cells of the tumor islands are not true ameloblasts in that these cells are not capable of producing enamel stroma, in particular because the tumor islands are embedded in a mature, fibrous connective tissue. An account on the terminology (with historical aspects) of the ameloblastoma was published by Baden in 1965.[6]

2. Clinical and radiographic profile

The SMA is traditionally considered a benign epithelial neoplasm with virtually no tendency to metastasize. It is slow-growing but locally invasive, with a high rate of recurrence if not removed adequately. It is of utmost importance to understand that the local biologic behavior of an SMA is that of a low-grade malignant tumor. It is located centrally or intraosseously in both jaws, and there are few or no clinical signs in the early stages. Later there is gradually increasing facial deformity, teeth in the area may become loose, and spontaneous fracture may occur in cases where only a rim of normal bone forms the base of the mandible. The affected part of the jaw is bony hard and bulky. Pain occurs with varying, often quite low, frequency. It is not known whether the cause of the pain is pressure from the tumor on peripheral nerves or secondary infection. Tumors that continue to enlarge may cause the surrounding bone to become so thin that crepitation or eggshell crackling may be elicited. Perforation of the bone, however, is a late feature. An unusually large ameloblastoma was reported by Partriella et al.[7]

Radiographically, the SMA may show considerable variation. The typical picture is of a multilocular destruction of bone (Fig 5-1), but unilocular appearances also occur. In the multilocular type the bone is replaced by a

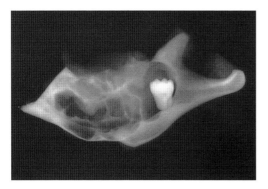

Fig 5-1 Radiograph of an operation specimen showing a large, multilocular, follicular SMA of the molar/ascending ramus region of the mandible containing a displaced, unerupted third molar.

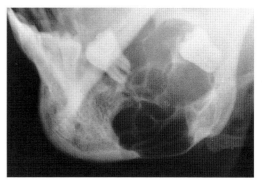

Fig 5-2 An SMA with typical multilocular, soap-bubble appearance and extensive bone destruction in the molar/ascending ramus area. Histology showed a mixed follicular/plexiform SMA.

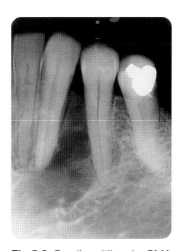

Fig 5-3 Small multilocular SMA in the canine/ first premolar area of the mandible.

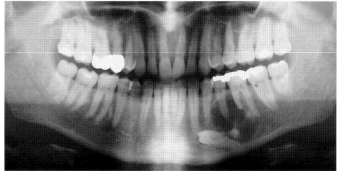

Fig 5-4 Unilocular SMA of the first and second premolar mandibular region. Notice the embedded supernumerary premolar at the periphery of the radiolucency and resorption of the mesial root of the mandibular first molar.

number of small, well-defined radiolucent areas, giving the whole lesion a honeycomb or soap-bubble appearance and ranging in size from extensive destruction of half the mandible (Fig 5-2) to a small lesion confined to the alveolar process (Fig 5-3). In the unilocular type (not to be misinterpreted as "unicystic" ameloblastoma) there is a well-defined area of radiolucency that forms a single compartment. If this type is associated with an unerupted tooth (Fig 5-4), the appearance closely resembles that of a dentigerous cyst or an odontogenic keratocyst. Ueno et al[8] found that among 97 cases of SMAs, 47% were unilocular and 37% were multilocular; 16% had a soap-bubble or a combination of soap-bubble and multilocular appearance. Figures 5-5 and 5-6 show the result of applying computed tomography (CT) software for three-dimensional reconstruction of a SMA located to the angle and ascending ramus of the mandible.

3. Epidemiological data

3.1 Prevalence, incidence, and relative frequency

Prevalence and incidence figures could not be derived form the study by Reichart et al.[9] Accurate figures of this type can only be obtained if every new case of SMA in a defined population is recorded in a tumor registry and the microscopic material is reviewed by a pathologist who is experienced with odontogenic tumors. A reasonable estimate of the incidence of ameloblastomas in a white population (in Swedes) was reported by Larsson and Almeren.[10] They found the annual incidence rate to be 0.6 new cases per one million people. A second study was that of Shear and Singh,[11] who investigated the incidence of ameloblastomas among the white and black populations in a well-defined region around Johannesburg, South Africa. Gardner[12] recalculated the figures in Shear and Singh's report and found the incidence for both sexes to be 2.29 new cases each year per one million people for blacks and 0.31 for whites. Relative frequency data, on the other hand, can be retrieved from several sources and show great variation, from 11.0% to 95.4%.

The article by Reichart et al[9] reviewed the biologic profile of 3,677 cases of ameloblastomas retrieved from the literature from 1960 to 1993, making it the most extensive review of ameloblastomas ever published. One of the aims of the article was to compare find-

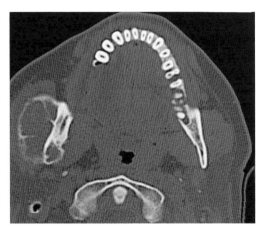

Fig 5-5 CT showing buccal, multilocular expansion of an ameloblastoma located in the molar/ascending ramus area.

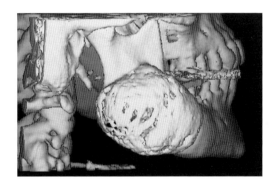

Fig 5-6 Three-dimensional reconstruction of the expanding ameloblastoma shown in Fig 5-5.

ings from recent years with those of the historical review by Small and Waldron,[13] who evaluated 1,046 cases of ameloblastomas. The retrospective study by Reichart et al[9] suffers, however, from several disadvantages, including the inconsistencies of the data provided in the 262 papers reviewed and the classifications used. The generally well-accepted concept developed during recent years of dividing ameloblastomas into three entities—solid/multicystic or conventional; unicystic; peripheral—was applied to the data collected. However, in certain instances, particularly regarding the elucidation of the mean age at diagnosis of the classic ameloblastoma (SMA), the outcome was less clear due to the circumstances involved in producing the review which have already been mentioned (see the following section).

3.2 Age

The mean age of patients at the time of diagnosis for all three types of SMA ($n = 2,280$, including reviews and case reports) was 35.9 years with a range of 4 to 92 years. On the basis of case reports alone ($n = 650$), the mean age at time of diagnosis was 37.4 years (with a range of 4 to 92 years) (Fig 5-7). The mean age of 39.2 years for men was significantly different ($P < 0.05$) from that of 35.2 years for women. The present authors agree

with the subsequent calculations made by Gardner[12] and find his estimate of 39 years for the mean age at diagnosis of the classic SMA, 22 years for the unicystic, and 51 years for the peripheral ameloblastoma to be reasonable at this time.

The mean age of patients with tumors of the maxilla was 47.0 years ($n = 171$) compared to tumors of the mandible with a mean age of 35.2 years ($n = 393$; $P < 0.001$). Ueno et al[8] reported a significant difference in mean age between SMAs with a unilocular radiographic appearance and SMAs with a multilocular/soap-bubble appearance (26.4 years versus 37.5 years). It should be stressed that the authors did not state whether cases of unicystic ameloblastomas were included in their material.

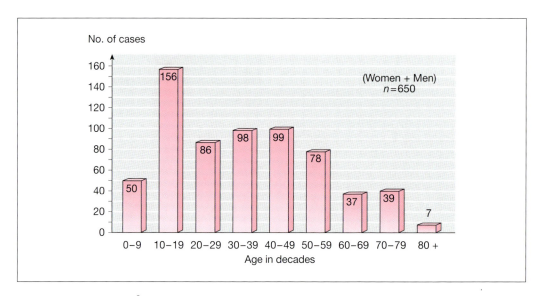

Fig 5-7 Age distribution[9] of 650 cases of ameloblastomas, including unicystic and peripheral variants. The peak in the 2nd decade most likely mirrors the inclusion of 102 cases of unicystic ameloblastomas (mean age: 22.1 years). Similarly, the rather large number of cases in the 5th and 6th decades may be ascribed to the inclusion of 63 cases of peripheral ameloblastomas (mean age: 51.0 years).

3.3 Gender

The distribution among men and women (n = 3,677)[9] was 46.7% women and 53.5% men (1:1.1).

3.4 Location

When case reports were evaluated the ratio between maxillary (n = 185) and mandibular (n = 404) ameloblastomas was 1:2.2.[9] If, however, case reports and reviews were considered together (n = 1,932), the ratio between maxillary and mandibular tumors was 1:5.8. This difference is due to the fact that maxillary tumors are reported more often in case reports. Based on the data reported by Reichart et al[9] the topographic location of ameloblastomas in the maxilla was 284 and in the mandible was 1,648 (Fig 5-8). When location and gender were cross-tabulated, a statistical significance (P < 0.05) was revealed. The incisor region and ramus of the mandible were affected more often in women than in men. In men the premolar region and the maxillary sinus were affected more frequently than in women, whereas the molar region was affected equally in both sexes.

3.5 SMA associated with unerupted teeth

Figures for the occurrence of unerupted teeth associated with SMAs can be retrieved from the review by Reichart et al.[9] Ueno et al[8] investigated 90 cases of SMAs with regard to the presence of impacted or unerupted teeth. They found that 34 cases (38%) were associated with impacted teeth, of which 82% involved the mandibular third molar, 15% the second molar, and 6% a premolar. In an additional case the tumor contained a fourth molar. None of the examined maxillary SMAs (n = 5) included impacted teeth.

4. Pathogenesis

It is generally agreed that most SMAs occur as growths arising from remnants of odontogenic epithelium, more specifically rests of the dental lamina (see chapter 3). It should be noted that residues from the dental lamina, if situated outside the bone in the soft tissues of the gingival and edentulous alveolar mucosa (together with the basal cell

Fig 5-8 Topographical distribution of 1,932 cases (case reports and reviews) of ameloblastomas (all variants) based on data from Reichart et al.[9] Figures represent percentages of the total number. Cases involving an entire quadrant are indicated between arrows. Cases located in the maxillary sinus (2.1%) and nasal cavity (0.7%) are not shown. Numbers at the top and bottom of the broken lines indicate cases involving both adjoining regions: anterior/premolar and premolar/molar.

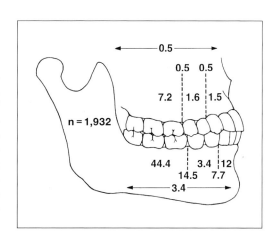

layer of the oral epithelium), may give rise to peripheral ameloblastoma (see chapter 6). It is also agreed that SMAs may arise as a result of neoplastic changes in the lining or wall of a non-neoplastic odontogenic cyst, in particular in dentigerous and odontogenic keratocysts. Opinions differ regarding the incidence of these so-called mural ameloblastomas. Baden[14] indicated an incidence varying from 17.8% to 30% and correlates with the preferred location for SMA—the mandibular third molar. As early as 1885, Malassez[4] suggested that intraosseous ameloblastomas may originate from "*les debris épithéliaux*" (epithelial rests of Malassez). Early (microscopic) ameloblastomas located between teeth, near the crest of the alveolar ridge, document such a histogenesis and have been reported, especially in literature from the mid-1950s and earlier. Similarly, several authors of reports appearing in the first half of the 20th century thought that the enamel organ was a likely origin of the SMAs.

5. Pathology

5.1 Macroscopy

The operation specimen will, depending on the treatment modality, consist of the tumor with a surrounding margin of normal bone. The tumor appears as a grayish white or grayish yellow mass replacing the bone. The tumor tissue cuts readily and contains no calcified material. Some lesions are completely solid, but in most cases cystic spaces are present. These are generally quite small and scattered randomly. Less frequently the cysts are larger and the whole lesion has the appearance of a multicystic lesion. The cyst content varies from straw-colored fluid to semisolid, gelatinous material. Sometimes the lesion consists of only a single cyst, in

which case there may be a close resemblance to a unicystic ameloblastoma or an odontogenic cyst. However, if one or more small nodules of growth protrude from an otherwise smooth lining, a preliminary diagnosis of a unicystic ameloblastoma (see chapter 8) must be considered. One or more teeth may be involved by the tumor.

5.2 Microscopy

5.2.1 Histologic definitions

According to the 1992 World Health Organization (WHO) definition, an SMA is "a polymorphic neoplasm consisting of proliferating odontogenic epithelium, which usually has a follicular or plexiform pattern, lying in a fibrous stroma."[15]

The definition used by the present authors is as follows:

A polymorphic neoplasm consisting of proliferating odontogenic epithelium, usually occurring in two main patterns. In the follicular type of growth the tumor consists of enamel organ–like islands or follicles of epithelial cells, while in the plexiform type the epithelium forms continuous anastomosing strands. In both types the epithelial tumor components are embedded in a mature, connective tissue stroma. Generally, a tumor shows one or the other pattern throughout. However, not infrequently both patterns are present in the same tumor.

5.2.2 Histopathologic findings

In the previously mentioned follicular pattern (Fig 5-9), the islands consist of a central mass of polyhedral cells, or loosely connected angular cells resembling stellate reticulum, surrounded by a layer of cuboidal or columnar cells resembling internal dental epithelium or preameloblasts. Cystic degeneration commonly occurs within the epithelial islands (Fig 5-10). In the plexiform pattern (Fig 5-11) the

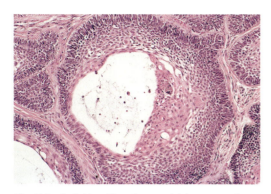

Fig 5-9 Solid/multicystic ameloblastoma showing a follicular pattern with central cystic degeneration and some squamous cell metaplasia (hematoxylin-eosin [H&E] ×80).

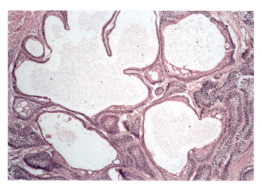

Fig 5-10 Solid/multicystic ameloblastoma with extensive cystic degeneration of follicular tumor islands (multicystic ameloblastoma) (H&E, ×25).

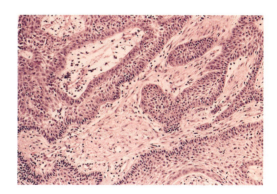

Fig 5-11 Solid ameloblastoma of plexiform type (H&E, ×80).

tumor epithelium is arranged as a network which is bound by a layer of cuboidal to columnar cells and includes cells resembling stellate reticulum. Cyst formation occurs but is usually due to stromal degeneration rather than to a cystic change within the epithelium. Reichart et al[9] found that in 397 case reports the follicular pattern was present in 32.5% of tumors and the plexiform pattern in 28.2%.

Coleman et al[16] and do Carmo and Silva[17] both used silver-staining nucleolar organizer region (AgNOR) counts in the investigation of possible differences in behavior between ameloblastomas and other odontogenic tumors. They concluded that AgNOR counts are not a good indicator of cell proliferation but represent variations in metabolic or transcriptional activity.

Histologic variants of the two main patterns of SMAs are described in the following sections. It should be emphasized that these variants are not tumor entities. It seems of no significance to prognosis or clinical management whether a tumor can be diagnosed as a follicular SMA, a plexiform SMA, or one of the numerous variations outlined here. However, in the past it was suggested that the granular cell SMA (see section 5.2.2.2) had a more aggressive behavior. This suggestion has not been substantiated and is to-

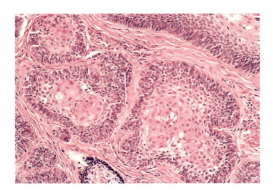

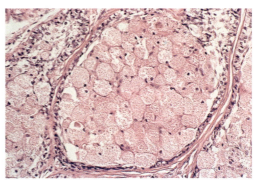

Fig 5-12 Follicular ameloblastoma showing acanthomatous changes (squamous metaplasia) of almost all tumor islands (H&E, ×80).

Fig 5-13 Follicular ameloblastoma with extensive granular transformation of the stellate reticulum–like cells (H&E, ×140).

day considered invalid. The clear cell SMA (see section 5.2.2.5), on the other hand, requires some attention because in at least some instances it is capable of locally destructive growth and both nodal and distant metastases. These tumors are today considered clear cell odontogenic carcinomas (see chapter 27).

5.2.2.1 Acanthomatous SMA (Fig 5-12).

This term is applied when there is extensive squamous metaplasia, sometimes with keratin formation, within the islands of tumor cells. The horny pearls may become calcified. Usually the general pattern of this tumor variant is of the follicular type. According to Reichart et al[9] the acanthomatous variant accounted for 12.1% of the reviewed 397 case reports and is the third most common histologic type. This variant must be distinguished from the squamous odontogenic tumor (see chapter 9), in which the peripheral cells of the tumor islands are flat rather than columnar.

5.2.2.2 Granular cell SMA (Fig 5-13).

This term is applied when the tumor, most often of the follicular type, shows an extensive granular transformation of the central stellate reticulum–like cells. In some lesions all cells of the tumor islands or nests are composed of granular cells. In a survey of 20 cases of granular cell SMAs, Hartman[19] found that this variant accounted for 5% of all ameloblastomas. The granular cells may be cuboidal, columnar, or rounded, and the cytoplasm is filled with acidophilic granules. The cytoplasmic granules have been identified ultrastructurally as lysosomal aggregates.[20–22] Kumamoto and Ooya[22] also performed immunohistochemical studies on six cases of granular cell SMAs and demonstrated that the granularity might be caused by increased apoptotic cell death and associated phagocytosis by neighboring neoplastic cells.

Altini et al[23] reported on two cases of what they termed "plexiform granular cell odontogenic tumor" (PGCOT). Both lesions consisted of interlacing strands of odontogenic epithelium, with each strand being two cell layers thick. The cells were large and polyhedral in shape, with granular acidophilic cytoplasm. No ameloblastoma-like tissue was found in either case. The authors suggested that these lesions might represent previously undescribed histologic variants of SMA. However, they could not exclude the possibility that the lesions represented a new entity. Siar and coworkers[24,25] described combined granular cell ameloblastoma and PG-COT, but the true nature of these lesions have yet to be clarified. Granular cells may occur in various odontogenic and nonodontogenic tumors.

Mirchandani and Sciubba[26] produced a comprehensive study of 44 oral granular cell lesions, including four granular cell ameloblastomas, presenting clinicopathologic, immunohistochemical, and ultrastructural findings. A similar but less intensive study was performed by Rühl and Akuamoa-Boateng.[27]

5.2.2.3 Desmoplastic SMA.
This term is used, especially in the follicular type of tumor, when there is a marked hyalinization (desmoplasia) of the connective tissue stroma (for details, see chapter 7).

5.2.2.4 Basal cell SMA (Fig 5-14).
In rare cases, an SMA may show a predominantly basaloid pattern. This variant occurs in only 2.02% of the reviewed case reports.[9] In a recent immunohistochemical study by Sandra et al[28] using monoclonal antiproliferating cell nuclear antigen (anti-PCNA) antibody and monoclonal anti–KI-67 antibody, the authors found that the basal cell SMA had the highest labeling indices for both PCNA and Ki-67, indicating that the basal cell type is the most actively proliferating type and therefore the most immature cells in an SMA.

5.2.2.5 Clear cell SMA.
SMAs may contain clear, periodic-acid–Schiff (PAS) positive cells most often localized to the stellate reticulum–like areas of the follicular SMA. It is important to realize that in recent years at least some clear cell SMAs have proved to be malignant tumors. Details about this rare entity are described in chapter 27.

5.2.2.6 Keratoameloblastoma (KA) and papilliferous KA.
In 1970, Pindborg[29] produced a radiograph and three photomicrographs of an unusual type of ameloblastoma consisting partly of keratinizing cysts (Fig 5-15) and partly of tumor islands with papilliferous appearance (Figs 5-16 and 5-17); he suggested the term *papilliferous keratoameloblastoma* (PKA) for this lesion. Later, Altini et al[30] described a similar tumor that differed from the one described by Pindborg in that it did not show the papilliferous epithelium nor the extensive necrosis and debris in the middle of the follicles. Altini et al raised the question as to whether both lesions represented the same tumor. In 1993, Siar and Ng[31] reported four cases resembling KAs to some extent, with the exception that papilliferous epithelial tumor islands were not found. The tumors were characterized by the simultaneous occurrence of areas of ameloblastoma with pronounced keratinization and cystic areas resembling odontogenic keratocysts. In 1997 Said-Al-Naief et al[32] added a fifth case to those reported by Siar and Ng.

KAs, PKAs, or possible hybrid lesion of the two are extremely rare neoplasms and an accurate evaluation of the clinical spectrum, radiology, and behavioral potential must await further case accrual.

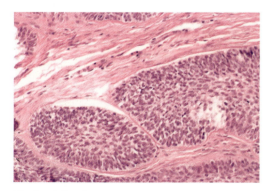

Fig 5-14 Solid ameloblastoma with tumor islands showing a basaloid pattern (H&E, ×140).

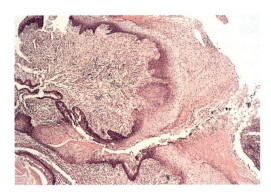

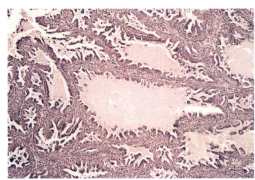

Fig 5-15 Papilliferous keratoameloblastoma. In this area of the tumor there are several keratinizing, irregular cysts with massive parakeratinization (H&E, ×60).

Fig 5-16 Papilliferous keratoameloblastoma (same tumor as shown in Fig 5-15). In this part of the tumor the islands show a papilliferous, epithelial lining of small cysts containing a homogenous eosinophilic content (H&E, ×60).

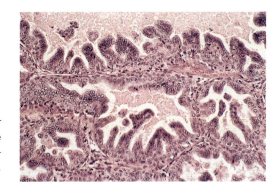

Fig 5-17 Higher magnification of the tumor shown in Fig 5-16. The papilliferous appearance is evident. The tumor stroma is restricted to delicate bands of fibrous connective tissue (H&E, ×140).

5.2.2.7 Mucous cell differentiation in SMA.
In a recent paper, Wilson et al[33] reported what was thought to be only the fourth case of an intraosseous, follicular ameloblastoma showing focal mucous cell differentiation. On the other hand, the presence of vacuolated and mucous cells in radicular and residual cysts has been well documented.[34]

5.2.2.8 Hemangiomatous ameloblastoma (HA).
Variations in the histomorphologic patterns of ameloblastomas do not appear to have a significant bearing on their biologic behavior or prognosis, with the possible exceptions of

the unicystic (see chapter 8), desmoplastic (see chapter 7), and hemangiomatous ameloblastoma (hemangioameloblastoma). The HA is a SMA in which part of the tumor contains spaces filled with blood or large endothelial-lined capillaries, first described by Kühn in 1932.[35]

Van Rensburg et al[36] recently reported a case of this rare tumor variant in a 26-year-old woman who had a gradually enlarging symptomatic swelling in the posterior region of the left mandible. Panoramic radiographs and CT revealed a mixed radiolucent-radiopaque lesion with buccolingual expansion and mild root resorptions of the second molar. On MRI the tumor contents displayed an intensity suggestive of bundles of vascular structures or blood vessels in various stages of thrombosis or slow flow. A vasoformative neoplasm or a tumor with a vascular stroma was considered the most likely diagnosis. Enucleation of the vascular tissue caused profuse bleeding. Histology revealed a plexiform ameloblastoma with a prominent vascular component consisting of numerous endothelial-lined channels and large blood-filled spaces with multiple thrombi located in the tumor stroma. The lesion was diagnosed as HA. The patient refused a planned subsequent radical operation.

The origin of the vascular component of the HA is not clear and several theories have been advanced; among them are excessive stimulation of angiogenesis during tumor development and trauma such as tooth extraction (in the preceding example, the second molar had been extracted 11 years earlier). It has further been suggested that the HA represents a collision tumor. Whether the vascular component of the HA is part of the neoplastic process, represents a separate neoplasm, or is a hamartomatous malformation remains to be seen. Lucas[37] believed that the unusual vascularity is not due to a neoplastic process. According to this author, there is an entire absence of vasoformative activity. In the process of formation of stromal cysts in the ordinary type of plexiform ameloblastoma, the blood vessels often persist and dilate instead of disappearing; thus, it is likely to represent a purely secondary change. Van Rensburg et al[36] concluded that findings on CT scans in association with an angiomatous/vascular stroma on MRI are suggestive of HA.

5.2.2.9 Extragnathic (tibial) adamantinoma (ETA).

The adamantinoma (an obsolete synonym for ameloblastoma) was first described by Fischer in 1913.[38] It is a rare, primary intraosseous epithelial neoplasm of low-grade malignancy with a marked predilection for the tibia, where 90% of cases arise in the middle third of the bone. Czerniak et al[39] distinguished two types of ETA: the classic form and the differentiated form. The classic form usually presents in older patients, grows beyond the cortex, and sometimes metastasizes. Histologically, the classic ETA is characterized by an abundance of epithelial cells which stain strongly for cytokeratin. The differentiated form, on the other hand, occurs at a young age (during the first two decades) and has an intracortical location. Histology shows that it has a uniform predominance of an osteofibrous dysplasia-like pattern, with only a scattered, inconspicuous epithelial cell component. The interesting relationship of osteofibrous dysplasia to the epithelial component of ETAs has recently been addressed in several reports.[40–43] The ETA was once thought to be related to the SMA of the jawbones because of some histologic resemblance to the latter; however, a relationship between the two has never been established. At one time the ETA was also thought to be endothelial, synovial, or mesenchymal in origin.

5.2.3 Histochemical/immunohistochemical findings

There have been few studies describing histochemical findings in ameloblastomas, whereas immunohistochemical demonstration of a great variety of important substances, antigens, and markers has been abundant, especially within the last two decades. A few of these reports have already been referred to in the preceding paragraphs. Almost all the publications have compared the findings in ameloblastomas to those of other odontogenic tumors, odontogenic cysts, and human fetal tooth germs. In summary, the following areas of ameloblastoma immunohistochemistry have been covered in the literature: cell surface carbohydrate composition (lectin histochemistry)[44,45]; blood group carbohydrates A, B, and H type 2[46,47]; involucrin expressivity[48]; expression of amelogenins, enamelin[49-51]; intermediate filaments (cytokeratins and vimentin)[52,53]; laminin-5[54]; osteolytic cytokines and adhesion molcules[55]; PCNA[56-58]; bone sialoprotein[59]; bone morphogenetic protein[60]; and bcl-2 protein.[61,62]

5.2.4 Ultrastructural findings

The first reports on the fine structure of SMAs appeared around 1960.[63,64] Moe et al[64] were the first to acknowledge that the peripheral cells of the solid, follicular ameloblastoma were ultrastructurally similar to the inner enamel epithelium. This viewpoint was subsequently supported by several studies. Kim et al[65] found that, in addition to the strong resemblance of the columnar cells of the tumor to the cells of the inner enamel epithelium at an early stage of differentiation, the stellate cells of the tumor epithelium were similar in many respects to the stellate reticulum of the normal enamel organ. In areas of metaplastic squamous cell changes, the authors found that these cells had ultrastructural features similar to those observed in basal cells and lower prickle cells of the oral mucosa, especially in the epithelium of the palatal mucosa. In a transmission electron microscopy (TEM) study of 12 plexiform and 9 follicular ameloblastomas, Nasu and Ishikawa[66] found that the follicular variant consisted of two cell types, one resembling the stellate reticulum and the other resembling the inner enamel epithelium of the normal enamel organ. The plexiform variant, on the other hand, did not show two cell types but resembled squamous epithelium. It should be mentioned that according to the clinical data given for the plexiform variant, at least 10 tumors may qualify for the tumor currently known as the plexiform, unicystic ameloblastoma (see chapter 8).

Lee et al[67] described the ultrastructure of a "simple" ameloblastoma (SMA), the occurrence of cells possessing single cilia which arose from a basal body and occasional cells containing Langerhans granules. In addition, the tumor stroma contained oxytalan fibers. Mucin-producing cells were reported by Mincer and McGinnis[68] to occur in a multicystic ameloblastoma. The discovery of these cells had earlier led Hodson[69] to propose a subclass of mucoepidermoid ameloblastoma. Occurrence of intracytoplasmic desmosomes in a maxillary ameloblastoma was reported by Cutler.[70] The presence of intracellular desmosomes could, according to the author, suggest a high degree of membrane polymorphism between tumor cells and thus indicate a more aggressive lesion. Occurrence of so-called hyaline bodies, ultrastructurally similar to those found in odontogenic cyst epithelium and cyst walls, have been demonstrated in a case of plexiform ameloblastoma by Takeda et al.[71]

Ultrastructural studies have concentrated on the epithelial components of SMAs as opposed to the tumor stroma. The stroma has been described as containing fibroblasts and collagen fibers, but Tothouse et al[72] also demonstrated the occurrence of myofibroblasts that showed formation of plaquelike structures on extended cell processes, which the authors identified as intracellular septate junctions. Smith and Bartov[73] confirmed the finding of abundant myofibroblasts in a case of recurrent SMA.

5.2.5 Ameloblastomas in tissue culture

The first attempt at studying primary cultures from explants of a follicular, solid ameloblastoma in roller tubes was done by Niizima,[74] who had previously done tissue culture studies of enamel epithelium.[75] Epithelial elements of squamous type, which formed widespread sheets, accounted for the major part of the outgrowth. The epithelial cells were similar in structure and behavior to those obtained from culture of the enamel organ, although in some respects—such as the vigorous movements of undulating membranes, pinocytosis, and the formation of perinuclear vacuoles—the tumor cells showed much more activity than did those of the normal tissue. During the last decade or so, investigators have tried to produce long-term cultures of human ameloblastomas. The ultrastructural three-dimensional growth of follicular ameloblastoma cells in collagen matrix in vitro was reported by Yasuda et al.[76] The result demonstrated that the cells developed in this short-term culture system had characteristics of ameloblastoma cells.

In 1998, Harada et al[77] succeeded in producing—by transfection with HPV-16DNA—an immortalized human ameloblastoma cell line which they designated AM-1. This cell line maintains epithelial cell morphology and expresses cytokeratins 8, 14, 18, and 19 but not 10 or 16. The expression of vimentin was weakly positive. Furthermore, bcl-2 protein, which prevents apoptosis, was consistently expressed. The behavior of these cells on a collagen matrix was investigated and showed that the cells grew in a monolayer over foci of collagen degradation and could invade the collagen gel at such sites, thus mimicking the behavior of in situ ameloblastoma cells. The authors concluded that AM-1 appears to be an appropriate model system which might be used in determining various mechanisms that influence the biology of ameloblastomas.

6. Notes on treatment and recurrence rate

No single standard type of therapy should be advocated for patients with SMAs. Rather, each case should be judged on its own merits. As stated previously, modern classifications divide the ameloblastomas into three or four entities. This classification is of utmost importance because the clinical behavior and treatment of these ameloblastomas differ. The solid/multicystic ameloblastoma requires radical surgical intervention. Unicystic ameloblastomas (see chapter 8) require only conservative surgical enucleation, unless infiltration from the epithelial cyst lining into the cyst wall has been demonstrated, in which case the treatment should follow that outlined for SMAs. Peripheral ameloblastomas should be treated conservatively. Two recent reports[78,79] can be recommended as an overview of the current status of the surgical management of ameloblastomas. Gardner[78] points out that the characteristic slow growth of the SMA is significant in that it may take years before a recurrence becomes evident. As a result, clinicians and patients tend to be lulled into a false sense of security, and consequently follow-up examinations may be neglected after the first few years. Recurrences may occur 5 to 10 years after surgery, and it is therefore imperative that the surgical sites be examined thoroughly (including radiographs) for at least 10 years and preferably longer. Recurrences following different treatment modalities have been reported by Reichart et al[9] and Gardner.[78]

References

1. Cusack JW. Report of the amputation of portions of the lower jaw. Dublin Hosp Rec 1827;4:1–38.

2. Broca PP. Recherches sur un nouveau groupe de tumeurs designées sous le nom d'odontomes. Gaz Hebd Sci Méd 1868;5:70–84.

3. Malassez L. Note sur la pathogénie des kystes dentaires dites périostiques. J Conn Med Prat (Paris) 1884;7:98–99;106–107;115–116.

4. Malassez L. Sur le role des debris épitheliaux paradentaires. Arch Physiol Norm Pathol 1885;5: 309–340 and 6:379–449.

5. Ivy RH, Churchhill HR. The need of a standardized surgical and pathological classification of the tumors and anomalies of dental origin. Trans Am Assoc Dent Sch 1930;240–258.

6. Baden E. Terminology of the ameloblastoma: History and current use. J Oral Surg 1965;23:40–49.

7. Partriella VM, Rogow PN, Baden E, Williams AC. Gigantic ameloblastoma of the mandible: Report of case. J Oral Surg 1974;32:44–49.

8. Ueno S, Nakamura S, Mushimoto K, Shirasu R. A clinicopathologic study of ameloblastoma. J Oral Maxillofac Surg 1986;44:361–365.

9. Reichart PA, Philipsen HP, Sonner S. Ameloblastoma: Biological profile of 3677 cases. Eur J Cancer B Oral Oncol 1995;31B:86–99.

10. Larsson Å, Almeren H. Ameloblastoma of the jaws. An analysis of a consecutive series of all cases reported to the Swedish Cancer Registry during 1958–1971. Acta Pathol Microbiol Scand [A] 1978;86:337–349.

11. Shear M, Singh S. Age-standardized incidence rates of ameloblastoma and dentigerous cyst on the Witwatersrand, South Africa. Community Dent Oral Epidemiol 1978;6:195–199.

12. Gardner DG. Critique of the 1995 review by Reichart et al. of the biologic profile of 3677 ameloblastomas. Oral Oncol 1999;35:443–449.

13. Small IA, Waldron CA. Ameloblastomas of the jaws. Oral Surg 1955;8:281–297.

14. Baden E. Odontogenic tumors. Pathol Annu 1971;6:487–509.

15. Kramer IRH, Pindborg JJ, Shear M. Histological Typing of Odontogenic Tumours. 2d ed. Berlin: Springer-Verlag, 1992.

16. Coleman HG, Altini M, Groeneveld HT. Nuclear organizer regions (AgNORs) in odontogenic cyst and ameloblastomas. J Oral Pathol Med 1996;25: 436–440.

17. Do Carmo MAV, Silva EC. Argyrophilic nucleolar organizer regions (AgNORs) in ameloblastomas and adenomatoid odontogenic tumours (AOTs). J Oral Pathol Med 1998;27:153–156.

18. Yamamoto G, Yoshitake K, Tada K, et al. Granular cell ameloblastoma. A rare variant. Int J Oral Maxillofac Surg 1989;18:140–141.

19. Hartman KS. Granular-cell ameloblastoma. Oral Surg Oral Med Oral Pathol 1974;38:241–253.

20. Narvarrette AR, Smith M. Ultrastructure of granular cell ameloblastoma. Cancer 1971;27:948–955.

21. Tandler B, Rossi EP. Granular cell ameloblastoma: Electron microscopic observations. J Oral Pathol 1977;6:401–412.

22. Kumamoto H, Ooya K. Immunohistochemical and ultrastructural investigation of apoptotic cell death in granular cell ameloblastoma. J Oral Pathol Med 2001;30:245–250.

23. Altini M, Hille JJ, Buchner A. Plexiform granular cell odontogenic tumor. Oral Surg Oral Med Oral Pathol 1986;61:163–167.

24. Siar CH, Ng KH, Chia TY. Combined granular cell ameloblastoma and plexiform granular cell odontogenic tumour. Singapore Dent J 1990;15:35–37.

25. Siar CH, Ng KH. Unusual granular cell odontogenic tumor. Report of two undescribed cases with features of granular cell ameloblastoma and plexiform granular cell odontogenic tumor. J Nihon Univ Sch Dent 1993;35:134–138.

26. Mirchandani R, Sciubba JJ. Granular cell lesions of the jaws and oral cavity: A clinicopathologic, immunohistochemical, and ultrastructural study. J Oral Maxillofac Surg 1989;47:1248–1255.

27. Rühl GH, Akuamoa-Boateng E. Granular cells in odontogenic and non-odontogenic tumours. Virchows Arch A Pathol Anat Histopathol 1989;415: 403–409.

28. Sandra F, Mitsuyasu T, Nakamura N, et al. Immunohistochemical evaluation of PCNA and Ki-67 in ameloblastoma. Oral Oncol 2001;37:193–198.

29. Pindborg JJ. Odontogenic tumors. In: Pathology of the Dental Hard Tissue. Copenhagen: Munksgaard, 1970:367–428.

30. Altini M, Slabbert HD, Johnston T. Papilliferous keratoameloblastoma. J Oral Pathol Med 1991; 20:46–48.

31. Siar CH, Ng KH. "Combined ameloblastoma and odontogenic keratocyst" or "keratinizing ameloblastoma." Br J Oral Maxillofac Surg 1993;31: 183–186.

32. Said-Al-Naief NAH, Lumerman H, Ramer M, et al. Keratoameloblastoma of the maxilla. A case report and review of the literature. Oral Surg Oral Med Oral Pathol Oral Radiol Endod 1997;84: 535–539.

33. Wilson D, Walker M, Aurora N, Moore S. Ameloblastoma with mucous cell differentiation. Oral Surg Oral Med Oral Pathol Oral Radiol Endod 2001;91:576–578.

34. Slabbert H, Shear M, Altini M. Vacuolated cells and mucous metaplasia in the epithelial linings of radicular and residual cysts. J Oral Pathol Med 1995;24:309–312.

35. Kühn A. Über eine Kombination von Adamantinom mit Hämangiom als zentrale Kiefergeschwulst. Dtsch Mschr Z 1932;50:49–56.

36. Van Rensburg LJ, Thompson IOC, Kruger HEC, Norval EJG. Hemangiomatous ameloblastoma: Clinical, radiologic, and pathologic features. Oral Surg Oral Med Oral Pathol Oral Radiol Endod 2001;91:374–380.

37. Lucas RB. A vascular ameloblastoma. Oral Surg Oral Med Oral Pathol 1957:10;863–868.

38. Fischer B. Über ein primäres Adamantinom der Tibia. Z Pathopsych 1913;12:422–433.

39. Czerniak B, Rojas-Corona RR, Dorfman HD. Morphologic diversity of long bone adamantinoma. The concept of differentiated (regressing) adamantinoma and its relationship to osteo-fibrous dysplasia. Cancer 1989;64:2319–2334.

40. Ueda Y, Blasius S, Edel G, Wuisman P, Bocker W, Roessner A. Osteofibrous dysplasia of long bones—a reactive process of adamantinomatous tissue. J Cancer Res Clin Oncol 1992;18:152–156.

41. Hazelbag HM, Van den Broek LJ, Fleuren GJ, Taminiau AH, Hogendoom PC. Distribution of extracellular matrix components in adamantinoma of long bone suggests fibrous-to-epithelial transformation. Hum Pathol 1997;28:183–188.

42. Sweet DE, Vinh TN, Devaney K. Cortical osteofibrous dysplasia of long bone and its relationship to adamantinoma. A clinicopathologic study of 30 cases. Am J Surg Pathol 1992;16:282–290.

43. Kumar D, Mulligan ME, Levine AM, Dorfman HD. Classic adamantinoma in a 3-year-old. Skeletal Radiol 1998;27:406–409.

44. Aguirre A, Takai Y, Meenaghan M, et al. Lectin histochemistry of ameloblastomas and odontogenic keratocysts. J Oral Pathol Med 1989;18:68–73.

45. Saku T, Shibata Y, Koyama Z, et al. Lectin histochemistry of cystic jaw lesions: An aid for differential diagnosis between cystic ameloblastoma and odontogenic cysts. J Oral Pathol Med 1991; 20:108–113.

46. Vedtofte P, Pindborg JJ, Hakomori S. Relationship of blood group carbohydrates to differentiation patterns of normal and pathological odontogenic epithelium. Acta Pathol Microbiol Immunol Scand [A] 1985;93:25–34.

47. Gardner DG, O'Neill PA. Inability to distinguish ameloblastomas from odontogenic cysts based on expression of blood cell carbohydrates. Oral Surg Oral Med Oral Pathol 1988;66:480–482.

48. Yamada K, Tatemoto Y, Okada Y, Mori M. Immunostaining of involucrin in odontogenic epithelial tumor and cysts. Oral Surg Oral Med Oral Pathol 1989;67:564–568.

49. Mori M, Yamada K, Kasai T, et al. Immunohistochemical expression of amelogenins in odontogenic epithelial tumours and cysts. Virchows Arch A Pathol Anat Histopathol 1991;418:319–325.

50. Saku T, Okabe H, Shimokawa H. Immunohistochemical demonstration of enamel proteins in odontogenic tumors. J Oral Pathol Med 1992;21: 113–119.

51. Snead ML, Luo W, Hsu DD-J, et al. Human ameloblastoma tumors express the amelogenin gene. Oral Surg Oral Med Oral Pathol 1992;74: 64–72.

52. Heikinheimo K, Hormia M, Stenman G, et al. Patterns of expression of intermediate filaments in ameloblastoma and human fetal tooth germ. J Oral Pathol Med 1989;18:264–273.

53. Heikinheimo K. Cell growth and differentiation of developing and neoplastic odontogenic tissues. Turku, Finland: University of Turku, 1993. Dissertation.

54. Salo T, Kainulainen T, Parikka M, Heikinheimo K. Expression of laminin-5 in ameloblastomas and human fetal teeth. J Oral Pathol Med 1999;28: 337–342.

55. Pripatnanont P, Song Y, Harris M, Meghji S. In situ hybridization and immunocytochemical localization of osteolytic cytokines and adhesion molecules in ameloblastomas. J Oral Pathol Med 1998;27:496–500.

56. Kim J, Yook JI. Immunohistochemical study on proliferating cell nuclear antigen expression in ameloblastomas. Eur J Cancer B Oral Oncol 1994;30B:126–131.

57. Funaoka K, Arisue M, Kabayashi I, et al. Immunohistochemical detection of proliferating cell nuclear antigen (PCNA) in 23 cases of ameloblastoma. Eur J Cancer B Oral Oncol 1996;32B: 328–332.

58. Piattelli A, Fioroni M, Santinelli A, Rubini C. Expression of proliferating cell nuclear antigen in ameloblastomas and odontogenic cysts. Oral Oncol 1998;34:408–412.

59. Chen J, Aufdemorte TB, Jiang H, et al. Neoplastic odontogenic epithelial cells express bone sialoprotein. Histochem J 1998;30:1–6.

60. Gao YH, Yang LJ, Yamaguchi A. Immunohistochemical demonstration of bone morphogenetic protein in odontogenic tumors. J Oral Pathol Med 1997;26:273–277.

61. Mitsuyasu T, Harada H, Higuchi Y, et al. Immunohistochemical demonstration of bcl-2 protein in ameloblastoma. J Oral Pathol Med 1997; 26:345–348.

62. Kumamoto H. Detection of apoptosis-related factors and apoptotic cells in ameloblastomas: Analysis by immunohistochemistry and an in situ DNA nick end-labelling method. J Oral Pathol Med 1997;26:419–425.

63. Kitamura K. The study on the ameloblastoma by electron microscope. J Osaka Univ Dent Sch 1958;3:17–34.

64. Moe H, Clausen F, Philipsen HP. The ultrastructure of the simple ameloblastoma. Acta Pathol Microbiol Scand 1961;52:140–154.

65. Kim SK, Nasjleti CE, Weatherbee L. Fine structure of cell types in an ameloblastoma. J Oral Pathol 1979;8:319–332.

66. Nasu M, Ishikawa G. Ameloblastoma. Light and electron microscopic study. Virchows Arch Pathol Anat 1983;399:163–175.

67. Lee KW, El-Labban NG, Kramer IRH. Ultrastructure of a simple ameloblastoma. J Pathol 1972;108:173–176.

68. Mincer HH, McGinnis JP. Ultrastructure of three histologic variants of the ameloblastoma. Cancer 1972;30:1036–1045.

69. Hodson JJ. Observations on origin and nature of the adamantinoma with special reference to certain muco-epidermoid variations. Br J Plast Surg 1957;10:38–59.

70. Cutler LS. Intracytoplasmic desmosomes in human oral neoplasms. Arch Oral Biol 1976;21: 221–226.

71. Takeda Y, Kikuchi H, Suzuki A. Hyaline bodies in ameloblastoma: Histological and ultrastructural observations. J Oral Pathol 1985;14:639–643.

72. Tothouse LS, Majack RA, Fay JT. An ameloblastoma with myofibroblasts and intracellular septate junctions. Cancer 1980;45:2858–2863.

73. Smith SM, Bartov SA. Ameloblastoma with myofibroblasts: First report. J Oral Pathol 1986;15: 284–286.

74. Niizima M. Tissue culture of an ameloblastoma. Z Zellforsch Mikrosk Anat 1957;46:127–138.

75. Niizima M. Enamel epithelium in tissue culture. Am J Anat 1956;99:351–389.

76. Yasuda K, Satomura K, Nagayama M. Behaviour of human ameloblastoma cell in collagen matrix in vitro: An ultrastructural study. J Oral Pathol Med 1991;20:438–442.

77. Harada H, Mitsuyasu T, Nakamura N, et al. Establishment of ameloblastoma cell line, AM-1. J Oral Pathol Med 1998;27:207–212.

78. Gardner DG. Controversies in the nomenclature, diagnosis and treatment of ameloblastoma. In: Wormington P, Evans JR, eds. Controversies in Oral and Maxillofacial Surgery. Philadelphia: WB Saunders, 1994:301–314.

79. Feinberg SE, Steinberg B. Surgical management of ameloblastoma. Current status of the literature. Oral Surg Oral Med Oral Pathol 1996;81: 383–388.

Chapter 6

Peripheral Ameloblastoma

1. Terminology

The peripheral ameloblastoma (PA)—also known as the extraosseous ameloblastoma, soft tissue ameloblastoma, ameloblastoma of mucosal origin, or ameloblastoma of the gingiva—has several of the same histologic characteristics as a solid/multicystic ameloblastoma (SMA), but it occurs in the soft tissues overlying the tooth-bearing areas of the maxilla and mandible. PAs do not invade the underlying bone. (This definition excludes five questionable cases reported as PAs in extragingival locations.[1-5]) Six cases of basal cell carcinomas (BCCs) arising in the gingiva have also been reported and are included in this chapter. Currently, there is general agreement that the PA and the BCC are essentially the same lesion and thus should be regarded as a single entity.[6-9] Sciubba[10] claimed that in spite of many histologic similarities between PA and BCC, the PA deserves to be a separate entity in a biologic context.

Several authors[11-13] refer to Kuru[14] as having reported on the peripheral ameloblastoma for the first time. However, what Kuru described was not a peripheral but rather an intraosseous SMA that penetrated through the alveolar bone, fused with the oral epithelium, and eventually presented itself clinically as a "peripheral lesion." Kuru's case and similar cases reported by Tongdee and Ganggavakin[15] and Stevenson and Austin[16]

should not be considered peripheral ameloblastomas. The cases reported by Gullifer[17] and Ch'in[18] likewise leave much to be desired in fulfilling the requirements of true PAs. The first completely documented case of a PA must be attributed to Stanley and Krogh.[19]

The tumor profile presented in this chapter is based on data from 160 cases of PAs published by Philipsen et al.[20]

2. Clinical and radiologic profile

The PA is a painless, sessile, firm, and exophytic growth, the surface of which is usually relatively smooth but in several cases has been described as "granular" or "pebbly." In other cases the surface exhibits a "papillary" or "warty" appearance. The color of the lesion varies between normal or pink and red or dark red. During mastication the PA may be traumatized, and the lesion may thus show an ulcerated surface or appear keratotic (frictional keratosis). The duration of the lesion is reported to be anywhere between 2 days and 20 years, and the size ranges from 0.3 to 4.5 cm in diameter with a mean of 1.3 cm.

In the vast majority of cases there is no radiologic evidence of bone involvement. Radiographically or at surgery a superficial ero-

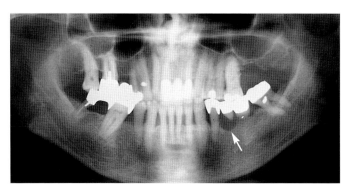

Fig 6-1 Orthopantomograph showing a peripheral ameloblastoma in the area of the left mandibular second premolar. Notice the shallow saucerization of the bone (*arrow*).

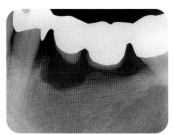

Fig 6-2 Intraoral radiograph of the same case as shown in Fig 6-1.

sion of the bone or a superficial bony depression—cupping, or saucerization—may be noticed (Figs 6-1 and 6-2), a finding that is thought to be caused by pressure resorption rather than resorption caused by neoplastic invasion.

PA is rarely made as the initial preoperative diagnosis. The most common diagnoses, depending on morphology, texture, and color of the lesion, are epulis (42.6%) and benign tumor (26.0%), followed in decreasing order by papilloma and pyogenic granuloma. When the PA arises on the edentulous alveolar mucosa in denture-wearing patients, it may be diagnosed as denture irritation hyperplasia. The correct diagnosis requires histologic evaluation.

3. Epidemiological data

3.1 Incidence, prevalence, and relative frequency

Information on the relative frequency of PAs is very scarce. Data from various sources[20] show that the PA comprises from 2% to 10% of all ameloblastomas. The PA is generally described as an exceedingly rare lesion. The following profile tends to indicate that the PA is actually more prevalent than hitherto anticipated.

3.2 Age

The age range of patients with PAs ($n = 135$) varies between 9 and 92 years at the time of diagnosis, with an overall mean of 52.1 years (Fig 6-3). The mean age of men is slightly higher (52.9 years) than that of women (50.6 years), with 63.7% of all cases occurring in the 5th, 6th, and 7th decades (men, 45.2%; women, 18.5%). Men reach a peak in the 5th and 6th decades, whereas women show two peaks, one in the 4th decade and one in the 7th. The mean age for SMAs[21] was reported to be 37.4 years. Thus, it is important to note that the PA occurs at a significantly higher age than its central "counterpart" (if this term is applicable). This may seem puzzling because most other peripheral odontogenic tumors, such as the adenomatoid odontogenic tumor or the calcifying epithelial odonto-

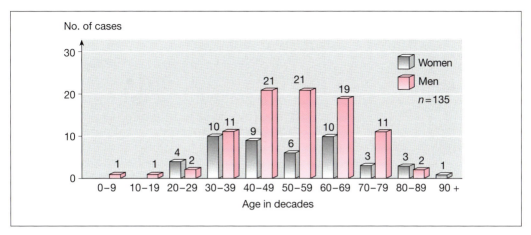

Fig 6-3 Distribution of 135 cases of PAs by age (in decades) and gender.

genic tumor, occur at a noticeably lower mean age than their corresponding (true) intraosseous counterparts.

3.3 Gender

When considering the distribution of PAs according to gender (n = 160), 104 (65.0%) occurred in men and 56 (35.0%) in women, the male:female ratio being 1.9:1. The corresponding figures for SMAs are 54.5% in men and 45.5% in women, giving a ratio of 1.2:1.[21]

3.4 Location

The soft tissues overlaying the tooth-bearing areas of the mandible are clearly the most common site for PAs (n = 135; as no statistically significant differences could be found between the Japanese and the non-Japanese location data, the data were pooled) as shown by the occurrence of 97 (71.9%) lesions in the mandible and 38 (28.1%) lesions in the maxilla. A detailed location analysis is shown in Fig 6-4. By far the most common site for PA development within the jaws was

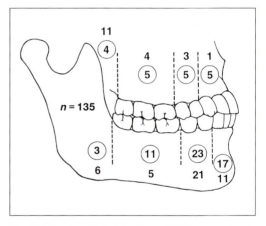

Fig 6-4 Anatomic distribution of 135 cases of PAs according to Japanese cases (n = 73, numbers circled) and non-Japanese cases (n = 62, numbers not circled).

the soft tissues of the mandibular premolar region with 32.6% of all lesions found here. Second was the anterior mandibular region, accounting for 20.7%. In the maxilla, however, the most common location was the soft palatal tissue of the tuberosity which accounted for 11.1% of all cases. The maxilla:mandible ratio was 1:2.5, a figure that should be compared to 1:5.4 for solid/multicystic ameloblastomas. It is of further interest that the majority of the mandibular PA cases were located on the lingual aspect of the gingiva.

3.5 Extragingival lesions reported as PAs

As mentioned earlier, five extragingival lesions have been reported under the term *peripheral ameloblastoma*. Four of the lesions involved the buccal mucosa and one, the floor of the mouth. The authors argued that because of the histologic similarity to ameloblastomas, and with consideration given to the pluripotentiality of the oral epithelium, these lesions could be considered to be examples of PA. Zhu et al[13] believed the term *peripheral ameloblastoma* should be used not only to describe a neoplasm arising in the soft tissues overlying a tooth-bearing region, but also to include those found in more remote locations such as the buccal mucosa, lips, palate, and other parts of the oral mucosa. The authors based their view on an animal experiment, where combined oral epithelium and dental papilla were cut from 17.5-day-old C3H mouse embryos and transplanted to the renal subcapsular space of 3-month-old syngeneic mice. After 3 weeks the formation of teeth and odontogenic keratocysts were apparent. These findings were later interpreted by Zhu and coworkers[13] as the oral epithelium having the potential to differentiate into ameloblasts and to form teeth and odontogenic lesions, an interpretation that may be difficult to accept regarding the development of PAs.

Extragingival lesions have not been included under the diagnosis of PA in this book. They most likely represent basal cell adenomas with a histopathologic resemblance to an ameloblastoma or the rare ameloblastoid variant of the squamous cell carcinoma. It is characteristic that the reported five extragingival cases all developed around the orifices of either the Stensen duct or the Wharton duct and could thus represent tumors of salivary gland origin.

3.6 Inclusion of the odontogenic gingival epithelial hamartoma (OGEH) under a peripheral ameloblastoma diagnosis

The OGEH, also referred to as a hamartoma of the dental lamina rests, is a rare, as yet incompletely defined, peripherally localized hamartomatous lesion initially described by Baden et al.[22] Details of the six cases reported so far are summarized in Table 2 in Philipsen et al.[20] The OGEHs occurred in one male and five female patients with a mean age of 57 years at the time of diagnosis. The maxilla:mandible ratio was 1:5 and the lesions were located in the anterior gingival (5 cases) and premolar (1 case) regions of the jaws. The lesions presented as asymptomatic, small rounded masses, often on the lingual aspect of the alveolar ridge.

Radiographically or at surgery a slight cupping of the adjacent bone was a common finding. Histologically the lesions showed islands, clusters, and thin bands of odontogenic epithelial cells scattered in a mature fibrous stroma which became loose and slightly myxomatous in the depth of the lesion. The epithelial cells sometimes occurred in a lobular pattern and tended to be arranged in an outer layer that was cuboidal or columnar shaped with closely packed central cells, oval to polyhedral in shape. Half of the cases reported revealed continuity between the lesional tissue and the overlying rete ridges of the oral epithelium, while in the other half no such connection could be found. In considering the histogenesis of the OGEH, two major sources of origin must be considered: the basal cell layer of the surface epithelium and remnants of the dental lamina. Following excision, no recurrences were reported in the five cases where follow-up data were available.

A comparison between the clinical and behavioral features of the OGEH with those of the PA leads to the assumption that they could likely be considered the same lesion. Data on age, clinical findings such as location, radiographic appearance, behavioral pattern, and histology appear to be identical. Whereas knowledge and understanding of the biologic profile of PA is well documented, the same cannot be said of the OGEH, the characteristics of which are based on only six reported cases. In 1989, Moskow and Baden[23] published a report of four cases of what they termed odontogenic epithelial hamartoma (OEH). Unfortunately, no data were given as to gender, age, or clinicoradiologic features. The authors described two variants of OEH, a peripheral or gingival type (formerly known as OGEH) and a second, intraosseous or central type not hitherto reported. The authors believed it is likely that OEH can occur wherever epithelial residues from the developing tooth and the dental lamina exist. Thus, both gingival and intraosseous lesions may occur. A final conclusion as to terminology, relationship to PA, and peripheral odontogenic fibroma awaits assessment of additional published cases of OEH.

4. Pathogenesis

When discussing the cellular origin of PAs that continue to provide an academic challenge, two major sources should be considered. Those lesions that are located entirely within the connective tissue of the gingiva show no continuity with the surface epithelium, and are separated from the surface epithelium by a band of collagenous tissue likely arise from remnants of the dental lamina located in the soft tissues overlying the tooth-bearing areas of the jawbones. These cell remnants, or Serres pearls, are often encountered in the normal tissues adjacent to PAs.

Alternatively, lesions may arise from the surface epithelium, in some cases at one or a few sites and in others multifocally.[24] The hypothesis that the continuity between the tumor and the surface epithelium is fortuitous and simply represents fusion of the underlying tumor with the surface epithelium seems unlikely because of its frequent appearance.[6]

5. Pathology

5.1 Macroscopy

The gross specimen consists of a firm to slightly spongy mass of pink to pinkish gray color. The cut surface may contain minute cystic spaces filled with clear, pale yellow fluid. As occasional areas of dystrophic calcification are very small, they are not disclosed by cutting through the specimen or detected on a radiograph of the operation specimen.

5.2 Microscopy

5.2.1 Histologic definitions

The 1992 edition of the WHO clasification[25] does not contain a histologic definition of the PA (and/or BCC) in spite of the fact that almost 50 published cases were available for analysis at the time of publication. It receives only a brief (three-line) mention under ameloblastoma ("other variations"), simply indicat-

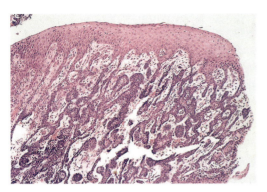

Fig 6-5 Photomicrograph showing epithelial tumor cell nests that are continuous with the oral epithelium (hematoxylin-eosin [H&E], ×20).

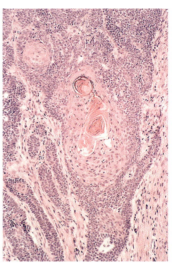

Fig 6-6
Follicular tumor islands showing acanthomatous features (H&E, ×160).

ing that "some ameloblastomas (peripheral ameloblastoma) appear to arise directly from the surface epithelium or from residues of the dental lamina lying outside the bone."

The histologic definition used by the present authors is as follows:

The peripheral ameloblastoma is a benign neoplasm (or hamartomatous lesion) confined to the soft tissue overlying the tooth-bearing areas of the jaws or alveolar mucosa in edentulous areas. The tumor consists of proliferating odontogenic epithelium that exhibits the same histomorphologic cell types and patterns as seen in the solid/multicystic ameloblastoma. The stroma is that of mature, fibrous connective tissue. Occurrence of calcifications, dentinoid, bonelike, or cementum-like masses are not characteristic histologic features of the PA.

5.2.2 Histopathologic findings

Most of the epithelial islands exhibit palisading of columnar basal cells, but a stellate reticulum is seldom conspicuous (Fig 6-5). A basaloid lesion without the classical follicular component but often exhibiting acan-

thomatous areas (Fig 6-6) is difficult to distinguish from the basal cell carcinoma. Some of the squamous cells in the acanthomatous nests may show "ghosting" (ghost cell formation and foreign body reaction to this material within the connective tissue), features generally associated with the calcifying ghost cell odontogenic cyst (see chapter 17).[6,26]

A number of cases of PAs exhibiting areas composed of clear cells have been reported.[24,27,28] In some parts of the tumors, vacuolated or clear cells occurred as discrete clusters or in direct transition from ameloblastic (often acanthomatous) tumor cells. These clear cells are cytomorphologically and histochemically identical to those reported to occur in the dental lamina and in several other lesions of odontogenic origin—notably the lateral periodontal cyst, the gingival cyst of adults, the calcifying ghost cell odontogenic tumor (see chapter 17), the calcifying epithelial odontogenic tumor (see chapter 10), and the clear cell odontogenic carcinoma (see chapter 27).

It is of the utmost importance for oral pathologists and oral surgeons to understand that, irrespective of the nomenclature, the peripheral ameloblastoma exhibits a different biologic behavior than the solid/multicystic ameloblastoma. This knowledge can help avoid the unnecessary, extensive, and sometimes mutilating surgery that has been performed in some cases.[20]

5.2.3 Malignant variants of PA

The nosology of odontogenic carcinomas has varied over the years since the first edition of the WHO classification in 1971. A recent nosologic approach was proposed by Eversole.[29] A total of six cases of malignant PAs (ameloblastic carcinomas) have been published[12,30–34] (see Table 3 in Philipsen et al[20]).

5.2.4 Differential diagnostic considerations

Three lesions may be considered by the pathologist in the differential diagnosis of PA. The first is the *peripheral odontogenic fibroma* (POF) (WHO or complex type, Gardner[35]). The proliferation of strands and islands of odontogenic epithelium in this tumor may be so extensive as to make the distinction from PA very difficult.[36] Siar and Ng[37] investigated the immunohistochemical characteristics of POF and PA in an attempt to elucidate their histogenesis but could not confirm or exclude an origin in the surface epithelium for the epithelial elements. The second lesion is the rare *peripheral variant of the squamous odontogenic tumor* (SOT). The SOT was recently reviewed[38] based on 36 cases from the literature, of which five were of the peripheral type. The oral pathologist should, however, not encounter severe problems when differentiating PA from SOT. The third lesion is the *odontogenic gingival epithelial hamartoma* discussed previously. The question of whether this lesion should be included under the histopathologic spec-

trum of the peripheral ameloblastoma awaits further clarification.

Of the three lesions, POF constitutes the most important differential diagnostic problem. It must be stressed, however, that although the differential diagnosis relating to PA is challenging, it remains an academic exercise because all the lesions concerned are benign neoplasms and/or hamartomatous lesions requiring only conservative treatment modalities.

6. Notes on treatment and recurrence rate

As noted by Gardner,[6] the term *peripheral ameloblastoma* is potentially dangerous in that this diagnosis may lead to unnecessarily aggressive treatment. Whereas the solid/multicystic ameloblastoma is a locally aggressive neoplasm capable of invasive behavior and destruction of bone—and thus requires extensive surgical treatment, the PA does not manifest such behavior. The current treatment of choice, conservative supraperiosteal surgical excision with adequate disease-free margins, is often confounded by the ominous connotation the term *ameloblastoma* has in the mind of the surgeon. A change in nomenclature to the term *peripheral ameloblastoid hamartoma*, which has been suggested by Richardson and Greer,[39] may, however, create confusion and the present authors do not subscribe to its use.

Recurrent PAs develop from the general site of the original lesion and are thought to be a sign of incomplete removal rather than aggressiveness. Although the recurrence rate is much lower (16%[28] to 19%[40]) than that of SMAs, long-term follow-up is mandatory, especially in light of the report of a benign-appearing PA recurring as an ameloblastic carcinoma.[12] There is at least one major factor responsible for the good prognosis of PAs. The cortical bone of the jaws, which represents a strong barrier to the infiltrative power of SMAs, is also an efficient barrier to invasion by PAs. Some authors have questioned, based on the benign behavior of PAs, whether they are truly analogous to SMAs.[20] The biologic behavior of the PA seems in line with that of a hamartoma or persistent hyperplasia rather than that of a neoplasia.

Since the first review in 1987,[40] the number of published cases of PAs has increased from 26 to 160 (at the end of 2000), making the fairly detailed profile in this chapter possible. This tumor must be viewed as a relatively innocuous lesion totally lacking the persistent invasiveness of the intraosseous ameloblastoma. There remain, however, unsolved PA-related problems, like tumor origin, the origin of "extragingival PA lesions," the relationship between OGEHs and PAs (one or two entities), and the malignant potentiality of PAs to mention a few.

It is highly recommended that clinicians report cases that involve data and/or information relevant to the areas where knowledge is lacking. It may be worth stressing that any published report should include all relevant data—age, gender, exact tumor location (preferably with clinical photographs), radiographic documentation, and histopathology (micrographic documentation that includes low as well as high magnifications), to mention but a few. It is the (sad) experience of the present authors that, in the past, a considerable number of publications that seemed to represent valuable contributions had to be excluded from a given review due to inadequate and insufficient case presentation.

References

1. Braunstein E. Case report of an extraosseous adamantinoblastoma. Oral Surg Oral Med Oral Pathol 1949;2:726–728.

2. Klinar K, McManis JC. Soft-tissue ameloblastoma. Report of a case. Oral Surg Oral Med Oral Pathol 1969;28:266–272.

3. Ramnarayan K, Nayak RG, Kavalam AG. Peripheral ameloblastoma. Int J Oral Surg 1985;14: 300–301.

4. Woo S-B, Smith-Williams JE, Sciubba JJ, Lipper S. Peripheral ameloblastoma of the buccal mucosa: Case report and review of the English literature. Oral Surg Oral Med Oral Pathol 1987;6:78–84.

5. Shibata T, Keneko N, Hokazono K, et al. An ameloblastoma-like neoplasm of the buccal mucosa. Report of a case. Int J Maxillofac Surg 1990;19:203–204.

6. Gardner DG. Peripheral ameloblastoma. A study of 21 cases, including 5 reported as basal cell carcinoma of the gingival. Cancer 1977;39:1625–1633.

7. Waldron CA. Comment on the basal cell carcinoma of the oral cavity. J Oral Surg 1972;30:66.

8. Simpson HE. Basal-cell carcinoma and peripheral ameloblastoma. Oral Surg Oral Med Oral Pathol 1974;38:233–240.

9. Moskow BS, Baden E. The peripheral ameloblastoma of the gingiva. Case report and literature review. J Periodontol 1982;53:736–742.

10. Sciubba JJ. Discussion of El-Mofty S, Gerard NO, Farish SE, Rodu B. Peripheral ameloblastoma: A clinical and histologic study of 11 cases. J Oral Maxillofac Surg 1991;49:970–975.

11. Kaneko Y, Ueno S. Peripheral ameloblastoma resembling a papilloma: Report of case. J Oral Maxillofac Surg 1986;44:737–739.

12. Baden E, Doyle JL, Petriella V. Malignant transformation of peripheral ameloblastoma. Oral Surg Oral Med Oral Pathol 1993;75:214–219.

13. Zhu EX, Okada N, Takagi M. Peripheral ameloblastoma: Case report and review of literature. J Oral Maxillofac Surg 1995;53:590–594.

14. Kuru H. Ueber das Adamantinom. Zentralbl Allg Pathol 1911;22:291–295.

15. Tongdee C, Ganggavakin S. Peripheral amelo-blastoma (report of a case and review of litera-ture). J Dent Assoc Thai 1978;28:31–38.

16. Stevenson ARL, Austin BW. A case of amelo-blastoma presenting as an exophytic gingival le-sion. J Periodontol 1990;60:378–381.

17. Gullifer W. Adamantinoma. Dental Cosmos 1936:78:1256–1259.

18. Ch'in K. Adamantinoma in Chinese. Chin Med J 1938;(Suppl II): 91–130.

19. Stanley HR, Krogh HW. Peripheral ameloblas-toma. Report of a case. Oral Surg Oral Med Oral Pathol 1959;12:760–765.

20. Philipsen HP, Reichart PA, Nikai H, Takata T, Kudo Y. Peripheral ameloblastoma: Biological profile based on 160 cases from the literature. Oral Oncol 2001;37:17–27.

21. Reichart PA, Philipsen HP, Sonner S. Ameloblas-toma: Biological profile of 3677 cases. Oral On-col 1995;31B:86–99.

22. Baden E, Moskow BS, Moskow R. Odontogenic gingival epithelial hamartoma. J Oral Surg 1968;26:702–714.

23. Moskow BS, Baden E. Odontogenic epithelial hamartomas in periodontal structures. J Clin Pe-riodontol 1989;16:92–97.

24. Anneroth G, Johansson B. Peripheral ameloblas-toma. Int J Oral Surg 1985;14:295–299.

25. Kramer IRH, Pindborg JJ, Shear M. Histological Typing of Odontogenic Tumours. 2d ed. Berlin: Springer-Verlag, 1992.

26. Pansino FA, Meara JW. Case report: Peripheral ameloblastoma. J Mich Dent Assoc 1975;57:129–130.

27. Ng KH, Siar CH. Peripheral ameloblastoma with clear cell differentiation. Oral Surg Oral Med Oral Pathol 1990;70:210–213.

28. Redman RS, Keegan BP, Spector CJ, Patterson RH. Peripheral ameloblastoma with unusual mi-totic activity and conflicting evidence regarding histogenesis. J Oral Maxillofac Surg 1994;52:192–197.

29. Eversole LR. Malignant epithelial odontogenic tumors. Semin Diagn Pathol 1999;16:317–324.

30. Edmondson HD, Browne RM, Potts AJC. Intrao-ral basal cell carcinoma. Br J Oral Surg 1982;20:239–247.

31. Lin S-C, Lieu C-M, Hahn L-J, Kwan H-W. Periph-eral ameloblastoma with metastasis. Int J Max-illofac Surg 1987;16:202–204.

32. McClatchey KD, Sullivan MJ, Paugh DR. Periph-eral ameloblastic carcinoma: A case report of a rare neoplasm. J Otolaryngol 1989;18:109–111.

33. Bucci E, Lo Muzio L, Mignogna MD, de Rosa G. Peripheral ameloblastoma: Case report. Acta Stomatol Belg 1992;89:267–269.

34. Califano L, Maremonti P, Boscaino A, et al. Pe-ripheral ameloblastoma: Report of a case with ma-lignant aspect. Br J Oral Maxillofac Surg 1996;34:240–242.

35. Gardner DG. Central odontogenic fibroma cur-rent concepts. J Oral Pathol Med 1996;25:556–561.

36. Gardner DG. The peripheral odontogenic fibro-ma: An attempt at clarification. Oral Surg Oral Med Oral Pathol 1982;54:40–48.

37. Siar CH, Ng KH. An immunohistochemical study of two cases of either peripheral odontogenic fi-broma (WHO type) or peripheral ameloblastoma. J Nihon Univ Sch Dent 1996;38:52–56.

38. Philipsen HP, Reichart PA. Squamous odonto-genic tumor (SOT): A benign neoplasm of the pe-riodontium. A review of 36 reported cases. J Clin Periodontol 1996;23:922–926.

39. Richardson JF, Greer RO. Ameloblastoma of mu-cosal origin. Arch Otolaryngol 1974;100:174–175.

40. Buchner A, Sciubba JJ. Peripheral epithelial odontogenic tumors: A review. Oral Surg Oral Med Oral Pathol 1987;63:688–697.

Chapter 7

Desmoplastic Ameloblastoma

1. Terminology

Two reports from Japan, the first in 1981[1] and the second in 1983,[2] first called attention to an unusual variant of the solid/multi-cystic ameloblastoma (SMA). However, Eversole and coworkers[3] are usually credited for the first English-language publication on the desmoplastic ameloblastoma (DA). This tumor is characterized by an unusual histomorphology, including extensive stromal collagenization or desmoplasia, leading to the proposed term *ameloblastoma with pronounced desmoplasia*, or desmoplastic ameloblastoma. A possible "transitional" form of DA, showing microscopic features of the desmoplastic variant together with areas typical of "classic" follicular or plexiform ameloblastoma, has been called a "hybrid" lesion of ameloblastoma and is described later in this chapter. The following data are based on a review of 100 cases (Philipsen et al[4]) supplemented with data from a recent report (Kishino et al[5]), bringing the total number of DA cases reviewed to 109.

2. Clinical and radiologic profile

DA is a benign, locally infiltrative epithelial neoplasm believed to be a variant or subtype of the SMA. A painless swelling represents the chief initial complaint in most cases. A characteristic feature is an almost equal distribution in location between the maxilla and mandible. The size of the tumor varies between 1.0 and 8.5 cm at its greatest diameter. A true peripheral variant of DA without bone involvement, and thus similar to the peripheral ameloblastoma (PA), has not been reported so far.

The radiographic features of DA differ in most cases from those of SMA. The radiographic features of SMA are classically described as uni- or multilocular radiolucencies with relatively well-defined borders. However, borders were well defined in only 7% of the DA cases where data were available. The content of the lesion was mixed radiolucent/radiopaque in 53% of the cases (Figs 7-1 to 7-3). Thus, in many cases the preoperative radiographic diagnosis was that of a fibro-osseous lesion. Resorption of tooth roots is a common finding (Fig 7-4). The fact that new bone formation has been reported in several cases of DAs may explain the mixed radiolucent/radiopaque appearance.[6-14] Takata et al[15] believed that the mixed radiologic appearance expresses the infiltrative pattern of the tumor. When the DA infiltrates the bone marrow spaces, as observed in their seven reported cases, remnants of the original nonmetaplastic or nonneoplastic bone remain in the tumor tissue. The infiltrative behavior of the DA may also explain one of the characteristic features of

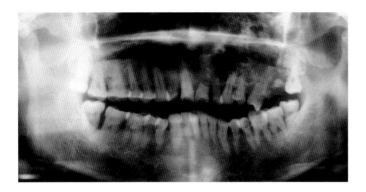

Fig 7-1 Orthopantomograph revealing a fibro-osseous–like DA occupying the entire left maxillary region in a 53-year-old man.

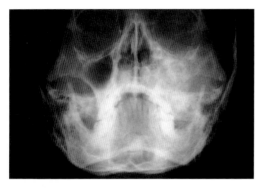

Fig 7-2 Radiograph of the patient in Fig 7-1, showing involvement of the entire left maxilla.

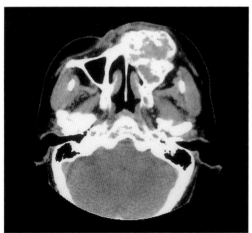

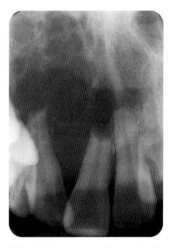

Fig 7-3 Computed tomography (CT) scan of the same patient. There is obliteration of the left maxillary sinus by a radiolucent/radiopaque tumor mass.

Fig 7-4 Intraoral radiograph showing marked root resorption of both lateral and central upper incisors. Note scattered radiopacities.

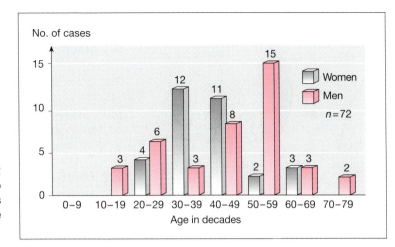

Fig 7-5 Distribution of 72 DA cases according to gender and age groups (where a specific age was identified).

this tumor, the ill-defined border. Takata et al's interpretation of the mixed radiologic appearance does not, however, explain why this feature is never found in the conventional SMA. An association between DA and an unerupted or impacted tooth has been found in only three cases (3.4%) so far[16,17] compared to 8.7% among SMA.[18]

3. Epidemiological data

3.1 Incidence, prevalence, and relative frequency

DAs account for 4% to 13% of all SMAs.[14–26] Data retrieved from different geographic regions[27] seem to suggest that the relative frequency of DA is slightly less in the Japanese population compared to American and European populations. However, to evaluate some true geographic differences in relative DA frequencies, more studies are needed. Ng and Siar[23] indicated a 3% rate for DA based on all odontogenic tumors.

3.2 Age

The age range of patients with DA varies between 17 and 72 years (n = 72) at the time of diagnosis (Fig 7-5), the overall mean age being 42.8 years (men, 42.9 years; women, 40.3 years) compared to 35.9 years (men, 39.2; women, 35.2) for SMAs. The age distribution in Fig 7-5 shows female peaks in the 4th and 5th decades; a single male peak appears in the 6th decade. Of all the tumors studied, 70.8% were within the age range of 30 to 59 years.

3.3 Gender

The male:female ratio was 1:0.9 (n = 109).

3.4 Location

Figure 7-6 shows the site distribution within the jawbones of 85 cases of DA (in which the site was identified). Note that 7 cases involved the entire maxillary quadrant. Given that 43 (50.6%) of the tumors were located in the maxilla and 42 (49.4%) in the mandible, the maxilla:mandible ratio was close to

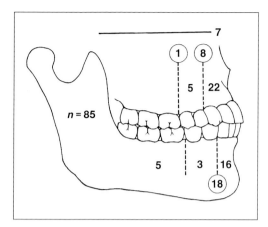

Fig 7-6 Anatomic distribution of DAs (*n* = 85) with known location. Circled numbers above and below the vertical broken lines indicate numbers of cases involving two adjacent areas of the jaw. Solid horizontal line at top indicates involvement of an entire maxillary quadrant.

1:1. This is in sharp contrast to the corresponding figures for SMAs which showed a ratio of 1:5.4.[18] Only 5 out of 85 cases (5.9%) of DA were found in the mandibular molar region as opposed to 39% of SMA cases.[18]

4. Pathogenesis

Although the biologic behavior of the DA is still unresolved, it is generally agreed that the tumor is a variant of SMA. It seems unlikely that the DA is derived from sources different from those of the SMA. Oxytalan fibers have been identified in the stromal tissue of one case reported by Kawai et al.[28] This finding was interpreted by the authors as indicating a tumor derivation from the epithelial rests of Malassez in the periodontal membrane of a related tooth.

5. Pathology

5.1 Macroscopy

The gross specimen most often consists of resected portions of the jaws. The tumor mass is often solid, whitish, and has a gritty or "frozen ice-cream"–like consistency.

5.2 Microscopy

5.2.1 Histologic definition

The relatively small number (approximately 20) of published cases of DAs available when the 1992 edition of the World Health Organization (WHO) classification[29] was published did not allow the authors to produce a detailed histologic definition for DA. The definition used by the present authors is as follows:
A benign but locally invasive variant of the solid/multicystic ameloblastoma consisting of proliferating, irregular, often bizarrely shaped islands (Figs 7-7 and 7-8) and cords of odontogenic epithelium of varying sizes embedded in a desmoplastic, connective tissue stroma.

5.2.2 Histopathologic findings

The occasional large tumor islands in DAs are often very irregular in shape with a pointed, stellate appearance. The morphology of these islands is often bizarre with an almost pathognomonic, "animal-like" configuration or outline. The epithelial cells at the periphery of the islands are cuboidal, occasionally with hyperchromatic nuclei. Columnar cells demonstrating reversed nuclear polarity are rarely conspicuous, although an occasional isolated island may exhibit focal ameloblast-like peripheral cells (Fig 7-9). The center of the epithelial islands appears hypercellular with spindle-shaped or squamatoid, occasionally keratinized, epithelial cells. Micro-

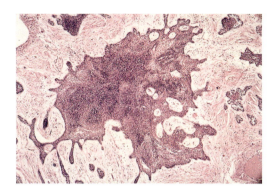

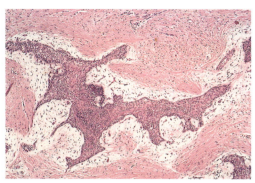

Fig 7-7 Photomicrograph showing a large epithelial tumor island with an irregular outline. The central part of the island is hypercellular (hematoxylin-eosin [H&E] ×50).

Fig 7-8 Higher magnification of the epithelial tumor island. Note the marked desmoplasia of the stroma (H&E, ×80).

Fig 7-9 Peripheral part of a tumor island. The cuboidal or low cylindrical (ameloblast-like) cells are present only focally. Toward the center there is hypercellularity of spindle-shaped or polygonal cells arranged in a whorled or fasciculated pattern. A stratum reticulare–like appearance is lacking (H&E, ×150).

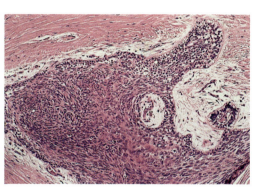

cysts that contain eosinophilic amorphous deposits or appear empty are commonly found within the tumor islands. Kawai et al[28] reported an unusual DA case where a large cavity lined by degenerated epithelial cells constituted a cystic part of the tumor. Foci of keratinization occur sporadically. True glandular differentiation with mucus cells has also been described in tumor nests.[15] Thus, the general histologic pattern of DA resembles, to some extent, that of a follicular SMA with acanthomatous features.

Extensive stromal desmoplasia is a constant and striking finding characterized by a moderately cellular fibrous connective tissue with abundant thick collagen fibers that seem to compress or "squeeze" the odontogenic epithelial islands from the periphery. The mechanism of desmoplasia is not understood. Myxoid changes of the stroma may be observed surrounding the odontogenic epithelium. Formation of metaplastic bone trabeculae (osteoplasia) rimmed by active osteoblasts has been described in several cases.[6–9,11,16,17] A peripheral fibrous condensation suggestive of a capsule is not characteristic.

5.2.3 Immunohistochemical findings

Using various immunohistochemical techniques, Siar and Ng[17] demonstrated that DA tumor cells showed variable expression of S-100 protein and desmin, similar to other types of SMAs. However, keratin immunoreactivity was inconstant and confined to tumor cells showing squamous differentiation. Vimentin was not expressed by either squamatoid or spindle-shaped cells. The authors concluded that the differences in the expression of these antigens among various ameloblastoma types may be attributed to diverse factors such as dedifferentiation or the rate of proliferation of the neoplastic cells, inherent cellular potentials, or extracellular mediators.

In a comparative immunohistochemical study, Becker et al[30] showed that the connective tissue stroma in a DA—contrary to that of an SMA—exhibited a strong positive reaction for collagen type VI. This was interpreted as indicating an active de novo synthesis of extracellular matrix protein. In other words, the desmoplastic stroma of DAs is not simple scar tissue but newly produced connective tissue. In contrast to SMAs, marked immunoexpression of transforming growth factor (TGF-β) was observed in 6 out of 7 DA cases.[15] The authors suggested that TGF-β produced by DA tumor cells plays a part in the prominent desmoplastic matrix formation.

6. Notes on treatment and recurrence rate

Current knowledge must lead to the recommendation that the same radical treatment modalities used for SMAs be used for DAs.

The biologic behavior of the DA, including recurrence rate, still cannot be fully appreciated due to the relatively few reported cases with sufficiently long follow-up periods. According to the 1992 WHO classification, "unicystic, peripheral, and possibly desmoplastic ameloblastoma have lower recurrence rates than other ameloblastomas."[29] However, even today, when as many as 109 cases of DAs are available for assessment, it is premature to estimate recurrence rates. The radiologic and histologic findings of poor encapsulation or total lack of a capsule require long-term follow-up, and the findings likely indicate that the DA has a potential for recurrence similar to SMAs, excluding some subtypes of the unicystic ameloblastoma. The answer can be found only when more information becomes available in the literature.

7. "Hybrid" lesion of ameloblastoma (HLA)

The HLA was first described by Waldron and El-Mofty[21] and is yet another tumor variant in which, histologically, areas of follicular or plexiform SMA coexist with areas characteristic of DAs. It is much too early to speculate whether desmoplastic changes occur secondarily in the stroma of a preexisting SMA, or whether areas of primary DA transform into an SMA. It has been suggested that the hybrid lesion should be considered a collision tumor. Melrose[31] wrote that the designation *hybrid tumor* serves no real purpose and, if taken literally, might overstate the significance of finding a DA in combination with islands of a SMA. Many more cases than the nine published so far[7,16,21,32]—with detailed clinical and radiologic data and corresponding histopathologic analysis—are needed to clarify the biologic behavior of this variant. Until then it is advisable to treat cases of HLA like those of SMAs.

References

1. Takigawa T, Matsumoto M, Sekine Y, et al. A case report of ameloblastoma proliferated like epulis of maxilla [in Japanese]. Nihon Univ Dent J 1981; 55:920–924.

2. Uji Y, Kodama K, Sakamoto A, Taen A. An ameloblastoma with interesting histological findings [in Japanese]. Jpn J Oral Maxillofac Surg 1983;29: 1512–1519.

3. Eversole LR, Leider AS, Hansen LS. Ameloblastomas with pronounced desmoplasia. J Oral Maxillofac Surg 1984;42:735–740.

4. Philipsen HP, Reichart PA, Takata T. Desmoplastic ameloblastoma (including "hybrid" lesion of ameloblastoma). Biological profile based on 100 cases from the literature and own files. Oral Oncol 2001;37:455–460.

5. Kishino M, Murakami S, Fukuda Y, Ishida T. Pathology of the desmoplastic ameloblastoma. J Oral Pathol Med 2001;30:35–40.

6. Okada Y, Sugimura M, Ishida T. Ameloblastoma accompanied by prominent bone formation. J Oral Maxillofac Surg 1986;44:555–557.

7. Philipsen HP, Ormiston IW, Reichart PA. The desmo- and osteoplastic ameloblastoma. Histologic variant or clinicopathologic entity? Case reports. Int J Oral Maxillofac Surg 1992;21: 352–357.

8. Yoshimura Y, Saito H. Desmoplastic variant of ameloblastoma: Report of a case and review of the literature. J Oral Maxillofac Surg 1990;48: 1231–1235.

9. Thompson IOC, van Rensburg LJ, Phillips VMJ. Desmoplastic ameloblastoma: Correlative histopathology, radiology and CT-MR imaging. J Oral Pathol Med 1996;25:405–410.

10. Tanimoto K, Takata T, Suei Y, Wada T. A case of desmoplastic variant of a mandibular ameloblastoma. J Oral Maxillofac Surg 1991;49:94–97.

11. Takemoto T, Yamashita T, Ito A, et al. A case of ameloblastoma of maxilla with bone tissue in the tumor [in Japanese]. Jpn J Oral Maxillofac Surg 1991;37:234–239.

12. Ishigami T, Sugihara K, Uchiyama T, et al. Ameloblastoma of the maxilla with bone tissue in the tumor: Report of a case [in Japanese]. Jpn J Oral Maxillofac Surg 1991;37:2103–2104.

13. Ludvikoya M, Michal M, Zamecnik M, et al. Desmoplastic ameloblastoma. Cesk Patol 1998; 34:94–98.

14. Ashman SG, Corio RL, Eisele DW, Murphy MT. Desmoplastic ameloblastoma. A case report and literature review. Oral Surg Oral Med Oral Pathol 1993;75:479–482.

15. Takata T, Miyauchi M, Ito H, et al. Clinical and histopathological analyses of desmoplastic ameloblastoma. Pathol Res Pract 1999;195: 669–675.

16. Higuchi Y, Nakamura N, Ohishi M, Tashiro H. Unusual ameloblastoma with extensive stromal desmoplasia. J Craniomaxillofac Surg 1991;19: 323–327.

17. Siar CH, Ng KH. Patterns of expression of intermediate filaments and S-100 protein in desmoplastic ameloblastoma. J Nihon Univ Sch Dent 1993;35:104–108.

18. Reichart PA, Philipsen HP, Sonner S. Ameloblastoma: Biological profile of 3677 cases. Oral Oncol 1995;31B:86–99.

19. Keszler A, Paparella ML, Dominguez FV. Desmoplastic and non-desmoplastic ameloblastoma: A comparative clinicopathological analysis. Oral Dis 1996;2:228–231.

20. Kaffe I, Buchner A, Taicher S. Radiologic features of desmoplastic variant of ameloblastoma. Oral Surg Oral Med Oral Pathol 1993;76:525–529.

21. Waldron CA, El-Mofty SK. A histopathologic study of 116 ameloblastomas with special references to the desmoplastic variant. Oral Surg Oral Med Oral Pathol 1987;63:441–451.

22. Lo Muzio L, Orabona P, Costalunga C, Della Valle A. Ameloblastoma desmoplastico. Presentazione di un caso clinico. Minerva Stomatol 1996;45: 285–288.

23. Ng KH, Siar CH. Desmoplastic variant of ameloblastoma in Malaysians. Br J Oral Maxillofac Surg 1993;31:299–303.

24. Lam KY, Chan ACL, Wu PC, et al. Desmoplastic variant of ameloblastoma in Chinese patients. Br J Oral Maxillofac Surg 1998;36:129–134.

25. Fukushima D, Kobayashi H, Takeda I, et al. A case of desmoplastic ameloblastoma of the maxilla. Bull Tokyo Dent Coll 1997;38:223–227.

26. Morita S, Arika T, Nakajima M, et al. A clinical, radiologic and pathologic study of desmoplastic ameloblastoma [in Japanese]. Jpn J Oral Maxillofac Surg 1994;40:988–996.

27. Lu Y, Xuan M, Takata T, et al. Odontogenic tumors: A demographic study of 759 cases in a Chinese population. Oral Surg Oral Med Oral Pathol 1998;86:707–714.

28. Kawai T, Kishino M, Hiranuma H, et al. A unique case of desmoplastic ameloblastoma of the mandible: Report of a case and brief review of the English language literature. Oral Surg Oral Med Oral Pathol Oral Radiol Endod 1999;87:258–263.

29. Kramer IRH, Pindborg JJ, Shear M. Histological Typing of Odontogenic Tumors. 2d ed. Berlin: Springer-Verlag, 1992.

30. Becker J, Reichart PA, Philipsen HP. Comparative immunohistochemical study of the follicular and the desmoplastic ameloblastoma. Pathol Int (in press).

31. Melrose RJ. Desmoplastic ameloblastoma. Pathol Rev 1999;4:21–27.

32. Takata T, Miyauchi M, Ogawa I, et al. So-called "hybrid" lesion of desmoplastic and conventional ameloblastoma: Report of a case and review of the literature. Pathol Int 1999;49:1014–1018.

Chapter 8

Unicystic Ameloblastoma

1. Terminology

Much confusion still exists when it comes to the terminology used for unicystic ameloblastomas (UAs). Some of the terms used for this lesion prior to 1977, when Robinson and Martinez[1] introduced the concept of UA, were cystic (intracystic) ameloblastoma, ameloblastoma associated with dentigerous cyst, cystogenic ameloblastoma, extensive dentigerous cyst with intracystic ameloblastic papilloma, mural ameloblastoma, dentigerous cyst with ameloblastomatous proliferation, and ameloblastoma developing in a radicular (or "globulomaxillary") cyst.

The present authors propose the following nomenclature, which will be used throughout this chapter. The term *unicystic* is derived from the macro- and microscopic appearance, the lesion being essentially a well-defined, often large monocystic cavity with a lining, focally but rarely entirely composed of odontogenic (ameloblastomatous) epithelium. The term *unilocular,* on the other hand, is drawn from the radiographic interpretation of a radiolucency having only one loculus or compartment. Much confusion stems from the fact that a unicystic ameloblastoma may appear not only as a unilocular but also as a multilocular bone defect.[2,3] The term *unicystic ameloblastoma* is, however, so well established, that a change in nomenclature could create even more confusion.

On removal of the cyst, whether in toto or as a cyst wall curettage, it is important for the surgeon and the pathologist to examine both the interior and exterior of the cyst sac. Careful macroscopic inspection of the specimen may reveal important diagnostic clues. The inner surface of the cyst (facing the lumen) may show one or several polypoid or papillomatous, pedunculated, exophytic masses, which in rare cases almost fill the entire cyst lumen. This subtype of UA has been called intracystic, luminal, or intraluminal ameloblastoma and corresponds to the plexiform UA, the histological equivalent coined by Gardner.[4] The present authors strongly support the use of the term *intraluminal UA* when describing this type of tumor, because it indicates precisely the location of the tissue proliferation.

In addition to the intraluminal excrescences, the cyst capsule may show one or several rounded and slightly protruding nodules that may also be seen macroscopically when viewing the cyst wall from the outside. These formations have been named mural or intramural nodules in the literature, thus creating confusion with the intraluminal excrescences already described. This is unfortunate because the latter represent thickenings of the cyst wall proper due to the occurrence of infiltrating and invading islands of SMA tissue. With regard to these nodules, the authors suggest using the terms *intramural nodules* and *intramural UA* for this

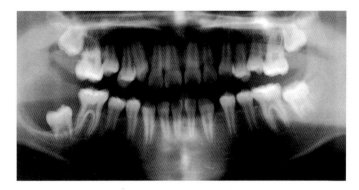

Fig 8-1 Orthopantomograph showing a well-defined unilocular UA (dentigerous variant) associated with an unerupted mandibular right second molar in a 10-year-old girl. The anlage of the right third molar is displaced by the expanding tumor.

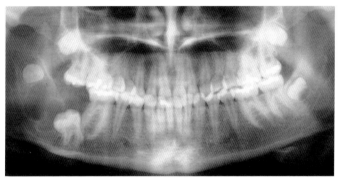

Fig 8-2 A 24-year-old man with a UA (dentigerous variant) appearing as a multilocular radiolucency occupying the mandibular right third molar and ramus area. The second molar is unerupted and the tooth germ for the third molar is markedly displaced.

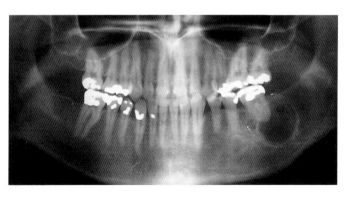

Fig 8-3 Orthopantomograph showing a unilocular UA (nondentigerous variant) mimicking a radicular cyst near the mandibular right first molar in a 45-year-old man.

subtype, as it is characterized by the occurrence of tumor tissue within the wall proper (*murus* is Latin for "wall").

The following profile and data are based on a critical review of 193 cases of UA from around the world.[5] (See Philipsen and Reichart[5] for specific details and a complete list of references.) In reviewing the literature it became evident that one feature divided the material into two categories: histologically verified UAs associated with an unerupted tooth (the dentigerous variant, $n = 90$) and UAs lacking an association with an unerupted tooth (the nondentigerous variant, $n = 101$). Two cases could not be diagnosed due to insufficient information.

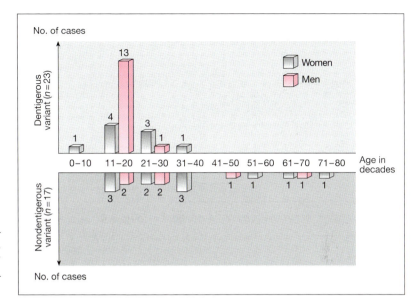

Fig 8-4 Age and gender distribution of 23 dentigerous and 17 nondentigerous variants of UA.

2. Clinical and radiologic profile

Local swelling, occasional pain, and signs of lip numbness, as well as discharge or drainage in cases of secondary infection, were common findings in both variants.

When the radiographic appearance of all UAs is divided into the two main patterns, unilocular (Fig 8-1) and multilocular (Fig 8-2), there is a clear predominance of the unilocular configuration in all studies where this feature was evaluated. This predominance was exceptionally marked for the dentigerous variant where the unilocular:multilocular ratio was 4.3:1.[2] For the nondentigerous type this ratio was 1.1:1 (Fig 8-3). Eversole et al[2] were able to identify six radiographic patterns for UA, ranging from well-defined unilocular to multilocular appearance. Root resorptions have been described in 40% to 70% of cases.[3,6] Li et al[3] recently made an interesting observation when they carefully examined seven UAs of the dentigerous variant. In none of these cases could they find a true dentigerous cyst–impacted tooth relationship. The

involved tooth crown was displaced by the cystic tumor rather than being projected into the cyst lumen. The interpretation of this finding is discussed further in section 4 of this chapter.

3. Epidemiological data

3.1 Prevalence, incidence, and relative frequency

No data are available concerning prevalence and incidence of UAs. The relative frequency has been reported as between 5% and 22% of all types of ameloblastomas.[7] Li et al[3] found 33 UAs among 175 cases of ameloblastomas (18.9%).

3.2 Age

The mean age at time of diagnosis differs considerably according to the UA variants

79

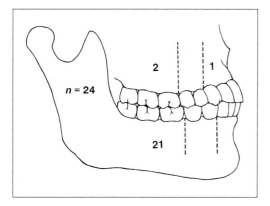

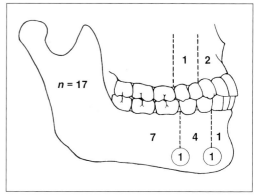

Fig 8-5 Location within the jaws of 24 dentigerous UA variants.

Fig 8-6 Location within the jaws of 17 nondentigerous UA variants. Circled numbers at the bottom of the broken lines indicate that the UA involved both adjoining regions.

(Fig 8-4). From the total number of cases reviewed, it was possible to obtain individual data from only a relative few. Those diagnosed as dentigerous (n = 23) occurred in much younger patients (mean 16.5 years with 78.3% occurring in the 1st and 2nd decades) than those diagnosed as nondentigerous (n = 17; mean 35.2 years with 29.4% occurring in the first two decades). Almost 20 years in mean age separated the two variants, mainly due to cases occurring in the 5th to 8th decades in the nondentigerous group.

3.3 Gender

In regard to gender distribution, the UA dentigerous variant shows a slight male predominance with a male:female ratio of 1.6:1. However, when the tumor is not associated with an unerupted tooth, the gender ratio is reversed to a male:female ratio of 1:1.8.

3.4 Location

The location of the UA within the jawbones shows a marked predominance for the mandible irrespective of the variant, the maxilla: mandible ratio being 1:7 versus 1:4.7 for the nondentigerous type (Figs 8-5 and 8-6). The posterior mandible, including the ascending ramus, is the region most often affected in both variants. An unerupted mandibular third molar was associated with UA in 58.3% of 24 dentigerous variants evaluated. If both second and third (mandibular) molars are included, they cover a total of 83.3% of the dentigerous UAs.

4. Pathogenesis

Some investigators believe the UA arises from preexisting odontogenic cysts, in particular a dentigerous cyst, while others maintain that it arises de novo. Robinson and Martinez[1] argued that as the epithelium of odontogenic cysts and ameloblastomas have a common ancestry, a transition from a non-neoplastic cyst to a neoplastic one could be possible, even though it occurs infrequently. Leider et al[8] proposed three pathogenic mechanisms for the evolution of UA:(1) the reduced enamel epithelium associated with a developing tooth undergoes ameloblastic transformation with subsequent cystic development; (2) ameloblastomas arise in dentigerous or other types of odontogenic cysts in which the neoplastic ameloblastic epithelium is preceded temporarily by a non-neoplastic stratified squamous epithelial lining; and (3) a solid ameloblastoma undergoes cystic degeneration of ameloblastic islands with subsequent fusion of multiple microcysts and develops into a unicystic lesion. Ackermann et al[9] stated that based on 57 cases of UAs there was absolutely no evidence that any other odontogenic cyst existed prior to the development of the lesions. Although these authors were not able to unequivocally exclude origin from preexisting odontogenic cysts in a few cases, they felt that all available evidence was against this possibility and strongly favored the idea that these lesions are cystic neoplasms de novo. Gold[10] disagreed, suggesting that the UA has a cystic origin and is derived from odontogenic keratocysts, lateral periodontal cysts, and dentigerous cysts. Li et al[11] made a comparison of proliferating cell nuclear antigen (PCNA) expression in the cystic tumor lining of UAs with published data on odontogenic cyst linings. They found that all areas of UA lining contained significantly more PCNA-positive cells than dentigerous cyst linings, even in areas where epithelial morphology was similar to that of the dentigerous cyst lining. This finding was interpreted as favorable to the concept that UAs are de novo cystic neoplasms.

It is difficult to produce convincing evidence for any of the theories presented. As alluded to earlier, Li et al[3] did not find a true dentigerous arrangement in any of their seven cases of the dentigerous variant. This finding was interpreted as an argument against the hypothesis that UA may originate from a preexisting dentigerous cyst. Similar observations were made by Philipsen et al[12] when they examined the dentigerous appearance characteristic of another odontogenic tumor, the follicular variant of the adenomatoid odontogenic tumor (AOT; see Fig 11-1). The lack of a true dentigerous cyst–impacted tooth relationship did not support the AOT originating from a preexisting dentigerous cyst but rather favored the "envelopmental" concept—that is, an unerupted tooth being embedded in an expanding tumor mass, whether cystic or solid. The most important point in this context is whether lesions that clinically and radiographically appear to be odontogenic cysts of any type may prove histologically to be one of several ameloblastoma variants (or other odontogenic tumors).

5. Pathology

5.1 Macroscopy

If removed in toto, the operation specimen is that of a partially or totally collapsed cystic sac. By careful examination of the inner and outer aspects of the cyst wall, it may be possible to spot characteristic UA features: one or several intraluminal papilloma-like tissue proliferations and/or intramural focal thickenings or nodules. Lack of these findings does not, however, contradict a diagnosis of UA. The diagnosis of UA can only be made histologically and cannot be predicted preoperatively on clinical or radiographic grounds. Examination of the entire lesion through sectioning at many levels is mandatory for securing the final diagnosis.

5.2 Microscopy

5.2.1 Histologic definitions

In the 1992 edition of the World Health Organization (WHO) classification,[13] a section on UA was added in view of its clinical importance. The classification distinguishes between three histologic subtypes of UA which correspond to subgroups 1, 1.2, and 1.3 in Table 8-1.

The histologic features of UA have been established by several authors,[3] all of whom recognize various subtypes determined by the pattern and extent of ameloblastomatous proliferation in relation to the cyst wall. The separation into four histologic subgroups (see Table 8-1) was chosen by the present authors as a basis for evaluating UA cases in a recent review[5] and is a modification of the classification suggested by Ackermann et al.[9] The minimum criterion for diagnosing a lesion as UA is the demonstration of a single (often macro-) cystic sac, with an odontogenic (ameloblastomatous) epithelium, which is usually present only in focal areas. It is often accompanied by an innocuous epithelium of varying histologic appearance that may mimic the lining of a dentigerous or radicular cyst.

Table 8-1 Histologic UA subgrouping (modified after Ackermann et al[9])

Subgroup	Interpretation
1	Luminal UA
1.2	Luminal and intraluminal UA
1.2.3	Luminal, intraluminal, and intramural UA
1.3	Luminal and intramural UA

The luminal type of tumor is called UA subgroup 1 (Figs 8-7 and 8-8) and is defined as having an epithelial lining of which parts may show transformation to cuboidal or columnar basal cells with hyperchromatic nuclei, nuclear palisading with polarization, cytoplasmic vacuolization with intercellular spacing, and subepithelial hyalinization. This definition was originally suggested by Vickers and Gorlin[14] (informally known as the V and G criteria) as representative of early ameloblastoma changes. UAs often show a combination of histologic features, so UA subgroup 1.2 (Figs 8-7 to 8-10) shows simple and intraluminal features. UA subgroup 1.2.3 (Figs 8-7 and 8-11) covers cases where there is an occurrence of intramural amelo-

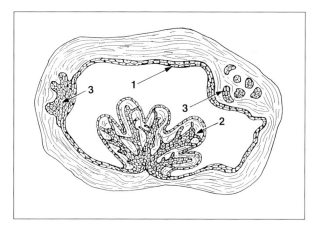

Fig 8-7 Histologic classification of UAs. 1 = a fibrous cyst wall lined by ameloblastomatous epithelium; 2 = an intraluminal "papillomatous" mass of plexiform, epithelial hyperplasia; 3 = intramural nodules with proliferating amelobastoma tissue. Different combinations of these features result in the four UA subgroups (1, 1.2, 1.2.3, and 1.3).

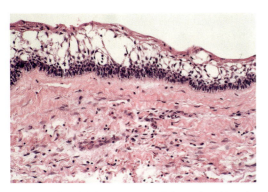

Fig 8-8 Ameloblastomatous lining of a UA subgroup 1 (hematoxylin-eosin [H&E], × 80).

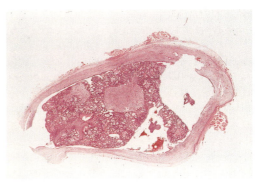

Fig 8-9 UA subgroup 1.2. The plexiform, intraluminal proliferation occupies a large portion of the cyst cavity (H&E, ×5).

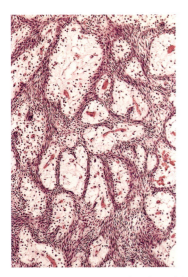

Fig 8-10 Higher magnification of the intraluminal proliferation in Fig 8-9. The V and G criteria for an early ameloblastoma are not fulfilled in this case. Notice the loosely structured and richly vascular connective tissue stroma (H&E, ×80).

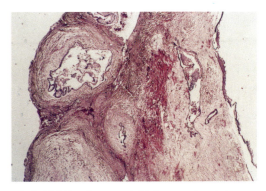

Fig 8-11 UA subgroup 1.3 intramural nodule containing ameloblastoma tissue of the follicular type. Each tumor island is surrounded by a thick fibrous layer of connective tissue, giving this subgroup a nodular appearance. There is pronounced cystic degeneration of the tumor islands (H&E, ×80).

blastoma tissue as well as subgroup 1.2 features. The last subgroup (1.3) exhibits a cyst with a luminal lining in combination with intramural nodules of SMA tissue. The intramural ameloblastoma tissue may be seen as an infiltration from the cyst lining or as free islands of follicular SMA, often with central cystic degeneration (see Fig 8-11). It is important to stress that these four subgroups all occur in both the dentigerous and the non-dentigerous variants. It should be added that UA subgroup 1.2 is sometimes referred to as the plexiform unicystic ameloblastoma.[8,15] Although this epithelial proliferation (or hyperplasia) does not exhibit the V and G criteria[14] as do most epithelial linings of UAs, Gardner[16] maintains that it represents SMA tissue.

5.2.2 Histopathologic findings

As shown in Table 8-2, where the histologic subgroups are distributed according to clinical variants, about two thirds of both variants showed intramural invasive SMA tissue (subgroups 1.2.3 and 1.3) with a slightly stronger tendency for occurrence in the non-dentigerous variant. It is also noteworthy that cases of UAs showing intraluminal proliferations (plexiform UA) occur more than twice as frequently in UAs of the dentigerous type.

5.2.3 Immunohistochemical findings

Several attempts have been made to distinguish the lining of UAs from that of odontogenic cysts. Although immunocytochemical expression of blood cell carbohydrates and epidermal growth factor receptor showed no consistent difference between odontogenic cysts and UAs, immunocytochemical markers for lectins (*Ulex europaeus agglutinin I* and *Bandeirea simplicifolia agglutinin I*) and proliferating cells (proliferating cell nuclear antigen and Ki-67) may assist in their differential diagnosis.[11,17,18] More immunocyto-

Table 8-2 Distribution (in percentage) of histologic UA subgroups according to clinical variants[5].

	Subgroups			
	1	1.2	1.2.3	1.3
Dentigerous	8	25	17	50
Nondentigerous	17	12	12	59

chemical studies are needed, with special attention to a comparison of the different subgroups. Studies aimed at resolving the question of whether the intraluminal exophytic masses (subgroup 1.2, or plexiform UA) are truly tumorous or merely represent a non-neoplastic, plexiform epithelial hyperplasia are also needed.

6. Notes on treatment and recurrence rate

Treatment planning depends on the final histopathologic diagnosis. The present authors are entirely in agreement with the viewpoints expressed by Ackermann et al[9] and Gardner[16] that UAs diagnosed as subgroups 1 and 1.2 may be treated conservatively (careful enucleation), whereas UAs belonging to subgroups 1.2.3 and 1.3 should be treated aggressively in the same manner as the classic SMA. Stoelinga and Bronkhorst[19] used Carnoy's solution after enucleation in the treatment of UA and reported no recurrences in five patients treated by this method. Their follow-up period in three of their cases was 2 to 2.5 years and consequently too short to be meaningful. Therefore, their results should not be interpreted as proof that the additional use of Carnoy's solution is more effective than enucleation alone. More studies with adequate follow-up periods (7 to 10 years or more) are needed.

A preoperative incisional biopsy is representative of the entire lesion in very few instances and will probably result in an incorrect classification of the lesion with a subsequent faulty diagnosis. As repeatedly mentioned, the true nature of these lesions becomes evident only when the entire specimen is available for microscopy. Thus, the authors strongly recommend abstaining from incisional biopsies. Operation specimens, whether a complete, cleanly enucleated UA or a curettage, should be subjected to multiple sampling or (preferably) serial sectioning to specifically search for cell and tissue configurations of an ameloblastomatous nature in intramural nodules. If invading tumor islands or strands are found intramurally, their presence indicates an aggressive surgical approach, possibly involving a second operation where bone adjacent to the initial operation site is removed. The patient must be followed closely for at least 10 years because recurrences often become apparent many years after surgery.

Recurrence rates for UAs after conservative surgical treatment (curettage or enucleation) are generally reported to be less than 25%, and a figure as low as 10.7% has been calculated for the UA subgroup 1.2.[15] Many reports in the literature indicate a less aggressive nature for UAs, but few are prospective studies that have examined individual histologic variants with respect to behavior and treatment.[20] In Li et al's study of 33 Chinese patients with UA,[3] the authors addressed the previously mentioned clinicopathologic correlation. In five of six recurrences, the initial enucleated UA contained intramural ameloblastoma islands (UA subgroups 1.2.3 and 1.3). Overall, tumors exhibiting intramural invasion had a higher recurrence rate (35.7%, the highest

rate reported to date) than other subgroups (6.7% for both 1 and 1.2). The authors further found that the average interval between initial treatment and obvious recurrence was approximately 7 years, and all their recurrences were recorded 4 years or more after initial surgery. Thus, inclusion of patients with less than 4 years of follow-up may result in an underestimation of the recurrence rate, so it may be somewhat optimistic when some authors[8,9,21] categorically claim that UAs have a recurrence rate of approximately 10% to 15% after enucleation. Due to inadequate follow-up, the largest of UA cases published to date (57 by Ackermann et al[9]) unfortunately lacks information about recurrence rates. There are indications that there may be a lower recurrence rate for cases diagnosed as UA subgroup 1.2 compared to UA subgroups 1.2.3 and 1.3. However, sufficient data to substantiate this assumption are not yet available. On the other hand, whatever true recurrence rate future studies may disclose, it is generally held that the UA has a lower recurrence rate than that of the classic SMA following the same conservative treatment. Commonly cited SMA recurrence rates of 50% to 90% should, however, be viewed cautiously.[5]

References

1. Robinson L, Martinez MG. Unicystic ameloblastoma. A prognostically distinct entity. Cancer 1977;40:2278–2285.

2. Eversole LR, Leider AS, Strub D. Radiographic characteristics of cystogenic ameloblastoma. Oral Surg Oral Med Oral Pathol 1984;57:572–577.

3. Li T-J, Wu Y-T, Yu S-F, Yu G-Y. Unicystic ameloblastoma. A clinicopathological study of 33 Chinese patients. Am J Surg Pathol 2000;24:1385–1392.

4. Gardner DG. Plexiform unicystic ameloblastoma. A diagnostic problem in dentigerous cysts. Cancer 1981;47:1358–1363.

5. Philipsen HP, Reichart PA. Unicystic ameloblastoma. A review of 193 cases from the literature. Oral Oncol 1998;34:317–325.

6. Roos RE, Raubenheimer EJ, van Heerden WFP. Clinico-pathological study of 30 unicystic ameloblastomas. J Dent Assoc S Afr 1994;49:559–562.

7. Reichart PA, Philipsen HP, Sonner S. Ameloblastoma: Biological profile of 3677 cases. Eur J Cancer B Oral Oncol 1995;31B:86–99.

8. Leider AS, Eversole LR, Barkin ME. Cystic ameloblastoma. Oral Surg Oral Med Oral Pathol 1985;60:624–630.

9. Ackermann GL, Altini M, Shear M. The unicystic ameloblastoma: A clinicopathologic study of 57 cases. J Oral Pathol 1988;17:541–546.

10. Gold L. Biologic behaviour of ameloblastoma. Clin Oral Maxillofac Surg North Am 1991;1:21–71.

11. Li TJ, Browne RM, Matthews JB. Expression of proliferating cell nuclear antigen (PCNA) and Ki-67 in unicystic ameloblastoma. Histopathology 1995;26:219–228.

12. Philipsen HP, Samman N, Ormiston IW, Wu PC, Reichart PA. Variants of the adenomatoid odontogenic tumor with a note on tumor origin. J Oral Pathol Med 1992;21:348–352.

13. Kramer IRH, Pindborg JJ, Shear M. The histological typing of odontogenic tumours. 2d ed. Berlin: Springer-Verlag, 1992.

14. Vickers RA, Gorlin RJ. Ameloblastoma: Delineation of early histopathologic features of neoplasia. Cancer 1970;26:699–710.

15. Gardner DG, Corio RL. Plexiform unicystic ameloblastoma. A variant of ameloblastoma with a low-recurrence rate after enucleation. Cancer 1984; 53:1730–1735.

16. Gardner DG. Some current concepts on the pathology of ameloblastomas. Oral Surg Oral Med Oral Pathol Oral Radiol Endod 1996;82: 660–669.

17. Li T-J, Browne RM, Matthews JB. Epithelial cell proliferation in odontogenic keratocysts: A comparative immunocytochemical study of Ki67 in simple, recurrent and basal cell naevus syndrome (BCNS) associated lesions. J Oral Pathol Med 1995;24:221–226.

18. Saku T, Shibata Y, Koyama Z, Cheng J, Okabe H, Yeh Y. Lectin histochemistry of cystic jaw lesions: An aid for differential diagnosis between cystic ameloblastoma and odontogenic cysts. J Oral Pathol Med 1991;20:108–113.

19. Stoelinga PJW, Bronkhorst FB. The incidence, multiple presentation and recurrence of aggressive cysts of the jaws. J Craniomaxillofac Surg 1988;16:184–189.

20. Li T-J, Kitano M, Arimura K, Sugihara K. Recurrence of unicystic ameloblastoma: A case report and review of the literature. Arch Pathol Lab Med 1998;122:371–374.

21. Gardner DG. Controversies in the nomenclature, diagnosis, and treatment of ameloblastoma. In: Worthington P, Evans JR. Controversies in Oral and Maxillofacial Surgery. Philadelphia:WB Saunders 1994:301–314.

Chapter 9

Squamous Odontogenic Tumor

1. Terminology

Pullon et al[1] first described a particular odontogenic tumor located in the periodontium as squamous odontogenic tumor (SOT) in 1975. The authors described a series of six tumors which "caused radiolucent areas of bone destruction adjacent to the roots of teeth."

According to the World Health Organization (WHO) classification of 1992,[2] the SOT belongs to the family of epithelial odontogenic tumors. The term *SOT* has been widely accepted, although others such as squamous odontogenic hamartoid lesion have been suggested. The following characterization of the SOT is based on a recent review of 36 cases published in 1996.[3] Two additional cases were published by Favia et al in 1997[4] and Ide et al in 1999.[5] The latter was of special significance since the SOT was associated with a squamous cell carcinoma. The authors suspected a malignant variant of the SOT.

A number of cases published in the literature discussed purported SOTs, which are considered to be other tumors by the present authors. Squamous odontogenic tumors, among others, were confused with peripheral ameloblastoma, desmoplastic ameloblastoma, and particularly squamous odontogenic tumorlike islands arising in the walls of odontogenic cysts.[3] SOT-like islands in cyst walls are non-neoplastic and represent reactive, inflammatory hyperplasias of the cyst epithelium. Therefore, the term suggested by Batsakis and Cleary[6]—*mural variant of SOT*—should be discouraged.

2. Clinical and radiologic profile

The squamous odontogenic tumor is a benign but locally infiltrative odontogenic neoplasm. It is slow growing with few clinical signs and symptoms. Mobility of the teeth, swelling of the alveolar process, and moderate pain are possible indicators of the underlying tumor. Most cases develop in the periodontal ligament of permanent teeth; therefore, the most common variant is the intrabony or central type of SOT. A rare peripheral variant has also been described.[3] Some SOTs are localized in edentulous areas, and multicentric occurrence has been reported.[3] This fact stresses the need for thorough clinical and especially radiologic examination of a patient with a neoplasm diagnosed as SOT. Of particular significance is the observation that SOTs occurring in the maxilla seem to be more aggressive than those in the mandible, a behavior common to several odontogenic tumors. A familial pattern of SOT was observed by Leider et al,[7] who reported multiple lesions in three siblings. SOT seems to be associated with im-

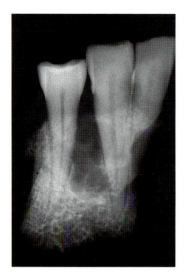

Fig 9-1 Radiograph of a resection specimen of SOT. A triangular, multilocular radiolucency is seen between the roots of a mandibular canine and first premolar. Differential diagnosis should include ameloblastoma and odontogenic myxoma.

pacted teeth only rarely in contrast to many other odontogenic tumors. Its association with squamous cell carcinoma (primary, intraosseous) is not clear.[5]

Radiology of the central variant of SOT shows a well-defined unilocular and triangu-lar radiolucency between the roots of adjacent teeth (Fig 9-1). Radiopacities seen in other odontogenic tumors are not found in SOTs. Embedded teeth have been found in a few SOT cases. Extensive SOT lesions may have a multilocular pattern involving the mandible or the maxillary sinuses. The peripheral variant of SOT may reveal some "saucerization" of the underlying bone which is explained as a pressure phenomenon rather than a result of neoplastic infiltration.

3. Epidemiological data

3.1 Prevalence, incidence, and relative frequency

Since the number of reported cases of SOT is still rather small, no data are available.

3.2 Age

The age of 39 patients with SOT[3-5] ranged from 8 to 74 years with a mean age of 38.7 years. Patients in the 3rd decade of life seem to be affected most frequently (Fig 9-2).

Fig 9-2 Distribution of SOT cases according to age and gender. There is a peak for both men and women in the third decade.

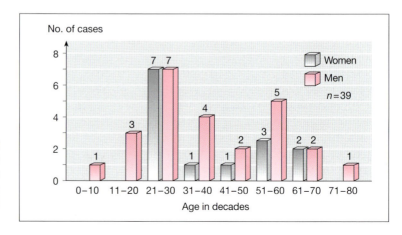

3.3 Gender

The gender ratio among the 39 SOT patients was 1:1.4 (women:men).[3]

3.4 Location

Figure 9-3 shows the location of SOTs (n = 28).[3-5] The central or intraosseous SOT, which is by far the most common variant, usually begins to develop in one periodontal location adjacent to the roots of erupted, permanent teeth. However, the coexistence of bilateral, posterior maxillary SOTs and a mandibular, primary carcinoma in association with an impacted third molar has also been reported. Recently another case of an intraosseous SOT associated with a squamous cell carcinoma and an impacted third molar has been described.[5]

4. Pathogenesis

The origin of the SOT is unclear; however, there are indications that it may arise from epithelial rests of Malassez located in the periodontal ligament. Peripheral SOTs may originate in the gingival surface epithelium as a "dropping off" phenomenon or from remnants of the dental lamina. In cases where the origin of the SOTs was supposed to be the surface epithelium, the tumors appeared histologically as pseudoepitheliomatous hyperplasias or peripheral ameloblastomas. Inflammatory stimuli do not seem to be involved in the initiation of proliferation of epithelial remnants, in contrast to SOT-like proliferations observed in odontogenic cysts. Some authors have considered that the SOT may have a hamartomatous nature.[3,4]

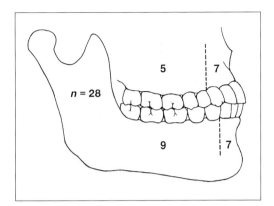

Fig 9-3 Location of tumors. In addition to the 28 single tumor sites shown, 5 SOTs had multiple locations in both the maxilla and the mandible, 4 were located in both the anterior and posterior maxilla, and 1 tumor had a bilateral, maxillary location (total n = 38).

5. Pathology

5.1 Macroscopy

No descriptions of the macroscopic appearance of SOTs are available.

5.2 Microscopy

5.2.1 Histologic definition

The present authors use the following definition for SOTs: A benign but locally infiltrative neoplasm consisting of islands of well-differentiated squamous epithelium in a fibrous stroma. The epithelial islands occasionally show foci of central cystic degeneration.

5.2.2 Histopathologic findings

Histologically, the SOT is composed of islands of well-differentiated squamous epithelium of varying size and shape (Fig 9-4).

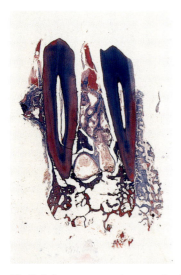

Fig 9-4 Low-power micrograph of the specimen shown in Fig 9-1. Between the roots of the canine and first premolar, multiple islands of odontogenic epithelium are seen. Some of these have undergone cystic degeneration (Mallory stain, ×1.2)

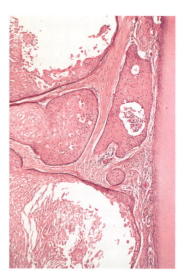

Fig 9-5 A higher magnification of the same specimen showing several epithelial nests and islands bordering a root surface (*right*). Some of the islands exhibit central cystic degeneration. Tumor islands are embedded in a sparse connective tissue stroma (hematoxylin-eosin [H&E], ×50).

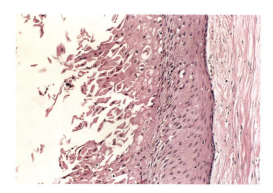

Fig 9-6 The interface between tumor islands and connective tissue stroma. Epithelial cells are flat and lose interepithelial contact toward the center of the islands (microcystic degeneration) (H&E, ×100).

Often the islands are rounded or oval, but they may also reveal irregular and cordlike structures (Fig 9-5), as is characteristic for the desmoplastic ameloblastoma. Individual tumor islands reveal a peripheral layer of low cuboidal or even flat epithelial cells. This is different from the high cylindrical epithelial cells observed in SMAs. Individual epithelial islands may undergo central microcystic degeneration of the spinous cells following single-cell keratinization (Fig 9-6). Some islands may become large and contain laminar calcified material. Mitotic activity of the epithelial tumor cells is not increased. Tumor islands are surrounded by mature connective tissue with little or no inflammatory reaction. Ghost cells or clear cells have not been found in SOTs.

The SOT may be mistaken for an acanthomatous or a desmoplastic ameloblastoma, a well-differentiated squamous cell carcinoma, or a pseudoepitheliomatous hyperplasia comparable to a keratoacanthoma. A histopathologic misinterpretation may thus lead to overtreatment or undertreatment.

5.2.3 Histochemical/immunohistochemical findings

Tatemoto et al[8] and Yamada et al[9] reported on immunohistochemical findings in cases of SOTs. Immunohistochemical staining of keratin proteins was performed using polyclonal antikeratin antiserum (TK, detecting 41- to 65-kd keratins) and monoclonal antibodies (KL1, 55 to 57 kd; PKK1, 40, 45 and 52.5 kd). Staining for PKK1-detectable keratin was negative in tumor islands; staining with KL1 and TK immunoreagents was confined to squamous epithelial cells.[8] The proliferative activity of the odontogenic epithelium of SOTs was also confirmed by heavy staining for keratin 13 and 16. The centers of the epithelial islands of the squamous differentiating cells revealed strong positive reactions for involucrin.[9] In the latter study, however, acanthomatous and follicular SMAs with foci of squamous differentiation were also positive for involucrin.

5.2.4 Ultrastructural findings

Pullon et al[1] were the first to describe ultrastructural features of the SOT. Neoplastic epithelial cells are arranged in nests or islands in a stroma of sparse collagen bundles. Individual islands are surrounded by a well-defined basal lamina. Squamous epithelial cells are surrounded by intercellular edema as seen in cells of the stratum spinosum of the oral mucosa. Desmosomes are numerous, and the cytoplasm contains abundant glycogen granules, a few mitochondria, and flattened cisternae of granular endoplasmic reticulum. Laminar structures (myelin bod-

ies) are also contained in the cytoplasm. In some areas the myelin bodies and glycogen granules take up a major portion of the cytoplasm and seem almost to replace the nucleus. Dense tonofilament bands are also observed in the cytoplasm. Nuclei are large and contain evenly distributed chromatin and an occasional nucleolus. Keratin formation and calcification are not observed.

6. Notes on treatment and recurrence rate

The SOT is generally considered a benign odontogenic neoplasm, and therefore most authors recommend conservative surgical procedures such as enucleation, curettage, or local excision. However, tumors located in the maxilla have to undergo a more radical treatment because of the aggressive potential of SOTs in this location. Recurrences have been described, but they seem to be rare and are probably due to incomplete removal of the tumor. When considering treatment, one also must be aware that SOTs may occur in a multicentric pattern.

Since the number of reported cases of SOTs is still rather small, the biologic profile of this entity is still not clear, especially its association with squamous cell carcinoma (primary, odontogenic). From the histopathologic point of view, ways to differentiate SOTs from acanthomatous and desmoplastic ameloblastomas have to be found. In addition, cases originating from the surface epithelium should be studied in great detail to confirm that they are true SOTs.

References

1. Pullon PA, Shafer W, Elzay RP, Kerr DA, Corio RL. Squamous odontogenic tumor. Oral Surg Oral Med Oral Pathol 1975;40:616–630.

2. Kramer IRH, Pindborg JJ, Shear M. Histological Typing of Odontogenic Tumours. 2d ed. Berlin: Springer-Verlag, 1992.

3. Philipsen HP, Reichart PA. Squamous odontogenic tumor (SOT): A benign neoplasm of the periodontium. J Clin Periodontol 1996;23:922–926.

4. Favia GF, Di Alberti L, Scarano A, Piattelli A. Squamous odontogenic tumour: Report of two cases. Oral Oncol 1997;33:451–453.

5. Ide F, Shimoyama T, Horie H, Shimizu S. Intraosseous squamous cell carcinoma arising in association with a squamous odontogenic tumour of the mandible. Oral Oncol 1999;35:431–434.

6. Batsakis JG, Cleary KR. Pathology consultation. Squamous odontogenic tumor. Ann Otol Rhinol Laryngol 1993;102:823–824.

7. Leider AS, Jonker AL, Cook HE. Multicentric familiar squamous odontogenic tumor. Oral Surg Oral Med Oral Pathol 1989;68:175–181.

8. Tatemoto Y, Okada Y, Mori M. Squamous odontogenic tumor: Immunohistochemical identification of keratins. Oral Surg Oral Med Oral Pathol 1989;67:63–67.

9. Yamada K, Tatemoto Y, Okada Y, Mori M. Immunostaining of involucrin in odontogenic epithelial tumors and cysts. Oral Surg Oral Med Oral Pathol 1989;67:564–568.

Chapter 10

Calcifying Epithelial Odontogenic Tumor

1. Terminology

In 1955, Pindborg[1] reported three cases of a benign but locally aggressive tumor which he called the calcifying epithelial odontogenic tumor (CEOT), today known as the intraosseous variant of CEOT. Pindborg followed his abstract with two more publications,[2,3] the latter reporting on the 24 cases known at the time. The tumor had been reported prior to 1955 under different names such as ameloblastoma of unusual type with calcification, calcifying ameloblastoma, malignant odontoma, adenoid adamantoblastoma, cystic complex odontoma, and a variant of the solid/multicystic ameloblastoma (SMA). The term *calcifying epithelial odontogenic tumor* has been generally accepted and adopted by the World Health Organization (WHO) since the publication of *Histological Typing of Odontogenic Tumours, Jaw Cysts, and Allied Lesions* in 1971.[4] For almost 40 years the CEOT has been known eponymously as the Pindborg tumor. The following profile of the CEOT is based on a literature review of 181 cases.[5]

2. Clinical and radiologic profile

The CEOT is a benign neoplasm located either intraosseously or extraosseously. When occurring intraosseously (by far the most common), it may occasionally show local invasiveness. The intraosseous CEOT often presents as a painless mass with slow growth. When located in the maxilla, patients may sometimes complain of nasal congestion, epistaxis, and headache.

The characteristic radiographic appearance is of an irregular unilocular or multilocular radiolucent area containing radiopaque masses of varying size and opacity (Figs 10-1 to 10-3). In many cases, especially in tumors of relatively short duration, the calcified concrements are minute and may be undetectable on radiographs.

When an unerupted tooth is associated with the tumor, the radiopacities tend to be located close to the tooth crown (Fig 10-4). At the periphery, the radiolucent margin may or may not be clearly demarcated from the normal bone. Clinically, the peripheral soft tissue, or extraosseous, CEOT appears most commonly as a painless, firm gingival mass with a preoperative clinical diagnosis that includes fibrous hyperplasia, peripheral giant cell granuloma, and epulis. The overlying mucosa may show ulceration due to local trauma. On surgical removal, an underlying bony depression or saucerization has been reported in a few cases.

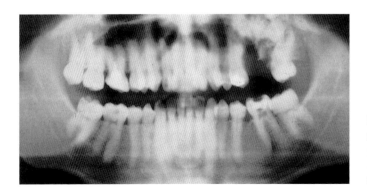

Fig 10-1 Orthopantomograph showing a CEOT in the left maxilla around the roots of the third molar with involvement of the left sinus.

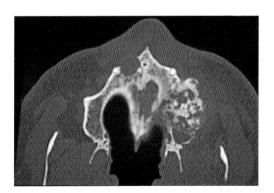

Fig 10-2 Computed tomography (CT) scan of the left maxillary sinus containing multiple, partly coalescent, radiopaque bodies.

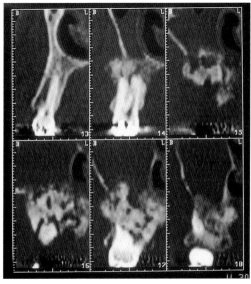

Fig 10-3 Transversal tomographs showing a mixed radiolucent/radiopaque CEOT lesion (same lesion as in Figs 10-1 and 10-2).

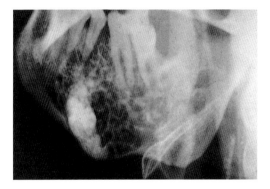

Fig 10-4 Radiograph of the left mandibular molar region showing an unerupted first molar with a pericoronally located CEOT.

3. Epidemiological data

3.1 Incidence, prevalence, and relative frequency

Information on incidence and prevalence of CEOTs is not available. Data from diagnostic biopsy services from various sources do, however, provide information about the relative tumor frequency (as a percentage of all odontogenic tumors), and it varies between 0.4% and 3%.[5-7] The CEOT has one of the lowest frequency rankings on a "hit list" of odontogenic tumors. The peripheral or extraosseous variant constitutes about 6% of the total number of CEOTs.

3.2 Age

The age range of all patients with CEOTs varies between 8 and 92 years at the time of diagnosis with a mean of 36.9 years ($n = 172$, Fig 10-5). However, if the tumors are divided

according to the two topographic variants, the age ranges and means are as follows: The intraosseous type has a range of 8 to 92 years (mean 38.9 years), and the extraosseous type has a range of 12 to 64 years (mean 34.4 years). Although the total number of reported cases of the extraosseous variant is still small (see Table 2 in Philipsen & Reichart[5] and Fig 10-5), the mean age seems to indicate that the peripheral variant is diagnosed a few years earlier than the intrabony type. This is not surprising since the peripheral type presents as a gingival mass (epulis), which lends itself to an earlier diagnosis than does an intraosseous lesion. Almost two thirds (64%) of the intraosseous variants are found in the 3rd, 4th, and 5th decades of life (see Fig 10-5).

When age and gender data from cases of white patients with intraosseous CEOTs are compared with a comparable number of Asian (Japanese and Chinese) patients with intrabony CEOT variants it is revealed that Asian CEOT cases seem to be diagnosed a few years earlier than their white counter-

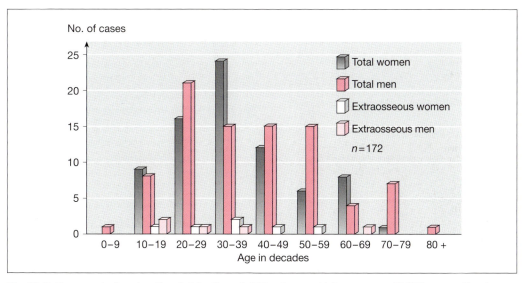

Fig 10-5 Bar graph showing the distribution of 172 extra- and intraosseous CEOTs according to age and gender.

parts—the difference being especially obvious for men.[5] An explanation for this difference cannot be offered at present.

3.3 Gender

The male:female ratio for 161 cases of the intraosseous variant with known gender is 80:81, or a nearly even distribution. If gender is distributed according to age groups (see Fig 10-5), the peak incidence for men is reached a decade earlier (3rd decade) than that for women (4th decade). Although the reported cases of extraosseous CEOTs are still few in number, the trend in gender distribution seems to follow that of the intraosseous variant (male:female = 6:5).

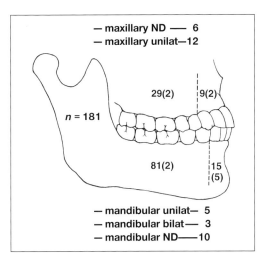

— maxillary ND —— 6
— maxillary unilat—12

29(2)   9(2)

n = 181

81(2)   15 (5)

— mandibular unilat— 5
— mandibular bilat — 3
— mandibular ND——10

Fig 10-6 Topographic distribution of extra- and intraosseous CEOTs within the jawbones. Numbers in parentheses indicate the number of extraosseous variants. ND = no details available; unilat = the tumor involves one quadrant (right or left); bilat = the tumor crosses the midline, involving two quadrants.

3.4 Location

As mentioned earlier, the CEOT appears in two clinicotopographic variants: the intraosseous (intrabony or central) and the extraosseous (peripheral). The former is by far the most common, accounting for 93.6% of all tumors. It may be further subdivided into cases with and without association with an unerupted tooth (or odontoma). Figure 10-6 shows the distribution of 181 cases of both variants within the jawbones. The intraosseous tumors are found primarily in the mandible (maxilla:mandible ratio, 1:2), and in 82% of the cases where the exact site of the tumor has been registered they are located in the premolar and molar regions. It is too early to assess the predilection site for the extraosseous variant.

Among 181 cases of CEOT, two patients presented with the rare phenomenon of two isolated tumors. Chomette et al[8] described a 40-year-old woman with two intraoral swellings, the first located in the left maxilla in the second and third molar region and the second in the left mandible in the third molar region. Radiographs showed two well-defined radiolucencies, both containing numerous small radiopacities, as well as an unerupted mandibular third molar.

After revising a case initially reported as the simultaneous occurrence of two ameloblastic fibromas in the same patient,[9] Busch and Hoppe[10] came to the conclusion that the 48-year-old man discussed actually had two CEOTs (and not two ameloblastic fibromas) located in the right maxilla and the left mandible.

3.5 CEOT in association with unerupted permanent teeth

The distribution of unerupted permanent teeth in association with the intraosseous variant of CEOT shows that 53% of these

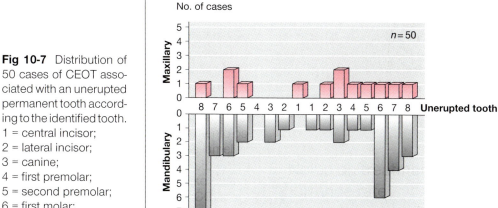

Fig 10-7 Distribution of 50 cases of CEOT associated with an unerupted permanent tooth according to the identified tooth.
1 = central incisor;
2 = lateral incisor;
3 = canine;
4 = first premolar;
5 = second premolar;
6 = first molar;
7 = second molar;
8 = third molar.

CEOTs have a definite association with an unerupted tooth (or odontoma). Based on 50 of the most recently reported cases of intraosseous CEOTs associated with unerupted teeth, 52% of the teeth were identified as mandibular molars (Fig 10-7).

4. Pathogenesis

Because the first few reported cases of CEOTs were all associated with an unerupted tooth, Pindborg[2] was initially of the opinion that the CEOT was of odontogenic origin and developed from the reduced enamel organ of the unerupted tooth. Later, Chaudhry and associates[11] emphasized that the tumor cells exhibit morphologic characteristics of squamous epithelium; they stated categorically that, in their case, the cells had been derived from the reduced enamel epithelium of the closely related unerupted tooth. With the appearance of reports of cases of intraosseous CEOTs without an associated unerupted tooth—and particular cases of the peripheral variant—it became evident that other sources than reduced enamel epithelium should be considered when discussing the histogenesis of CEOTs. The peripheral location strongly suggests the possibility that the tumor arises from rests of the dental lamina or from the basal cells of the oral epithelium. To conceptualize a unified source of origin for the diverse locations of CEOTs, one must look for a widespread occurrence of odontogenic epithelium. Of the possible candidates only one matches the requirements of widespread distribution: epithelial remnants of the dental lamina complex. Disintegration of the complex system of dental laminae gives rise to a countless number of epithelial remnants persisting in the jawbones and gingiva after completion of normal odontogenesis. This argument also seems relevant for the histogenesis of several other odontogenic tumors and hamartomatous lesions.

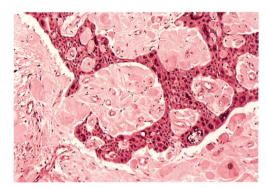

Fig 10-8 Photomicrograph showing anastomosing sheets of epithelial, eosinophilic cells with cellular and nuclear polymorphism (hematoxylin-eosin [H&E], ×80).

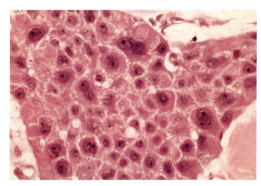

Fig 10-9 Higher magnification of epithelial sheet shown in Fig 10-8. Note the nuclear polymorphism and intercellular bridges (H&E, ×150).

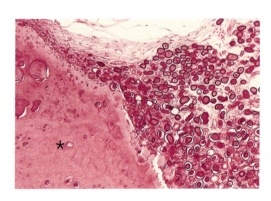

Fig 10-10 Calcified amyloid-like bodies revealing Liesegang rings. * = root dentine (H&E, ×80).

5. Pathology

5.1 Macroscopy

The intraosseously located CEOT is often easily enucleated, and the tumor size varies from 1 to 4 cm in diameter. The mass varies in color from grayish white or yellow to tan-pink. Bisecting the specimen usually reveals calcified particles that make a crunching sound during cutting. The tumor may be solid or contain minute cystic spaces. If associated with an unerupted tooth, the crown (or hard dental structures of an odontoma) can be found embedded in the tumor mass.

5.2 Microscopy

5.2.1 Histologic definitions

According to the 1992 WHO classification,[12] a CEOT is "a locally invasive epithelial neoplasm characterized by the development of intraepithelial structures, probably of an amyloid-like nature, which may become calcified and which may be liberated as the cells break down."

The definition used by the present authors is as follows:
A locally invasive epithelial neoplasm consisting of sheets and strands of polyhedral, pleomorphous cells with well-defined cell borders often showing intercellular bridges (Figs 10-8 and 10-9). A characteristic feature is an amyloid-like material that may become calcified (Fig 10-10), is formed intraepithelially, and may be liberated as the cells break down.

5.2.2 Histopathologic findings

The basic histologic pattern of CEOTs, usually described as characteristic and unique, is an unusual and variable combination of odontogenic epithelium and calcified structures. There is no fundamental difference in histomorphology between the intraosseous and extraosseous variants of CEOT except for the minimal amount or total lack of calcified material in the latter. Ai-Ru et al[7] suggested in their report of 9 cases of CEOTs that the histologic features be subtyped into four main patterns. This classification has, however, not been widely used.

The use of fine-needle aspiration biopsy in the diagnosis of CEOT was recently reported.[13] Cytologic smears were characterized by clusters, sheets, and rare isolated pleomorphic cells of the squamoid type; blocks of amorphous material encircled by fibroblasts; and occasional calcifications. A cytologic diagnosis of CEOT was made, which was confirmed by histopathologic examination. Evaluation of DNA ploidy by semiautomated image cytometry produced an aneuploid histogram.

5.2.2.1 Occurrence of amyloid-like material in CEOT

Though investigated intensively during the past 40 years or more using histochemical, immunologic, and ultrastructural methods, the true nature of the eosinophilic (amyloid-like, pseudoamyloid) tumor cell product occurring in CEOT is still creating controversy. The biologic and biochemical significance, as well as the origin of this material, is far from being understood. An origin from light chain fragments of immunoglobulin molecules has been proposed for some forms of systemic amyloid.[14] Another type is possibly associated with endocrine tumors such as the medullary carcinoma of the thyroid derived from the endocrine polypeptide cells of the amine precursor uptake decarboxylation (APUD) system. Obviously, these sources do not apply to the CEOT amyloid. Mori and Makino[15] found that most of the calcified and homogeneous acellular materials were positive for protein reactions, which resembled those observed in enamel matrix. In a thorough histochemical and immunologic study,[16] the authors were unable to determine the precise nature of this material, but suggested that the CEOT protein appeared to be a distinct protein moiety derived from immune amyloid or amyloid of unknown origin.

The homogeneous substance seen histologically appears in the electron microscope as either a fibrillar or granulofibrillar material. Yamaguchi et al[17] supported the amyloid concept, but agreed with Page and coworkers[18] that the material with a beta protein configuration is likely similar to enamel matrix. It is interesting that although there are few case reports of intraosseous CEOTs with minimal or no calcification,[19-21] it is the general view that lack of calcification is more common in the peripheral or extraosseous variant.

5.2.2.2 Cementum-like components of CEOT stroma

In the scanty fibrous connective tissue stroma of CEOTs, studies have demonstrated the presence of cementum-like components.[22-24] The mechanism of formation of the cementum-like material is still unclear. It should, however, be remembered that the majority of calcified homogenous masses of CEOT stroma is thought to be dystrophic calcification. In the study by El-Labban[23] it was found that the outer layer of the calcified lamellar bodies consisted of typical banded calcified collagen with an arrangement like that seen in cemental Sharpey fibers. Slootweg[24] suggested that the amyloid-like material is an inductive stimulus for the stroma cells to differentiate toward production of a collagenous matrix that is destined to mineralize and resembles cementum.

5.2.2.3 Occurrence of clear cells

Variations in the typical histo- and cytomorphologic CEOT appearance occasionally occur. Sheets of classic polyhedral epithelium with abundant eosinophilic cytoplasm may alternate with zones of epithelium characterized by large cells with clear, foamy cytoplasm and distinct cell borders. Yamaguchi et al[17] believed that the clear tumor cells represent a feature of cytodifferentiation rather than a simple degenerative phenomenon. Fifteen cases of documented examples of clear cell CEOT (CCCEOT) (Figs 10-11 and 10-12) have been published so far (see Table 5 in Philipsen and Reichart[5]). Overall ages ranged from 14 to 68 years with a mean of 41.5 years. The mean age for the intraosseous CCCEOT is, however, consid-

erably higher (46.3 years) than for the extraosseous variant (34.3 years). The male:female ratio for the intraosseously located clear cell type is 1:2 compared to 1:1 for the extraosseous variant.

It should be remembered that not only clear cell CEOT but also several other odontogenic tumors such as SMAs[25,26] (see chapter 5), calcifying ghost cell odontogenic tumors[27] (see chapter 17), and occasionally adenomatoid odontogenic tumors (AOTs)[28] (see chapter 11) may show clear cell differentiation. It is not yet known whether clear cell variants of odontogenic tumors behave biologically different from the classic CEOT, although the two cases of clinically aggressive clear cell ameloblastoma reported by Waldron et al[29] may indicate that such a possibility does exist. Primary jaw tumors of putative odontogenic origin, composed principally of clear cells, have recently been described under the diagnosis of clear cell odontogenic tumor (CCOT).[30,31]

The CCOT is a rare tumor but is established in the 1992 WHO classification[12] under the definition of a benign but locally invasive neoplasm originating from odontogenic epithelium and characterized by sheets and islands of uniform, vacuolated, and clear cells. CCOT can be distinguished from the clear cell variant of CEOT because it lacks the characteristic calcifications and the amyloid-like deposition.

It should be mentioned that certain odontogenic lesions of developmental origin—like the lateral periodontal cyst and the gingival cyst of adults—contain conspicuous foci of clear cells in their epithelial lining identical to those described here. The fact that cellular remnants of the dental lamina complex contain clear cells as a typical feature strongly suggests that the previously mentioned cysts arise from clear cell rests of the dental lamina. Thus, it seems logical to the present authors to suggest that the CEOT originates from the dental lamina or its remnants.

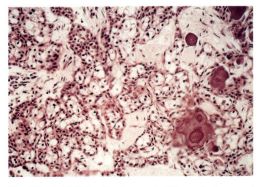

Fig 10-11 CEOT with clear cell differentiation and scattered calcified bodies (H&E, ×60).

The distinction of an extraosseous CEOT clear cell variant from some clear cell salivary gland tumors, metastatic renal cell carcinoma, and odontogenic lesions (such as the clear cell odontogenic carcinoma and peripheral ameloblastoma with clear cell differentiation) represents a diagnostic challenge. The same can be said about the identification of an intraosseous clear cell CEOT when only a small incisional biopsy specimen is available. Although the gingiva is not a typical location for a salivary gland neoplasm, mucoepidermoid carcinoma, acinic cell carcinoma, clear cell carcinoma of the salivary gland, and clear cell variant of oncocytoma must be considered in the microscopic differential diagnosis. Recently, Milchgrub et al[32] reported a unique salivary gland neoplasm under the term *hyalinizing clear cell carcinoma of the salivary gland* (HCCC), which also may be confused with the clear cell variant of CEOT. The differential diagnosis should include a glycogen-rich adenocarcinoma, either metastatic or derived from a mucoepidermoid or an acinic cell adenocarcinoma. These considerations are valid for the intraosseous as well as for the extraosseous CEOT. A recent article by Maiorano et al[33] summarizes the problem of clear cell occurrence in the heterogeneous group of lesions, which may be either odontogenic, salivary gland, or metastatic in origin.

5.2.2.4 Occurrence of Langerhans cells in CEOT

Asano et al[21] and Takata et al[34] described yet another histologic variant of the intraosseous CEOT in two Japanese patients. In both cases the tumor chiefly consisted of scattered small islands of epithelial cells. In some nests there were a few, occasionally several, clear cells positive for S-100 protein, lysozome, MT1, LN-3, and OKT6 antibodies, but not for keratin antibody. Almost no calcification of homogenous eosinophilic materials was observed. Ultrastructurally, the S-100–positive cells were identified as Langerhans cells based on the finding of rod- and tennis racket–shaped Birbeck granules. With only two published cases presently available, it is obviously too early to speculate on the importance of the presence of Langerhans cells on tumor behavior and prognosis. Langerhans cells belong to the mononuclear phagocyte system, are of bone marrow origin, and are often found in the skin and oral mucosa. It has been clearly ascertained that Langerhans cells function as antigen-presenting cells and as allogenic stimulatory cells to primed T lymphocytes in the epithelium.[35,36] As there are several reports suggesting some correlation between tumor regression and the number of Langerhans cells, Takata and coworkers[34] theorized that the Langerhans cells in CEOTs may play a role either in antigen presentation or in regression of the tumor.

5.2.2.5 Combined epithelial odontogenic tumor

In 1983 Damm et al[37] first described the presence of CEOT-like areas within two cases of adenomatoid odontogenic tumors and named them combined epithelial odontogenic tumors (CEOT/AOTs). A total of 24 cases of the histologic CEOT/AOT variant have now been reported.[38] There is nothing to indicate that a CEOT/AOT lesion reflects a true combination of two distinct and separate odontogenic tumor entities, and there are no reported cases of AOT in which CEOT-like areas predominate. Lastly, all published cases of the CEOT/AOT variant show a biologic behavior identical to that of an AOT, that is, a truly benign (hamartomatous) odontogenic lesion (see also chapter 11).

5.2.2.6 Occurrence of myoepithelial cells in CEOT

Ultrastructural findings in a case of CEOT disclosed that the tumor sheets and islands consisted of two cell populations.[39] One population constituted the classic polyhedral epithelial cells, and the other comprised cells arranged peripherally with elongated profiles and juxtaposed to the tumor epithelial cells. The latter cells exhibited a large number of cytoplasmic fine filaments with occasional electron-dense areas similar to those seen in the smooth muscle–type cell. These cells were found to extend basally around the tumor epithelium in most of the epithelial islands examined. They showed a lamina densa continuous with that of the neighboring epithelial cells and demonstrated a large number of hemidesmosomes. However, desmosomes between these cells and the tumor epithelial cells were not present. The ultrastructural characteristics of these cells were interpreted to be those of myoepithelial cells. This cell type, although found in tumors of glandular origin, has not been described previously in any of the odontogenic tumors and its occurrence in CEOT has so far not been confirmed in other electron microscopic studies of this tumor.

6. Notes on treatment and recurrence rate

When first described,[1] the CEOT was considered to be a locally invasive tumor, and some subsequent publications supported this concept. This view was based on evidence suggestive of bone marrow involvement from radiographs and histological sections.[2] However, Vap et al[40] maintained that the tumor is not of a very aggressive disposition; rather, it is an expansile lesion that does not extend into the intertrabecular spaces as does the solid ameloblastoma. Franklin and Pindborg[6] reported a recurrence rate of 14%, which was mostly attributable to inadequate treatment.

It is evident that long-term follow-up infor-

mation is required for the CEOT in order to choose the best treatment modality and assess the incidence of recurrence. Some authors have seen recurrences even after several decades and recommend a radical line of treatment. Others consider conservative surgery as the treatment of choice. In its ability to recur if treatment is not adequate, the CEOT is similar to the solid/multicystic ameloblastoma, and although its growth pattern may be slower, some believe that the two should be treated with an identical approach. Methods of treatment have ranged from simple enucleation or curettage (shelling) to homimandibulectomy or hemimaxillectomy. Eleven cases of clear cell CEOT with limited follow-up information do not allow conclusions to be drawn regarding the biologic behavior, treatment, and prognosis of this variant. However, as reported,[29,30] the occurrence of clear cells may prove to be a sign of increased tumor aggressiveness, indicating the need for a more radical surgical approach.

Correlation between the prognosis of CEOT and occurrence of Langerhans cells also needs further investigation. In view of the biologic behavior of the CEOT, destructive procedures such as a wide resection or hemiresection of the mandible seem unwarranted. Enucleation with a margin of macroscopic normal tissue is therefore the recommended treatment for lesions involving the mandible. CEOT of the maxilla, however, should be treated more aggressively, as maxillary tumors generally tend to grow more rapidly than their mandibular counterparts and do not usually remain well confined. This behavior is dramatically documented in a recent report by Bouckaert et al[41] where a large, maxillary CEOT was diagnosed in a 54-year-old black man. The tumor appeared to have developed from the left anterior maxilla and wall of the left maxillary sinus, expanding to the ethmoid sinus, eroding the cribriform plate into the anterior cranial fossa, and invading the left orbit with displacement of the eye. The situation was further complicated by the presence of an abscess located in the anterior cranial fossa with surrounding brain edema. The patient was treated with methylprednisolone to alleviate the edema. He showed dramatic recovery, asked to be discharged, and was then lost to follow-up.

Treatment should be individualized for each lesion because the radiographic and histologic features may differ from one lesion to another. Although it has not been established in the literature, 5 years should be the absolute minimum follow-up necessary to assess the cure for CEOT. Although many more cases are needed to evaluate the prognosis for the extraosseous or peripheral variant of the CEOT, none of the 11 cases published so far has shown signs of recurrence after conservative enucleation.

Although an unsubstantiated case of malignant CEOT in a 92-year-old patient was cited by Franklin and Pindborg,[6] the first well-documented case was reported by Basu et al.[42]

References

1. Pindborg JJ. Calcifying epithelial odontogenic tumors. Acta Pathol Microbiol Scand 1955;suppl 111:71.

2. Pindborg JJ. A calcifying epithelial odontogenic tumor. Cancer 1958;11:838–843.

3. Pindborg JJ. The calcifying epithelial odontogenic tumors. Review of literature and report of an extra-osseous case. Acta Odontol Scand 1966;24: 419–430.

4. Pindborg JJ, Kramer IRH. Histological Typing of Odontogenic Tumours, Jaw Cysts, and Allied Lesions. Berlin: Springer-Verlag, 1971.

5. Philipsen HP, Reichart PA. Calcifying epithelial odontogenic tumour: Biological profile based on 181 cases from the literature. Oral Oncol 2000; 36:17–26.

6. Franklin CD, Pindborg JJ. The calcifying epithelial odontogenic tumor. A review and analysis of 113 cases. Oral Surg Oral Med Oral Pathol 1976; 42:753–765.

7. Ai-Ru L, Zhen L, Jian S. Calcifying epithelial odontogenic tumors: A clinico-pathologic study of nine cases. J Oral Pathol 1982;11:399–406.

8. Chomette G, Auriol M, Guilbert F. Histoenzymological and ultrastructural study of a bifocal calcifying epithelial odontogenic tumor. Characteristics of epithelial cells and histogenesis of amyloid-like material. Virchows Arch A Pathol Anat Histopathol 1984;403:67–76.

9. Domarus H, Hoppe W. Ein multilokuläres ameloblastische Fibrom. Dtsch Zahnarztl Z 1976;31: 260–263.

10. Busch HP, Hoppe W. Multilokulärer kalzifizierender epithelialer odontogener Tumor (CEOT). Dtsch Z Mund Kiefer Gesichtschir 1988;12:193–194.

11. Chaudhry AP, Holte NO, Vickers RA. Calcifying epithelial odontogenic tumor. Report of a case. Oral Surg Oral Med Oral Pathol 1962;15:843–848.

12. Kramer IRH, Pindborg JJ, Shear M. Histological Typing of Odontogenic Tumours. 2d ed. Berlin: Springer-Verlag, 1992.

13. Fulciniti F, Vetrani A, Zeppa P, et al. Calcifying epithelial odontogenic tumor (Pindborg's tumor) on fine-needle aspiration biopsy smears: A case report. Diagn Cytopathol 1995;12:71–75.

14. Glenner GC, Page DL. Amyloid, amyloidosis and amyloidgenesis. Int Rev Exp Pathol 1976;15:1–32.

15. Mori M, Makino M. Calcifying epithelial odontogenic tumor: Histochemical properties of homogeneous acellular substances in the tumor. J Oral Surg 1977;35:631–638.

16. Franklin CD, Martin MV, Clark A, et al. An investigation into the origin and nature of "amyloid" in a calcifying epithelial odontogenic tumour. J Oral Pathol 1981;10:417–429.

17. Yamaguchi A, Kokubu JM, Takagi M, Ishikawa G. Calcifying epithelial odontogenic tumor: Histochemical and electron microscopic observations on a case. Bull Tokyo Med Dent Univ 1980;27: 129–135.

18. Page DL, Weiss SW, Eggleston JC. Ultrastructural study of amyloid material in the calcifying epithelial odontogenic tumor. Cancer 1975;36: 1426–1435.

19. Mopsik ER, Gabriel SA. Calcifying epithelial odontogenic tumor (Pindborg tumor). Report of two cases. Oral Surg Oral Med Oral Pathol 1971;32: 15–21.

20. Wallace BJ, MacDonald GD. Calcifying epithelial odontogenic tumour ("Pindborg tumor"): A case report. Br J Plast Surg 1974;27:28–30.

21. Asano M, Takahashi T, Kusama K. A variant of calcifying epithelial odontogenic tumor with Langerhans cells. J Oral Pathol Med 1990;19:430–434.

22. Maranda G, Gourgi M. Calcifying epithelial odontogenic tumor (Pindborg tumor). Review of the literature and case report. J Can Dent Assoc 1986; 52:1009–1012.

23. El Labban NG. Cementum-like material in a case of Pindborg tumour. J Oral Pathol Med 1990;19: 166–169.

24. Slootweg PJ. Bone and cementum as stromal features in Pindborg tumor. J Oral Pathol Med 1991; 20:93–95.

25. Müller H, Slootweg P. Clear cell differentiation in an ameloblastoma. J Maxillofac Surg 1986;14: 158–160.

26. De Aguiar MCG, Gomez RS, Silva EC, de Araujo VC. Clear-cell ameloblastoma (clear-cell odontogenic carcinoma). Report of a case. Oral Surg Oral Med Oral Pathol 1996;81:79–83.

27. Ng KH, Siar CH. Clear cell change in a calcifying odontogenic cyst. Oral Surg Oral Med Oral Pathol 1985;60:417–419.

28. Philipsen HP, Reichart PA, Nikai H. The adenomatoid odontogenic tumour (AOT): An update. Oral Med Pathol 1998;2:55–60.

29. Waldron CA, Small IA, Silverman H. Clear cell ameloblastoma: An odontogenic carcinoma. J Oral Maxillofac Surg 1985;43:701–717.

30. Hansen LS, Eversole LR, Green TL, Powell NB. Clear cell odontogenic tumor: A new histologic variant with aggressive potential. Head Neck Surg 1985;8:115–123.

31. Koppang HS, Bang G, Hansen SL, Gilhuus Moe O, Aksdal E. Hellzelliger odontogener Tumor. Kasuistischer Beitrag. Dtsch Z Mund Kiefer Gesichtschir 1988;12:356–360.

32. Milchgrub S, Gnepp DR, Vuitch F, Delgado R, Albores-Saavedra J. Hyalinizing clear cell carcinoma of salivary gland. Am J Surg Pathol 1994; 18:74–82.

33. Maiorano E, Altini M, Favia G. Clear cell tumors of the salivary glands, jaws, and oral mucosa. Semin Diagn Pathol 1997;14:203–212.

34. Takata T, Ogawa I, Miyauchi M, Ijuhin N, Nikai H, Fujita M. Noncalcifying Pindborg tumor with Langerhans cells. J Oral Pathol Med 1993; 22:378–383.

35. Lasser A. The mononuclear phagocyte system. A review. Hum Pathol 1983;14:108–126.

36. Shelley W, Juhlin L. Langerhans cells from a reticuloendothelial trap for external contact allergens. Nature 1976;261:46–47.

37. Damm DD, White DK, Drummond JF, et al. Combined epithelial odontogenic tumor: Adenomatoid odontogenic tumor and calcifying epithelial odontogenic tumor. Oral Surg Oral Med Oral Pathol 1983;55:487–496.

38. Philipsen HP, Reichart PA. Adenomatoid odontogenic tumour: Facts and figures. Oral Oncol 1999;35:125–131.

39. El-Labban NG, Lee KW, Kramer IRH. The duality of the cell population in a calcifying epithelial odontogenic tumour (CEOT). Histopathology 1984;8:679–691.

40. Vap DR, Dahlin DC, Turlington EG. Pindborg tumor: The so-called calcifying epithelial odontogenic tumor. Cancer 1970;25:629–636.

41. Bouckaert MMR, Raubenheimer EJ, Jacobs FJ. Calcifying epithelial odontogenic tumor with intracranial extension: Report of a case and review of the literature. Oral Surg Oral Med Oral Pathol Oral Radiol Endod 2000;90:656–662.

42. Basu MK, Matthews JB, Sear AJ, Browne RM. Calcifying epithelial odontogenic tumour: A case showing features of malignancy. J Oral Pathol 1984;13:310–319.

Chapter 11

Adenomatoid Odontogenic Tumor

1. Terminology

The tumor that meets today's diagnostic criteria for an adenomatoid odontogenic tumour (AOT) has been known for more than 90 years. The present authors agree with Unal and coworkers[1] that Steensland's report from 1905 of an "epithelioma adamantinum" represents the earliest identification of an AOT for which sufficient documentation is available. A variety of terms has been used to describe this lesion, of which *adenoameloblastoma* was in common use for many years because the tumor was considered a histologic variant of the solid/multicystic ameloblastoma. Unal et al[1] produced a list of related terms that was used from 1905 to 1969.

In 1969, Philipsen and Birn[2] presented a review based on 76 cases of AOTs that proved the tumor to be an entity clearly distinguishable from the SMA. They introduced the term *adenomatoid odontogenic tumor*, which was adopted by the World Health Organization (WHO) in 1971.[3] It is now the generally accepted nomenclature.[4] A comprehensive study appeared in 1991[5] reviewing 500 cases of AOTs. This report was followed by studies on AOT variants[6] and ultrastructural aspects.[7] Since the early 1990s approximately 250 to 300 published cases have been added to the previous 500. The following profile of the AOT is based on a review by Philipsen and Reichart.[8]

2. Clinical and radiologic profile

The AOT is a benign, non-neoplastic (hamartomatous) lesion with a slow but progressive growth. It occurs in both intraosseous and peripheral forms (Fig 11-1).

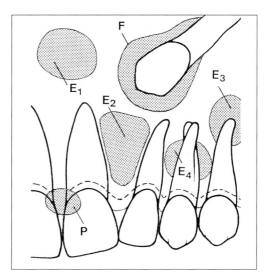

Fig 11-1 Schematic of AOT variants. In the intraosseous follicular type variant (F) the tumor is located around the crown and often—as shown here—covers part of the root of an unerupted tooth (envelopmental). Among extrafollicular types, E_1 = no relation to tooth structures either erupted or unerupted; E_2 = interradicular, adjacent roots diverge apically due to tumor expansion; E_3 = superimposed on the root apex (radicular/periapical); E_4 = superimposed at the midroot level. The extraosseous peripheral epulis type variant (P) exhibits slight erosion of the bone crest.

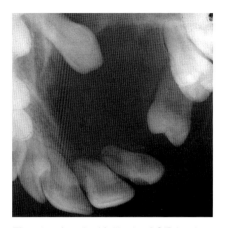

Fig 11-2 A typical follicular AOT that has developed around an unerupted left maxillary canine.

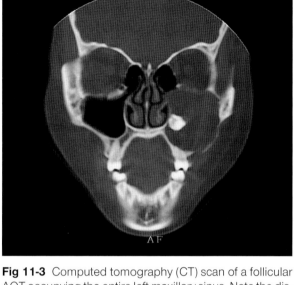

Fig 11-3 Computed tomography (CT) scan of a follicular AOT occupying the entire left maxillary sinus. Note the displaced unerupted third molar close to the nasal cavity.

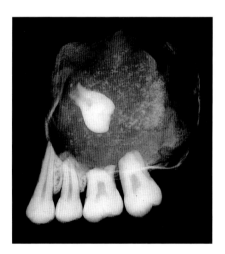

Fig 11-4 Operation specimen from the tumor shown in Fig 11-3. It exhibits a cloud of minute radiopacities surrounding the unerupted third molar. Note the unusual finding of root resorption of the first and second premolars and molars.

Radiographically, the intrabony variants comprise a follicular and an extrafollicular type. The follicular type shows a well-defined, unilocular (round or ovoid) radiolucency associated with the crown and often part of the root of an unerupted tooth, mimicking a dentigerous or follicular cyst (Figs 11-2 to 11-4). In fact, 77% of follicular type AOTs are initially diagnosed as dentigerous cysts.[2]

The extrafollicular type is not associated with an unerupted tooth, and the well-defined, unilocular radiolucency is found between (Fig 11-5), above, or superimposed on the roots of erupted permanent teeth (Fig 11-6). These locations often lead to a tentative preoperative diagnosis of a residual, radicular, "globulomaxillary," or lateral periodontal cyst, depending on the actual intraosseous site of the lesion. In approximately two thirds of the intrabony variants, the radi-

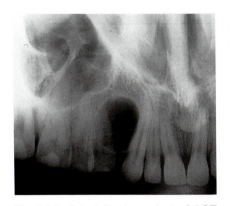

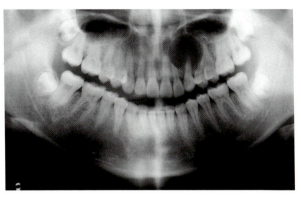

Fig 11-5 Extrafollicular variant of AOT (type E_2 in Fig 11-1) between the roots of the maxillary right canine and first premolar.

Fig 11-6 Orthopantomograph demonstrating an extrafollicular variant of AOT (type E_3 in Fig 11-1) superimposed on the apical half of the maxillary left canine root. Tumor growth has caused the roots of the adjacent lateral incisor and first premolar to deviate.

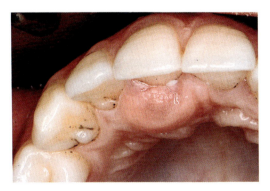

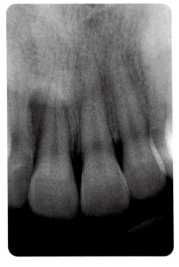

Fig 11-8 Intraoral radiograph of the tumor shown in Fig 11-7. A bony pocket (saucerization) along the palatal aspect of the maxillary right central incisor root is evident.

Fig 11-7 Clinical appearance of a peripheral variant of AOT. Epulis-like growth is seen on the palatal gingiva of the maxillary right central incisor.

olucency shows discrete radiopaque foci with a flocculent pattern. If the AOT contains minimal quantities of calcified deposits, intraoral periapical radiographs are superior to orthopantomographs in detecting the characteristic (although not pathognomonic) radiopacities.[9] Growth of the intrabony variants commonly results in cortical expansion. Displacement of neighboring teeth due to tumor expansion is much more common than root resorption.

The peripheral variant (Figs 11-7 and 11-8) appears as a gingival fibroma or epulis-like growth attached to the labial or (more rarely) the palatal gingiva. This type of AOT may show slight erosion ("saucerization") of the alveolar bone crest, but radiographic changes are often difficult to detect.

3. Epidemiological data

3.1 Incidence, prevalence, and relative frequency

Information on incidence and prevalence of the AOT is still not available. Surveys of oral pathology biopsy services from various sources do, however, provide information about relative tumor frequencies. The relative frequency of the AOT extracted from 12 oral biopsy surveys[8] shows that AOTs account for 2.2% to 7.1% of all odontogenic tumors, which gives it a ranking of fourth or fifth among the odontogenic tumors. It is surpassed only by odontomas, myxomas, and solid/multicystic ameloblastomas. Based on these figures, it is hardly reasonable to maintain that the AOT is a particularly rare odontogenic tumor.

3.2 Age

The age range of patients with AOTs varies between 3 and 82 years at the time of diagnosis.[8] No less than 68.6% of the tumors are diagnosed in the 2nd decade of life (Fig 11-9), and more than half of the cases (53.1%)

occur within the teens (13 to 19 years). This age distribution, with a very tall peak in the 2nd decade, makes the AOT unique among odontogenic tumors.

3.3 Gender

The female:male ratio for all age groups and AOT variants together is 1.9:1 (see Fig 11-9). If geographic/ethnic aspects are accounted for in the gender distribution, differences appear between Asian and non-Asian cases. Asian AOT cases (reported from Japan, India, China [including Hong Kong], Thailand, Taiwan, Sri Lanka, and Malaysia) show a female:male ratio of 2.3:1. If cases reported from Sri Lanka and Japan are considered separately they show ratios of 3.2:1 and 3.0:1, respectively.[10,11] This marked female predominance may reflect real ethnogeographic variations, but the question needs further investigation.

3.4 Location

The AOT appears, as mentioned earlier, in three clinicotopographic variants: follicular, extrafollicular, and peripheral (see Fig 11-1).

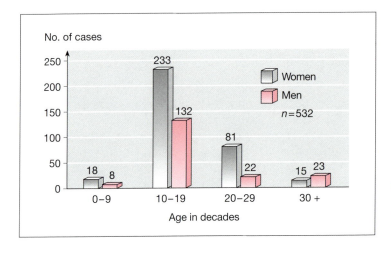

Fig 11-9 Distribution of all types of AOT variants (n = 532) according to gender and age.

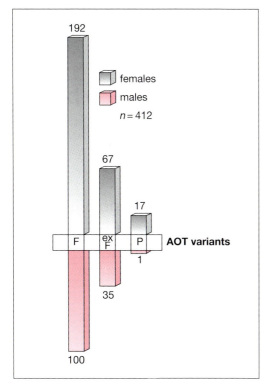

Fig 11-10 Distribution of AOT variants by gender (*n* = 412). F = follicular; exF = extrafollicular; P = peripheral. Based on data from Philipsen and Reichart,[8] Table 2.

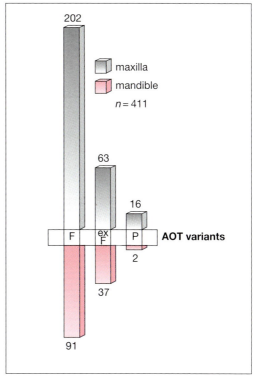

Fig 11-11 Distribution of AOT variants according to location (*n* = 411).

The follicular and extrafollicular variants are both intrabony or central tumors and account for 95.6% of all AOTs (of which 71.3% are of the follicular type). The follicular variant is close to three times as frequent as the extrafollicular variant in both men and women. Distribution of AOT variants by gender is shown in Fig 11-10. The two central variants together are more commonly found in the maxilla than in the mandible, with a total ratio of 2.1:1. The rare peripheral type occurs almost exclusively in the anterior maxilla, with this location accounting for 88.9% of such tumors. Distribution of AOT variants according to location is shown in Fig 11-11.

The distribution of unerupted permanent teeth found in association with the follicular AOT (Fig 11-12) shows that all four canines account for 59% and the maxillary canines alone for 40%. Unerupted first and second molars are the teeth most rarely involved in AOTs, only four cases having been reported. Association between central AOTs and unerupted deciduous teeth is exceedingly rare, only two cases having been published.[11]

The peripheral variant is still the most rarely reported type, constituting only 4.4% of all AOT cases. Of the 18 cases reported so far (see Table 4 in Philipsen and Reichart[8]), the mean age at the time of operation was 13.0 years; this is 3 and 10 years

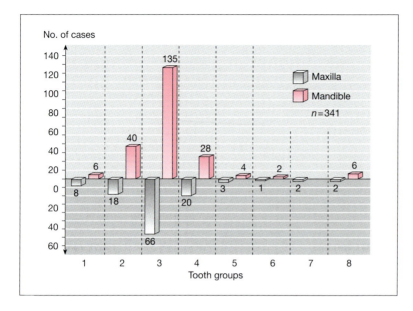

No. of cases

Tooth groups

Maxilla

Mandible

n=341

Fig 11-12 Distribution of unerupted permanent teeth associated with follicular AOT according to maxillary and mandibular tooth groups (n = 341).

earlier than the corresponding mean ages for AOT of follicular and extrafollicular types, respectively. The distribution by gender (female:male = 14:1) makes this type of AOT unique. The anterior maxillary gingiva is by far the most common location of the peripheral AOT variant. Two cases found in infants were recently reported.[1,12]

4. Pathogenesis

The fact that all AOT variants show identical histology[5] strongly points toward a common origin, and most authors agree on an odontogenic source. Based on present knowledge of the biology of the AOT, Philipsen et al[6] have strongly argued in favor of AOT being derived from the dental lamina or its remnants. Until more is known about the fate of the numerous epithelial remnants persisting in the jawbones and gingiva after completion of odontogenesis, clinicians are not in a po-

sition to answer questions such as why the follicular variant—and in particular the one associated with unerupted permanent canines—is so much more frequent than the other variants.

5. Pathology

5.1 Macroscopy

The intrabony AOT variants are roughly spherical in shape with a well-defined fibrous capsule. The cut surface may reveal a solid tumor mass or show one large or several small cystic spaces containing a yellowish, semisolid material. In the follicular type, a crown and often part of the root of an unerupted tooth is found embedded in the tumor mass or projecting into a cystic cavity. Estimation of the total protein level in aspirated fluid from cystic spaces in two intrabony AOTs[6] revealed a total protein content

110

of 5.2 g/100 ml and 7.0 g/100 ml. According to Toller,[13] if the protein level in cystic fluid is 5.0 g/100 ml or more, then the cyst epithelium is likely to be nonkeratinized. A cystic cavity, if present within an AOT, is always lined by nonkeratinized stratified squamous epithelium. Thus, the biochemical data of the two AOT cases mentioned here are in agreement with Toller's findings.

5.2 Microscopy

5.2.1 Histologic definitions

The 1992 WHO classification[4] defines the AOT as "a tumor of odontogenic epithelium with ductlike structures and with varying degrees of inductive change in the connective tissue. The tumor may be partly cystic, and in some cases the solid lesion may be present only as masses in the wall of a large cyst. It is generally believed that the lesion is not a neoplasm."

The definition used by the present authors is as follows:
A hamartomatous lesion of odontogenic epithelium producing solid nodules of cuboidal or columnar cells, here and there forming convoluted bands arranged in complicated patterns. Throughout the lesion the cells form structures of tubular or ductlike appearance. The lesion may be partly cystic with the solid tumorous tissue constituting part of a large cyst wall. The fibrous connective tissue stroma is rather sparse and may contain dysplastic dentinoid as well as calcified material that may be quite extensive.

5.2.2 Histopathologic findings

Irrespective of tumor variants, the histology of AOTs is identical and exhibits a remarkable consistency. At low magnification the most striking pattern is that of multisized solid nodules of cuboidal or columnar epithelial cells forming nests or rosettelike structures with minimal stromal connective tissue. Between the epithelial cells of nodules and in the center of the rosettelike configurations, eosinophilic amorphous material (often described as "tumor droplets") as well as calcified bodies are present (Figs 11-13 and 11-14). Spindle-shaped or polygonal, closely opposed epithelial cells with dark eosinophilic cytoplasm and round hyperchromatic nuclei fill in the spaces between the epithelial nodules. Conspicuous within the

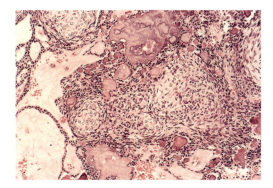

Fig 11-13 Tumor nodule composed of spindle-shaped or cuboidal epithelial cells forming rosettelike structures. There are several calcified bodies with Liesegang pattern. Note the cribriform pattern of tumor cell strands at the nodule periphery (hematoxylin-eosin [H&E], x50).

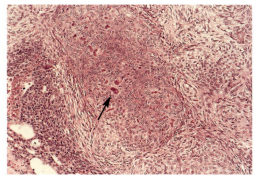

Fig 11-14 Cell-rich portion of an AOT with a whorled cell arrangement. Note the several eosinophilic tumor droplets (*arrow*) (H&E, x100).

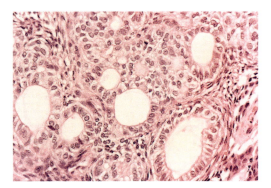

Fig 11-15 Characteristic tubular or ductlike structures lined by a single row of cuboidal or low columnar epithelial cells (H&E, x150).

cellular areas are structures of tubular or ductlike appearance (Fig 11-15). The duct-like spaces are lined by a single row of low columnar epithelial cells, the nuclei of which are polarized away from the lumenal surface. The lumen may be empty or contain a variable amount of eosinophilic material or cellular debris. The ducts vary considerably in diameter and may not always be present. However, due to the overall distinctive histomorphology of the AOT, the diagnosis can usually be secured without the presence of ductlike structures. In addition to forming ducts, the cuboidal to columnar cells form convoluted cords or bodies in complicated patterns that often exhibit invaginations.

Another characteristic cellular pattern is nodules composed of polyhedral, eosinophilic epithelial cells of squamous appearance exhibiting well-defined cell boundaries and prominent intercellular bridges. Their nuclei may occasionally show very mild (degenerative) pleomorphism. These islands may contain pools of amorphous amyloid-like material and globular masses of calcified substances (Fig 11-13). Occurrence of one or several nodules in this cellular arrangement in AOTs has led a number of authors to suggest the existence of a combined calcifying epithelial odontogenic tumor

(CEOT)/AOT lesion. However, the presence of CEOT-like foci within an AOT does not influence its biologic behavior or growth potential. A total of 24 cases of the histologic CEOT/AOT variant have been reported so far.[8] There is nothing to indicate that a CEOT/AOT lesion reflects a true combination of two distinct or separate entities, and there are no reported cases of AOT in which CEOT-like areas predominate. CEOT-like areas occurring in AOTs should be considered a normal feature within the continuous histomorphologic spectrum of AOT. Areas in AOTs mimicking calcifying ghost cell odontogenic cysts,[14] developing odontomas,[15,16] or other odontogenic tumors or hamartomas also should be regarded as histologic variants of AOTs.

Yet another epithelial pattern is found between and connecting the cell-rich nodules and particularly at the tumor periphery. This pattern is composed of strands of epithelium, one to two cells in thickness, forming a trabecular or cribriform configuration. Occasional foci of mitotic activity among AOT tumor cells may be traced, although they are not a prominent feature. Epithelial atypia has not been reported. In rare instances melanin pigmentation of both tumor and stroma cells and the presence of melanocytes may be found in AOTs,[17,18] as in several other odontogenic tumors or hamartomas.

The occurrence of a hyaline, dysplastic dentinoid material or calcified osteodentin in AOTs has been described by several authors.[4,8] Dentin or dentinoid containing dentinal tubules is exceedingly rare.[8] As the stroma is that of a fibrous, mature connective tissue without ectomesenchymal features, the production of dysplastic dentinoid is likely the result of a metaplastic process and is not to be interpreted as an epithelioectomesenchymal induction phenomenon. Calcified material in varying amounts occurs in most lesions. Irregular calcified bodies are common; they often exhibit a concentric or

Liesegang pattern that most likely represents dystrophic calcification of tissue elements in areas of loose connective tissue stroma (CEOT/AOT-like areas; Fig 11-13). Scattered throughout the tumor tissue are small or large masses of calcified bodies or globules often found adjacent to rows of tall columnar cells resembling ameloblasts.

The connective tissue stroma of the AOT is generally loosely structured and contains thin-walled congested vessels characteristically showing marked degenerative (fibrinoid) changes of the endothelial lining, vessel wall, and perivascular connective tissue.

5.2.3 Histochemical findings

Histochemical studies of the AOT have mainly focused on the nature of the hyaline or eosinophilic deposits (tumor droplets) and the calcified structures.[5] However, previous conventional and inadequate histochemical techniques failed to disclose whether these structures are of epithelial or mesenchymal origin. The controversy over the occurrence (or nonoccurrence) of amyloid, amyloid-like, or pseudoamyloid substances in AOTs is not surprising since the interpretation of amyloid-like substances is far from being uniform.

5.2.4 Immunohistochemical findings

In recent years a number of studies have added to the knowledge about the immunohistochemistry of AOTs. Tatemoto et al[19] demonstrated coexpression of keratin and vimentin in the tumor cells at the periphery of the ductal, tubular, or whorled structures. Whereas tumor cells were positive for keratin stains, mineralized and hyaline material were negative. Mori et al[20] and Saku et al[21] both studied enamel proteins in AOTs and found amelogenin and enamelin in small mineralized foci in both tumor cells and hyaline droplets.

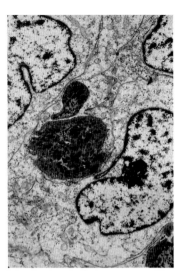

Fig 11-16 Electron micrograph showing the extracellular location of tumor droplets of varying electron density (transmission electron microscopy [TEM], x8,000).

5.2.5 Ultrastructural findings

Although almost all ultrastructural studies have been focused on the follicular type of AOTs, it is unlikely that ultrastructural differences should exist between the three variants given their identical histology. The epithelial nature of the AOT has been confirmed through findings of well-developed gap junctions, desmosomes, and desmosome-like junctions. Tight junctions have not been described. Tonofilaments are present in varying amounts. Three ultrastructurally different types of epithelial tumor cells have been recognized as corresponding to the three cell populations seen with light microscopy.[7] The material found in the ductlike spaces has a granulofibrillar appearance. This material is separated from the adjacent tumor cells by a basal lamina–like zone, a finding that lends support to earlier theories suggesting that the ducts are formed as a result of degeneration of the stromal tissue. Hemidesmosomes are found between the cells and this

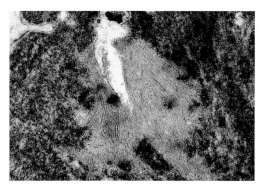

Fig 11-17 Finer details of the granulotubular components of tumor droplets (TEM x100,000).

matrix. Tumor cells demonstrating squamous cell metaplasia (representing CEOT-like areas) are polygonal, contain an abundance of tonofilament bundles, and possess well-formed desmosomes. El-Labban[22] reported that the eosinophilic amorphous masses are heterogeneous and consist of three types of fibrils: thin collagen fibrils, electron-dense fibrils, and amyloid filaments. A recent study[7] disclosed that the most conspicuous feature of the amorphous (noncalcified) eosinophilic material (tumor droplets) is concentrically arranged tubular structures, the surface of which may be coated with a fine granular material (Figs 11-16 and 11-17). The authors suggested that the tumor droplets probably represent some form of enamel matrix. Amyloid filaments or collagen fibrils were not encountered in this study.

6. Notes on treatment and recurrence rate

As all variants of AOT reveal an entirely benign biologic behavior and in almost all reported cases are well encapsulated, conservative surgical enucleation or curettage has proven the treatment modality of choice. In only 3 (all Japanese) of 750 AOT cases has the tumor recurred,[8] and in only one instance was extension of the recurring tumor into the intracranial space recorded.[23]

References

1. Unal T, Cetingul E, Gunbay T. Peripheral adenomatoid odontogenic tumour: Birth of a term. J Clin Pediatr Dent 1995;19:139–142.

2. Philipsen HP, Birn H. The adenomatoid odontogenic tumour. Ameloblastic adenomatoid tumour or adeno-ameloblastoma. Acta Pathol Microbiol Scand 1969;75:375–398.

3. Kramer IRH, Pindborg JJ. Histological Typing of Odontogenic Tumours, Jaw Cysts, and Allied Lesions. Berlin: Springer-Verlag, 1971.

4. Kramer IRH, Pindborg JJ, Shear M. Histological Typing of Odontogenic Tumours. 2d ed. Berlin: Springer-Verlag, 1992.

5. Philipsen HP, Reichart PA, Zhang KH, et al. Adenomatoid odontogenic tumor: Biologic profile based on 499 cases. J Oral Pathol Med 1991; 20:149–158.

6. Philipsen HP, Samman N, Ormiston IW, Wu PC, Reichart PA. Variants of the adenomatoid odontogenic tumor with a note on tumor origin. J Oral Pathol Med 1992;21:348–352.

7. Philipsen HP, Reichart PA. The adenomatoid odontogenic tumour: Ultrastructure of tumour cells and non-calcified amorphous masses. J Oral Pathol Med 1996;25:491–496.

8. Philipsen HP, Reichart PA. Adenomatoid odontogenic tumour: Facts and figures. Oral Oncol 1998; 35:125–131.

9. Dare A, Yamaguchi A, Yoshiki S, Okano T. Limitation of panoramic radiography in diagnosing adenomatoid odontogenic tumors. Oral Surg Oral Med Oral Pathol 1994;77:662–668.

10. Mendis BRRN, MacDonald DG. Adenomatoid odontogenic tumour. A survey of 21 cases from Sri Lanka. Int J Oral Maxillofac Surg 1990;19: 141–143.

11. Toida M, Hyodo I, Okuda T, Tatematsu N. Adenomatoid odontogenic tumor: Report of two cases and survey of 126 cases in Japan. J Oral Maxillofac Surg 1990;48:404–408.

12. Kearns GJ, Smith R. Adenomatoid odontogenic tumour: An unusual cause of gingival swelling in a 3-year-old patient. Br Dent J 1996;181:380–382.

13. Toller PA. Protein substances in odontogenic cyst fluids. Br Dent J 1970;128:317–322.

14. Zeitoun IM, Dhanrajani PJ, Mosadomi HA. Adenomatoid odontogenic tumor arising in a calcifying odontogenic cyst. J Oral Maxillofac Surg 1996;54:634–637.

15. Miles AEW. A cystic complex composite odontome. Proc R Soc Med 1951;44:51–55.

16. Dunlap CL, Fritzlen TJ. Cystic odontoma with concomitant adenoameloblastoma (adenoameloblastic odontoma). Oral Surg Oral Med Oral Pathol 1972;34:450–456.

17. Warter A, George-Diolombi G, Chazal M, Ango A. Melanin in a dentigerous cyst and associated adenomatoid odontogenic tumor. Cancer 1990;66: 786–788.

18. Aldred MJ, Gray AR. A pigmented adenomatoid odontogenic tumor. Oral Surg Oral Med Oral Pathol 1990;70:86–90.

19. Tatemoto Y, Tanaka T, Okada Y, et al. Adenomatoid odontogenic tumour: Co-expression of keratin and vimentin. Virchows Arch A Pathol Anat Histopathol 1988;413:341–347.

20. Mori M, Yamada K, Kasai T, et al. Immunohistochemical expression of amelogenins in odontogenic epithelial tumours and cysts. Virchows Arch A Pathol Anat Histopathol 1991;418:319–325.

21. Saku T, Okabe H, Shimokawa H. Immunohistochemical demonstration of enamel proteins in odontogenic tumors. J Oral Pathol Med 1992;21:113–119.

22. El-Labban NG. The nature of the eosinophilic and laminated masses in the adenomatoid odontogenic tumor: A histochemical and ultrastructural study. J Oral Pathol Med 1992;21:75–81.

23. Takigami M, Uede T, Imaizumi T, et al. A case of adenomatoid odontogenic tumour with intracranial extension. No Shinkei Geka 1988;16:775–779.

Section Three

Benign Neoplasms and Tumor-like Lesions Showing Odontogenic Epithelium With Odontogenic Ectomesenchyme, With or Without Dental Hard Tissue Formation

Introduction to Mixed Odontogenic Tumors

There has been considerable debate about whether and how the so-called mixed odontogenic tumors are interrelated. In recent years Philipsen et al,[1] Takeda,[2] and Tomich[3] have reviewed the different aspects of interrelationship between benign mixed odontogenic tumors.

Philipsen et al[1] clearly pointed out that, based on their findings, complex and compound odontomas should be regarded as two separate entities. This is in contrast to some authorities in the field[4] who suggested that complex and compound odontomas should—for therapeutic reasons—be considered the same. Clinical and radiologic data convincingly show that the lesions are different in important respects (relative frequency, location) and that separation seems to be justified irrespective of the fact that both odontomas can receive the same (conservative) treatment. Therefore, Philipsen et al[1] advocated that the two types be registered as separate entities in future studies and case reports.

When discussing the relationship between members of the benign mixed odontogenic tumors, the following entities have to be addressed: ameloblastic fibromas (AFs), ameloblastic fibrodentinoma (AFDs), ameloblastic fibro-odontomas (AFOs), and the two types of odontomas (complex and compound).

Cahn and Blum[5] proposed the "continuum concept" based on the assumption that an AF will, over time, mature and finally result in the formation of an odontoma. This concept, however, was not widely accepted, because residual or recurrent cases of AF have never shown further steps of differentiation or maturation into a dental hard tissue–forming odontogenic tumor of more advanced histodifferentiation. Another reason was that AFs are known to occur at ages beyond completion of odontogenesis, that is, after the age of 20 years. Philipsen et al[1] agreed with the authors of the 1992 World Health Organization (WHO) classification[6] that AFs—and in particular those 22.3% of cases occurring after the age of 20—are true benign neoplasms. All the cases of AF developing during the entire period of odontogenesis (childhood and adolescence), however, may represent non-neoplastic, hamartomatous lesions which over time may develop into AFOs and finally into mineralized complex odontomas. Both AFOs and odontomas go through stages of mineralization and calcification; none of them arise as calcified lesions *de novo*. On these grounds Philipsen et al[1] proposed some hypothetical considerations on the pathogenesis and relationship between mixed odontogenic tumors and odontomas: A neoplastic line of development (I) and a hamartomatous line (II) should be considered along which mixed odontogenic tumors may develop. In this context the authors fully support the view of Hansen and Ficarra[7] that some ameloblastic fibromas may represent the early stage of a developing complex odontoma (DCO) line. Based on these assumptions there may be two lesions with the histologic criteria of AFs: the neoplastic AF and the early, primitive, or first stage of a DCO. Final proof for this hypothesis is missing because at present there is no way to differentiate between the histology of the neoplastic and the hamartomatous lesion with the histologic features of the AF.

Philipsen et al[1] suggested that line I would only include the AF and possibly the closely related AFD. Presently there is no proof that this tumor line would develop further than the stage where dentinlike or dentinoid substances are produced in the ectomesenchymal tumor component.

Line II would comprise the hamartomatous or developing complex odontoma line, including a variety of stages of the complex odontoma. The ameloblastic fibro-odontoma was not considered to be a member of the neoplastic line but to represent a stage preceding the complex odontoma of the DCO line. The likelihood that AFOs which are characterized by irregularly arranged odontogenic tissues—including odontogenic epithelium, ectomesenchyme, abortive dentin, and enamel—will develop into compound odontomas seems very small. Available data point at the complex odontoma being the terminal stage of the line of hamartomatous lesions. Comparisons of age distribution at the time of diagnosis of ameloblastic fibro-odontomas and complex odontoma show that a higher age is common in the cases of complex odontomas.

There is general agreement that the compound odontoma is a malformation. Age and distribution of location support the hypothesis that the pathogenesis of the compound odontoma differs from that of the complex odontoma. Philipsen et al[1] did not agree with the 1992 WHO classification[6] which claimed that the distinction between compound and complex odontomas is arbitrary based on a preponderance of toothlike structures in the former in contrast to a preponderance of haphazardly arranged soft and hard odontogenic tissues in the latter, rather than on any absolute difference. Philipsen and coworkers suggested that the formation of compound odontomas may be the result of "multiple schizodontia" of unknown cause but probably due to a locally hyperactive dental lamina. The finding that 56% of maxillary supernumerary teeth are located in the anterior maxilla may lend support to this hypothesis. Although transitional cases of odontomas showing microscopic features of both types of odontomas do exsist, the clinical data and histologic evaluation will, in most cases, lead to a diagnosis of either a complex or a compound odontoma.

The concept expressed by Philipsen et al[1] and summarized here does not form the basis for the presentation of mixed odontogenic tumors in chapters 12–16, as all data stem from retrospective studies. Thus, the authors intend to follow the currently accepted classification expressed both in the WHO classification of 1992[6] and in the forthcoming WHO volume *Tumours of the Head and Neck.*

Comments

The two lesions described in chapters 17 and 18 do not belong to the mixed odontogenic tumor family (chapters 12 to 16). Moreover, chapter 17 ("Calcifying Ghost Cell Odontogenic Cysts/Tumors" [Odontogenic Ghost Cell Lesions]) requires some introductory notes.

Gorlin et al [8,9] first identified the calcifying odontogenic cyst (COC) as a specific odontogenic lesion. Controversy and confusion later ensued after the lesion was shown to be of extreme diversity in its clinical and histopathologic features, as well as in its biologic behavior. Today, several non-neoplastic (simple cystic), benign neoplastic, and malignant variants have been described (for references, see chapter 17). In chapter 17 the authors have combined the four published classification attempts[10-13] into one comprehensive classification (see Table 17-1). Because current research activities in this field are considerable, further attempts to classify these complex lesions are inevitable. In the forthcoming WHO volume *Tumours of the Head and Neck,* three odontogenic ghost cell tumors are described

comprising *calcifying cystic odontogenic tumor* (corresponds to 2Aaα in Table 17-1 of the present book), *dentinogenic ghost cell tumor* (corresponds to 2Abβ in Table 17-1 of the present book), and *ghost cell odontogenic carcinoma* (described in chapter 28 of the present book).

References

1. Philipsen HP, Reichart PA, Praetorius F. Mixed odontogenic tumours and odontomas. Considerations on interrelationship. Review of the literature and presentation of 134 new cases of odontomas. Oral Oncol 1997;33:86-99.

2. Takeda Y. Ameloblastic fibroma and related lesions: Current pathologic concept. Oral Oncol 1999;35:535-540.

3. Tomich CE. Benign mixed odontogenic tumors. Semin Diagn Pathol 1999;16:308-316.

4. Regezi JA, Kerr DA, Courtney RM. Odontogenic tumors. Analysis of 706 cases. J Oral Surg 1978;36: 771-778.

5. Cahn LR, Blum T. Ameloblastic odontoma, case report critically analyzed (letter). J Oral Surg 1952;10: 169-170.

6. Kramer IRH, Pindborg JJ, Shear M. Histological Typing of Odontogenic Tumours. 2d ed. Berlin: Springer-Verlag, 1992.

7. Hansen LS, Ficarra G. Mixed odontogenic tumors, analysis of 23 new cases. Head Neck Surg 1988; 10:330-430.

8. Gorlin RJ, Pindborg JJ, Clausen FP, Vickers RA. The calcifying odontogenic cyst—A possible analogue of the cutaneous epithelioma of Malherbe. Oral Surg Oral Med Oral Pathol 1962;15:1235–1243.

9. Gorlin RJ, Pindborg JJ, Redman RS, et al. The calcifying odontogenic cyst. A new entity and possible analogue of the cutaneous epithelioma of Malherbe. Cancer 1964;17:723–729.

10. Toida M. So-called calcifying odontogenic cyst: Review and discussion on the terminology and classification. J Oral Pathol Med 1998;27:49–52.

11. Praetorius F, Hjørting-Hansen E, Gorlin RJ, Vickers RA. Calcifying odontogenic cyst. Range, variations and neoplastic potential. Acta Odontol Scand 1981;39:227–240.

12. Buchner A. The central (intraosseous) calcifying odontogenic cyst: An analysis of 215 cases. J Oral Maxillofac Surg 1991;49:330–339.

13. Hong SP, Ellis GL, Hartman KS. Calcifying odontogenic cyst. A review of ninety-two cases with reevaluation of their nature as cysts or neoplasms, the nature of ghost cells, and subclassification. Oral Surg Oral Med Oral Pathol 1991;72:56–64.

Chapter 12

Ameloblastic Fibroma

1. Terminology

In 1891 Kruse[1] first described cystic tumors of the mandible, which are known today as ameloblastic fibromas (AFs). In 1981, Slootweg[2] published a comprehensive review of this entity in which he described 55 cases of AFs, 54 of which were retrieved from the literature covering the period between 1946 and 1978. In 1997 Philipsen et al[3] reviewed "mixed odontogenic tumors," including AFs. Based on a worldwide literature review, a total of 122 cases of AFs were evaluated.

Since 1997 a number of new cases have been described in the literature. Dallera et al[4] reported on six cases of AFs with follow-up. Piesold and Meerbach[5] reported a case of a maxillary AF. Other single case reports were published by Brethaux-Bardinon et al,[6] Bocklage et al,[7] and Mosby et al.[8] Mosqueda-Taylor et al[9] reported a series of 349 cases of odontogenic tumors from Mexico; among these, five cases of AFs were registered (1.4%). In an earlier study from Canada[10] seven cases of AFs were included, although with no details on age, gender, and location.

The AF is generally considered to be a true mixed odontogenic tumor in which both the epithelial and ectomesenchymal components are neoplastic. While there is no hard tissue formation in AFs, other lesions belonging to the family of mixed odontogenic tumors are characterized by hard tissue formation such as calcification and mineralization. These lesions are the ameloblastic fibrodentinoma, the ameloblastic fibro-odontoma, and the odontomas. The interrelationship between these lesions has been discussed recently by several authors.[3,11]

2. Clinical and radiologic profile

The AF is a painless, slow-growing expansile lesion of the jaws. Since the clinical symptoms are mild, about 20% of AFs are discovered accidentally on radiographs.[3] Impacted, unerupted teeth are associated with AFs in three quarters of the cases. Also, AFs may develop in areas of congenitally missing teeth.[12] In opercula of unerupted first and second permanent molars, AFs could be detected microscopically in 7 out of 74 specimens.[13] The size of the tumor varies between 1 and 10 cm in diameter; in Philipsen et al,[3] 9 of 16 lesions were considered large, with the greatest diameter more than 4 cm.

Radiologically, the tumor is characterized as a well-defined, uni- or multilocular radiolucency, often with a radiopaque border as observed in cysts. While smaller lesions reveal unilocular patterns, large lesions tend to have a multilocular appearance. The latter configuration is observed in 75% of the cases. Since the majority of cases of AF are

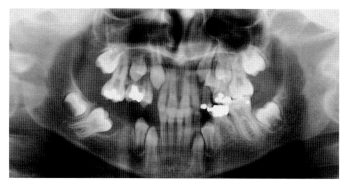

Fig 12-1 AF of the right mandible in association with an impacted first molar. The anlage of the second premolar is missing on both sides. The lesion appears as a follicular cyst.

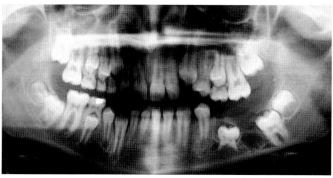

Fig 12-2 AF of the left mandible. The second deciduous molar is impacted and the anlage of the second premolar is missing. The cystic lesion is located mesial to the first mandibular molar which also has not erupted.

associated with impacted teeth, dentigerous cysts have to be considered in differential diagnosis (Figs 12-1 and 12-2).

3. Epidemiological data

3.1 Prevalence, incidence, and relative frequency

Figures indicating the relative frequency of AFs range between 1.5% and 4.5%.[3]

3.2 Age

AFs are most frequently observed during the first two decades of life (Fig 12-3), and 77.7% of all cases of AFs are diagnosed before the age of 20. Mean age of 121 cases of AFs was 14.8 years with a range of 0.5 to 62 years.[3] If all cases diagnosed after age 30 are excluded, the average is 12.4 years.

3.3 Gender

According to a review by Philipsen et al[3] the male:female ratio was 1.4:1.

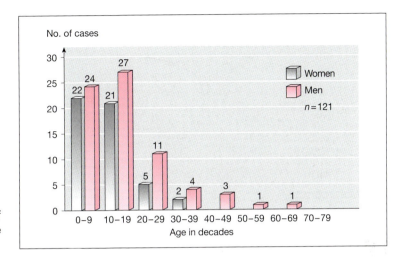

Fig 12-3 Distribution of AFs according to age and gender.

3.4 Location

Most AFs are located in the posterior mandible (Fig.12-4). If cases involving more than one quadrant are excluded, 69% of AFs occur in the posterior mandible. Also, the posterior mandible is affected more often than the maxilla by a factor of 3.1. It should be noted that AFs seem to occur as central variants and only recently has the first case of a *peripheral* AF been described.[14]

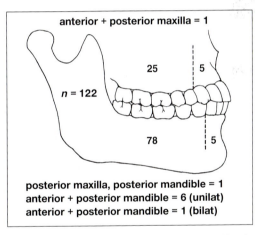

Fig 12-4 Location of 122 cases of ameloblastic fibromas.

4. Pathogenesis

According to the World Health Organization (WHO, 1992),[15] the AF is clearly a neoplasm of odontogenic origin with an epithelial and an ectomesenchymal component. Morphologically, the AF is similar to the normal tooth anlage before hard tissue formation has started. Due to the similarity of the AF to dental follicular tissue, the latter may be misinterpreted as an odontogenic tumor.[16]

Pathogenetically, the epithelial components—the ameloblast-like cell—are too primitive to induce the cells of the ectomesenchyme. Little is currently known about the interactions between epithelium and the ectomensenchymal tumor stroma, and it is unknown why, in contrast to physiologic tooth formation, the step of induction of odontoblastic differentiation is lacking in the AF.[17] However, as has been discussed in the introduction to these chapters, the present authors entertain the theory that two variants of the AF exist: a neoplastic type with no induction phenomena and a hamartomatous type showing inductive capabilities.

5. Pathology

5.1 Macroscopy

The cut surface of AFs is usually round or oval, well circumscribed, and of a grayish white color. The soft mass appears to be surrounded by a thin, transparent, capsule-like border.

5.2 Microscopy

5.2.1 Histologic definitions

The 1992 WHO classification[15] does not include a definition of the AF as an entity. The authors pooled the AF with "related lesions" which also covers the ameloblastic fibrodentinoma, and the ameloblastic fibro-odontoma. The suggested definition for this group of lesions was "Neoplasm composed of proliferating odontogenic epithelium embedded in a cellular ectomesenchymal tissue that resembles the dental papilla, and with varying degrees of inductive change and dental hard tissue formation."

The definition used by the present authors is as follows:

AF comprises two subtypes: a neoplasm and a hamartomatous lesion. The two variants are histopathologically undistinguishable, both being composed of proliferating epithelial odontogenic epithelium embedded in a cellular, odontogenic ectomesenchymal tissue that resembles the dental papilla. Induction does not take place in the neoplastic subtype.

5.2.2 Histopathologic findings

The epithelial tumor component is arranged in strands, cords, and islands of proliferating odontogenic epithelium. The strands often reveal a double or triple layer of cuboidal cells, thus resembling the dental lamina of early tooth development. In contrast, the islands often show a peripheral row of high cuboidal or columnar ameloblast-like cells (Figs 12-5 and 12-6). The centers of individual tumor islands may enclose a number of cells resembling stellate reticulum. The

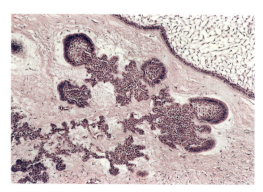

Fig 12-5 Strands and islands of odontogenic epithelium in a cell-rich ectomesenchyme (hematoxylin-eosin [H&E], x60).

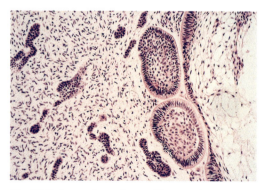

Fig 12-6 Several smaller and larger islands of epithelium in ectomesenchymal tissue (H&E, x80).

amount and density of the epithelial component of the AF may vary within the same tumor. Cyst formation within the epithelium is uncommon, and cysts usually remain small.

The ectomesenchymal cells are rounded or angular, and there is little collagen which is represented by a few delicate collagen fibrils. The degree of cellularity varies within the same tumor and among tumors.

Occasionally, some parts of the ectomesenchymal component may reveal a loose myxomatous structure (Fig 12-7) with weakly positive metachromatic substance. There may be a cell-free zone bordering the epithelial islands and strands, and in rare instances juxtaepithelial hyalinization of the type seen in solid/multicystic ameloblastomas may occur. Occasionally hyalinization may be more diffuse. The AF does not reveal a definite capsule histologically. In some cases of AFs, melanin granules have been found in the epithelial tumor component.[3]

While the histopathologic diagnosis of odontogenic tumors is usually made from representative biopsy tissue, fine-needle aspiration has also been applied for diagnostic purposes.[7] Papanicolaou-stained slides revealed branching epithelial structures and a hypercellular stroma. Stromal portions of the aspirate were composed of plaques and streaming uniform cells with distinct cellular borders and hyperchromatic, slightly spindled or round nuclei. Cytologic atypia, mitotic activity, and necrosis were not observed.

Another variant of AF, the *granular cell ameloblastic fibroma,* was described in 1962,[13] and until 1991 only 16 cases had been reported. Characteristically, the ectomesenchymal component is dominated by granular cells. Proliferative activity of the odontogenic epithelium and differentiation toward enamel organlike structures are not present. Foci of dystrophic calcification have been found among the granular cells. Ultrastructural studies of this variant of AF have revealed the granular cells to be similar to those in the granular cell myoblastoma and the congenital granular cell tumor. Further ultrastructural and immunohistochemical studies have shown that the granular cells have a strong association with the precursors of Langerhans cells. The histologic, immunohistochemical, and ultrastructural findings, combined with a characteristic mean age at the time of diagnosis of 47 years as opposed to the 1st and 2nd decades for AF, have led most authors to consider the granular cell AF a variant of the odontogenic fibroma (see chapter 19) rather than a variant of the ameloblastic fibroma.[3]

In the *papilliferous ameloblastic fibroma*, a rare variant of AF, a marked proliferation of the epithelium with a plexiform arrangement and cyst formation have been described.

In rare cases the AF may transform into an ameloblastic fibrosarcoma (see chapter 29).

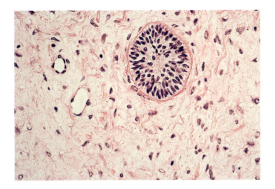

Fig 12-7 Higher magnification of an epithelial island. High columnar ameloblast-like cells are seen at the periphery of the island. The ectomesenchymal cells are slender or angular (H&E, ×100).

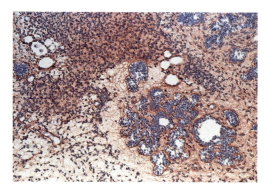

Fig 12-8 Collagen type I concentrated in tumor regions with high cellularity. Staining is weak and diffuse in the matrix surrounding the epithelial islands (APAAP, ×125).

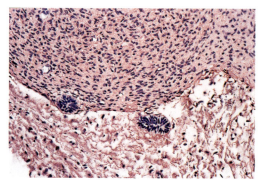

Fig 12-9 The ectomesenchymal component of the AF. An amorphous staining pattern is seen for procollagen type III, in contrast to the adjacent subepithelial connective tissue where fiber bundles positive for procollagen type III are found (APAAP, ×200).

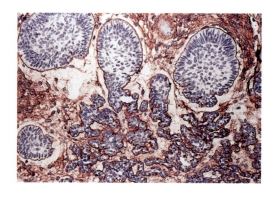

Fig 12-10 Marked staining for collagen type VI in the ectomesenchymal component. The zone of hyalinization is only faintly positive with epithelial islands being surrounded by a distinct rim of collagen type VI (APAAP, ×125).

5.2.3 Histochemical/immunohistochemical findings

Sano et al[18] assessed the growth potential of ameloblastic fibromas and related lesions by MIB-1 immunohistochemistry. MIB-1 is a monoclonal antibody against proliferation-associated nuclear antigen; it recognizes the epitope of Ki-67 antigen. In their study, the authors showed that MIB-1 labeling indices in the epithelial component ranged from 2.9% to 7.5%, whereas those in the ectomesenchymal component ranged from 1.5% to 13.5%. In particular, labeling indices were high for recurrent AFs and ameloblastic fibrosarcomas compared to AFs. These findings suggested that evaluation of growth potential in the AF could help to understand tumor aggressiveness.

In another study Becker et al[17] studied the difference between the ectomesenchymal and adjacent connective tissue proper of AFs. While the ectomesenchymal component of ameloblastic fibromas revealed marked staining for collagen types I and VI, the surrounding mature connective tissue remained almost unstained. Procollagen type III, on the other hand, was less prominent in the ectomesenchyme, in contrast to the strong staining pattern observed for collagen type I in the adjacent connective tissue. The authors demonstrated that the characteristics of the extracellular matrix composition allows for a clear distinction between the ectomesenchyme of the AF and the adjacent connective tissue of mesodermal origin. Findings also indicated that epithelial cells of AFs invade the adjacent normal mesenchyme, possibly inducing de novo formation of ectomesenchymal stroma (Figs 12-8 to 12-10). Other immunohistochemical studies concentrated on proliferating cell nuclear antigen (PCNA).[15,19]

5.2.4 Ultrastructural findings

Ultrastructural studies of AFs have focused on the epithelium-ectomesenchymal interface.[22,23] Changes in the basal lamina region were consistent with an attempted inductive stimulation with some similarities to normal odontogenesis. Ameloblastic fibromas revealed differing degrees of thickening of the lamina densa by a granulofilamentous material. However, the granulofilamentous zone was not wide enough to account for the hyaline, cell-free bands seen histologically.

6. Notes on treatment and recurrence rate

Recurrences of AFs have been described. Trodahl[20] recorded a recurrence rate of 43.5% in a series of 24 cases of AFs. Zallen et al[21] estimated a cumulative recurrence rate of 18%; these authors suggested a modified block resection rather than a simple enucleation. Gundlach[24] also stated that enucleation of the AF would not be sufficient in most cases. Most authors agree that the nonaggressive biologic behavior of AFs does not justify radical initial treatment, although large tumors, and those of the maxilla may have to be treated more radically. As with other odontogenic tumors, "reappearance" may not represent true recurrence but rather residual tumor tissue, as the result of inadequate initial surgery. Therefore, the tendency to "recur" does not always indicate aggressive behavior of the AF.

References

1. Kruse A. Über die Entwicklung cystischer Geschwülste im Unterkiefer. Arch Pathol Anat 1891; 124:137–189.

2. Slootweg PJ. An analysis of the interrelationship of the mixed odontogenic tumors—ameloblastic fibroma, ameloblastic fibro-odontoma, and the odontomas. Oral Surg Oral Pathol Oral Med 1981; 51:266–276.

3. Philipsen HP, Reichart PA, Prætorius F. Mixed odontogenic tumours and odontomas. Considerations on interrelationship. Review of the literature and presentation of 134 new cases of odontomas. Oral Oncol 1997;33:86–99.

4. Dallera P, Bertoni F, Marchetti C, et al. Ameloblastic fibroma—a follow up of six cases. Int J Oral Maxillofac Surg 1996;25:199–202.

5. Piesold J, Meerbach W. Ameloblastisches Fibrom im Oberkiefer. Mund Kiefer Gesichtschir 1997;1: 174–178.

6. Brethaux-Bardinon M-P, Ferkadji N, Deffez J-P. A propos des fibromes améloblastiques. Rev Stomatol Chir Maxillofac 1994;95:75–77.

7. Bocklage JT, Ardeman T, Schaffner D. Ameloblastic fibroma: A fine-needle aspiration case report. Diagn Cytopathol 1997;17:280–286.

8. Mosby EL, Russell D, Noren S, Scott Barker BF. Ameloblastic fibroma in a 7-week-old infant: A case report and review of the literature. J Oral Maxillofac Surg 1998;56:368–372.

9. Mosqueda-Taylor A, Ledesma-Montes C, Caballero-Sandoval S, et al. Odontogenic tumors in Mexico. A collaborative retrospective study of 349 cases. Oral Surg Oral Med Oral Pathol Oral Radiol Endod 1997;84:672–675.

10. Daley T, Wysocki GP, Pringle GA. Relative incidence of odontogenic tumors and oral and jaw cysts in a Canadian population. Oral Surg Oral Med Oral Pathol 1994;77:276–280.

11. Takeda Y. Ameloblastic fibroma and related lesions: Current pathologic concept. Oral Oncol 1999;35:535–540.

12. Schmidt-Westhausen AM, Philipsen HP, Reichart PA. Das ameloblastische Fibrom—ein odontogener Tumor im Wachstumsalter. Dtsch Zahnärztl Z 1991;46:66–68.

13. Philipsen HP, Thosaporn W, Reichart PA, Grundt G. Odontogenic lesions in opercula of permanent molars delayed in eruption. J Oral Pathol Med 1992;21:38–41.

14. Kusama K, Miyake M, Moro I. Peripheral ameloblastic fibroma of the mandible, report of a case. J Oral Maxillofac Surg 1998;56:399–401.

15. Kramer IRH, Pindborg JJ, Shear M. Histological Typing of Odontogenic Tumours. 2d ed. Berlin: Springer Verlag, 1992.

16. Kim J, Ellis GL. Dental follicular tissue: Misinterpretation as odontogenic tumors. J Oral Maxillofac Surg 1993;51:762–767.

17. Becker J, Reichart PA, Schuppan D, Philipsen HP. Ectomesenchyme of ameloblastic fibroma reveals a characteristic distribution of extracellular matrix proteins. J Oral Pathol Med 1992;21:156–159.

18. Sano K, Yoshida S, Ninomiya H, et al. Assessment of growth potential by MIB-1 immunohistochemistry in ameloblastic fibroma and related lesions of the jaws compared with ameloblastic fibrosarcoma. J Oral Pathol Med 1998;27:59–63.

19. Yamamoto K, Yoneda K, Yamamoto T, et al. An immunohistochemical study of odontogenic mixed tumors. Oral Oncol 1995;31:122–128.

20. Trodahl JN. Ameloblastic fibroma. A survey of cases from the Armed Forces Institute of Pathology. Oral Surg Oral Med Oral Pathol 1972;33:547–558.

21. Zallen RD, Preskar MH, McClary SA. Ameloblastic fibroma. J Oral Maxillofac Surg 1982;40:513–517.

22. Csiba A, Lapis K. Ultrastructure de l' ameloblastome fibromateux. Bull Group Int Rech Sci Stomatol 1972;15:233–250.

23. Farman AG, Gould AR, Merrell E. Epithelium—connective tissue junction in follicular ameloblastoma and ameloblastic fibroma: An ultrastructural analysis. Int J Oral Maxillofac Surg 1986;15:176–186.

24. Gundlach KK. Odontogene Tumoren. Mund Kiefer Gesichtschir 2000;4(Suppl 1): S187–S195.

Chapter 13

Ameloblastic Fibrodentinoma

1. Terminology

The ameloblastic fibrodentinoma (AFD) has up until now been called dentinoma and was first described by Straith in 1936.[1] He defined the AFD as "a very rare neoplasm composed of odontogenic epithelium and immature connective tissue, and characterized by the formation of dysplastic dentine."

In a 1997 review of mixed odontogenic tumors,[2] 25 cases of AFDs were retrieved from the literature. Ulmansky et al[3] published two cases in 1994, and two more cases were reported by Akal et al[4] in 1997.

The concept of a dentinoma being an individual entity has been questioned by some authors, and doubt has been expressed as to the exact nature of such lesions. In particular, the so-called immature dentinoma[5] has been considered different from the AFD based on histologic features. The interrelationship between ameloblastic fibromas, ameloblastic fibro-odontomas, and the odontomas is discussed in the introduction to this section.

2. Clinical and radiologic profile

The AFD has been described as a slow-growing, often asymptomatic tumor which may become quite large. It may be associated with unerupted teeth in some cases. Although few cases of AFDs have been re-

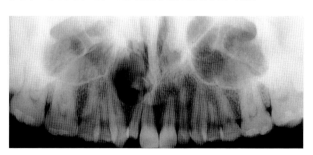

Fig 13-1 Radiograph of an early AFD. A small, well-delineated translucency with minor early calcifications is seen above the right permanent maxillary lateral incisor.

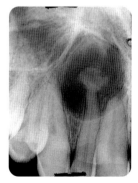

Fig 13- 2 Periapical radiograph of the cystic lesion shown in Fig 13-1. It appeared to have developed from the permanent maxillary right lateral incisor. An irregular radiopacity is seen overlying the apex of the tooth. Histopathology revealed the presence of an ameloblastic fibrodentinoma.

129

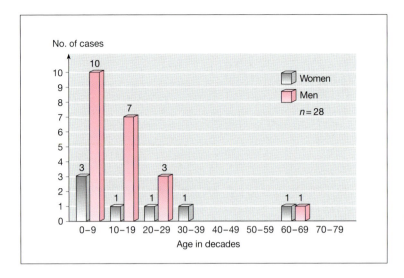

Fig 13-3 Distribution of ameloblastic fibrodentinomas by age and gender.

ported to date, the tumors seem to behave biologically as do ameloblastic fibromas or ameloblastic fibro-odontomas.

Radiologically, the AFD appears as a fairly well-delineated radiolucency with varying degrees of radiopacity, depending on the amount of dentin produced—either osteodentin or the rare tubular type of dentin (Figs 13-1 and 13-2). In cases of AFDs associated with embedded teeth, the tumor and the tooth crown are usually in close contact.

3. Epidemiological data

3.1 Prevalence, incidence, and relative frequency

Due to the rather small number of reported cases of AFDs in the literature, data are not available.

3.2 Age

The age at the time of diagnosis falls within the 1st and 2nd decades; 75% of AFDs (n=28) are diagnosed before the age of 20. Figure 13-3 shows the age distribution of AFDs according to age groups and gender. The mean age of 24 cases was 13.6 years (range, 4 to 63 years).[2]

3.3 Gender

The AFD shows a male predilection, the male:female ratio being 3:1 (n=28).[2-4]

3.4 Location

The majority (71.4%) of AFDs are located in the posterior mandible (n = 29).[2-4] The distribution of AFDs according to location is shown in Fig 13-4. A case of a *peripheral* AFD occurring in the gingiva has been described,[6] but it seems that the majority of cases occur as a central, intraosseous tumor.

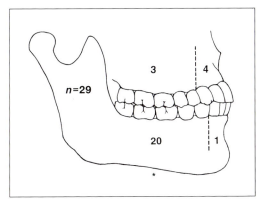

Fig 13-4 Location of AFDs. One case (indicated by an asterisk) involved both the anterior and posterior mandible.

4. Pathogenesis

The AFD is a member of the mixed odontogenic tumor family and, as such, is clearly of odontogenic origin. It has been considered by some to be an intermediate stage between the ameloblastic fibroma and the ameloblastic fibro-odontoma in terms of histologic differentiation (the hamartomatous line described earlier by the present authors). In the 1992 World Health Organization (WHO) classification[7] it was stated that "until more experience has been gained it may be worthwhile to separately identify the differing patterns or types of ameloblastic fibroma and related lesions, even though some of these may later prove to be nothing more than stages in the evolution of a single type tumour."

5. Pathology

5.1 Macroscopy

Macroscopy of ameloblastic fibrodentinomas has not been described in the literature.

5.2 Microscopy

5.2.1 Histologic definitions

The WHO definition[7] of AFD is "a neoplasm similar to ameloblastic fibroma, but also showing inductive changes that lead to formation of dentine."

The definition used by the present authors is as follows:
A hamartomatous lesion similar to the ameloblastic fibroma, but also showing inductive changes that lead to formation of dentinoid.

5.2.2 Histopathologic findings

Histopathologically, the AFD has the same epithelial and ectomesenchymal components as the ameloblastic fibroma. It is composed of strands and islands of odontogenic

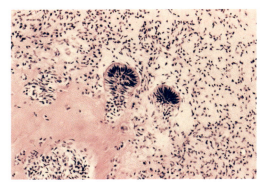

Fig 13-5 Two islands of odontogenic epithelium embedded in cell-rich ectomesenchyme. An area of abortive dentinoid with a number of entrapped ectomesenchymal cells is also observed (hematoxylin-eosin [H&E], ×50).

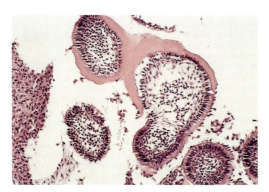

Fig 13-6 Islands of odontogenic epithelium. Two islands show formation of dentinoid at their periphery (H&E, ×70).

epithelium in a cell-rich primitive ectomesenchyme resembling the dental papilla. Dentinoid or osteodentin is deposited, often preceded by a zone of hyalinization. Abortive or poorly mineralized dentin may contain entrapped odontogenic epithelial and ectomesenchymal cells. Active odontoblasts are rare; as a consequence tubular dentin is rarely seen in AFDs. Enamel matrix is not induced by the presence of osteodentin or dentinoid structures (Figs 13-5 and 13-6).

The ameloblastic fibrodentinosarcoma (see chapter 30), a very rare malignant odontogenic neoplasm, is thought to result from malignant transformation of the ectomesenchymal component of the AFD.[8]

5.2.3 Ultrastructural findings

Van Wyk and van der Vyver[9] described ultrastructural features of the AFD, including early formation of dentinoid. The authors observed a spectrum of abortive features at the epithelium-ectomesenchymal interface.

6. Notes on treatment and recurrence rate

The recommended treatment of AFD is surgical excision. Recurrences have not been described.

References

1. Straith FE. Odontoma: A rare type. Dent Dig 1936; 42:196–199.

2. Philipsen HP, Reichart PA, Praetorius F. Mixed odontogenic tumours and odontomas. Considerations on interrelationship. Review of the literature and presentation of 134 new cases of odontomas. Oral Oncol 1997;33:86–99.

3. Ulmansky M, Bodner L, Praetorius F, Lustmann J. Ameloblastic fibrodentinoma: report on two new cases. J Oral Maxillofac Surg 1994;52:980–984.

4. Akal ÜK, Günhan Ö, Güler M. Ameloblastic fibrodentinoma. Report of two cases. Int J Oral Maxillofac Surg 1997;26:455–457.

5. Takeda Y. So-called "immature dentinoma": A case presentation and histological comparison with ameloblastic fibrodentinoma. J Oral Pathol Med 1994;23:92–96.

6. Grodjesk JE, Doblinsky HB, Schneider LC. Ameloblastic fibrodentinoma in the gingiva: Report of case. J Oral Med 1980;35:59–61.

7. Kramer IRH, Pindborg JJ, Shear M. Histological Typing of Odontogenic Tumours. 2d ed. Berlin: Springer-Verlag, 1992.

8. Altini M, Smith I. Ameloblastic dentinosarcoma—a case report. Int J Oral Surg 1976;5:142–147.

9. van Wyk CW, van der Vyver PC. Ameloblastic fibroma with dentinoid formation/immature dentinoma. J Oral Pathol 1983;12:37–46.

Chapter 14

Ameloblastic Fibro-odontoma

1. Terminology

The ameloblastic fibro-odontoma (AFO) has been described using a variety of terms such as *immature ameloblastic odontoma*[1]; however, Hooker[2] described it as an entity under the name *ameloblastic odontoma*. It is a rare odontogenic tumor composed of morphologic features characteristic of ameloblastic fibromas on the one hand and complex odontomas on the other. Ameloblastic fibro-odontomas show relatively uniform clinical and biologic behavior. A literature review of 50 cases of AFOs was published by Slootweg[3] in 1981; Philipsen at al[4] published an updated review with a total number of 86 cases; and in the 1990s an additional 8 cases were reported.[5–11] The ameloblastic fibro-odontoma is a member of the family of mixed odontogenic tumors. The interrelationship between AFOs and associated lesions is covered in the introduction to this section.

2. Clinical and radiologic profile

The AFO is a well-circumscribed, painless, slow-growing, and expanding tumor with no propensity for bony invasion. It tends to produce swelling and has a central location in the jaws. In the majority of cases (83%) the AFO is associated with an unerupted tooth. Frequently the noneruption of the associated tooth has led to the tumor's diagnosis. The size of the tumor varies from lesions that can only be detected microscopically to large calcified masses of several centimeters' diameter.

Radiologically the AFO presents as a uni- or multilocular radiolucency with a well-delineated radiopaque border. The central part of the tumor reveals radiopacity, the density of which resembles that of dental hard tissue as observed in odontomas. The radiopacities may be irregular in shape and density. In some AFOs the radiopacities appear as homogenous, rounded, calcified masses. In cases of association with an unerupted tooth, the AFO is usually located coronally to the crown of the tooth. Resorption of the roots of neighboring teeth has been reported. Occlusal radiographs may reveal the thinning and perforation of the cortical bone and the degree of displacement of associated teeth (Figs 14-1 to 14-3).

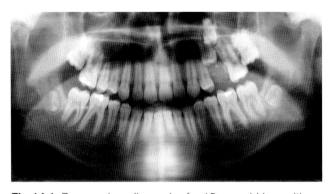

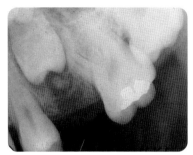

Fig 14-1 Panoramic radiograph of a 15-year-old boy with an AFO in the left maxilla. The second premolar and the first molar are retained, the latter being located high up in the maxillary sinus. A radiolucent area with a central radiopacity is seen coronal to the second retained premolar.

Fig 14-2 Periapical radiograph of the area of the maxillary left second premolar shown in Fig 14-1. Within a small radiolucent area overlying the crown of the second premolar, an irregular calcified mass is evident. The AFO inhibited the permanent tooth from erupting.

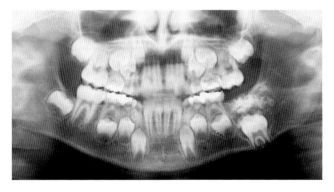

Fig 14-3 Panoramic radiograph showing a large, irregular, calcified mass overlying the impacted mandibular left first molar. Histologically, this lesion was diagnosed as an AFO.

3. Epidemiological data

3.1 Prevalence, incidence, and relative frequency

Figures indicating the relative frequency of AFOs vary between 0.3% and 3.7%.[12] This rate rises to 7% if patients under the age of 16 are considered separately.

3.2 Age

The first two decades are characteristic for the occurrence of AFOs (Fig 14-4), with 98.9% of cases (n=94) occurring before the age of 20. The mean age of 86 cases was 9.0 years (range, 1 to 22 years).[4] As such the AFO is a tumor of childhood and adolescence.

3.3 Gender

A review of 94 cases (see Fig14-4) has revealed a male:female ratio of 1.4:1.

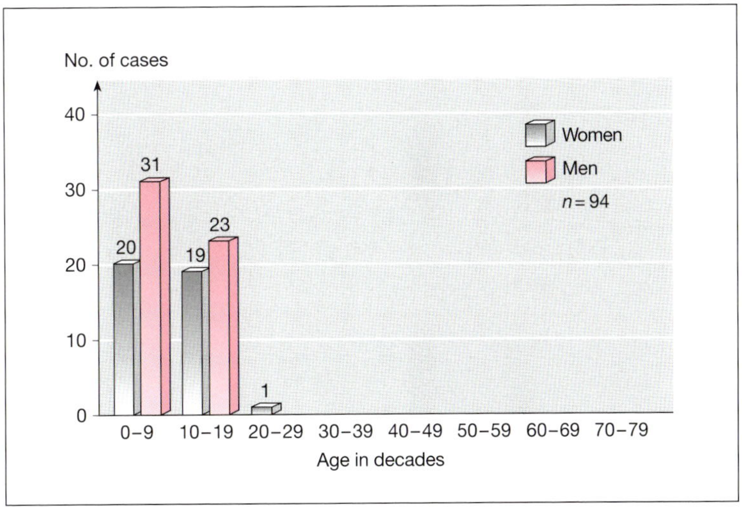

No. of cases

Fig 14-4 Distribution of 94 cases of AFO by age and gender. Note that only one patient was older than 20.

3.4 Location

About half (53.2%) of AFOs are found in the posterior mandible (Fig 14-5). The posterior mandible is affected 2.4 times more often than the entire maxilla. The AFO seems to occur exclusively as a central intraosseous tumor.

The occurrence of multiple AFOs in a father, his two sons, and a daughter was reported by Schmidtseder and Hausamen.[13] In addition to multiple AFOs, esophageal stenosis, hepatopathy, dyspepsia, and increased susceptibility to infection were observed. A dominant autosomal inherited disorder was suspected.

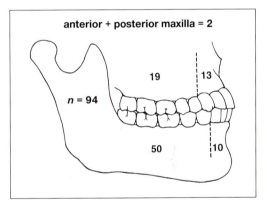

Fig 14-5 Location of 94 cases of AFO. The majority of tumors appeared in the posterior mandible.[4]

4. Pathogenesis

The AFO is another member of the mixed odontogenic tumor family, making it of odontogenic origin. Compared to the ameloblastic fibroma and the ameloblastic fibrodentinoma, the inductive changes in the AFO are more advanced and enamel is present in addition to dentin.

5. Pathology

5.1 Macroscopy

Macroscopically, the AFO appears as a circumscribed solid mass of varying size with a smooth surface. The cut surface of the soft part of the tumor may appear pinkish white

135

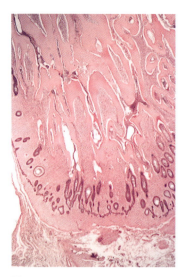

Fig 14-6 Photomicrographic overview of a complex odontoma. Note the surrounding connective tissue capsule (hematoxylin-eosin [H&E], ×30).

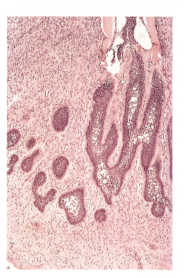

Fig 14-7 Peripheral zone of the lesion shown in Fig 14-6. This isolated area resembles an ameloblastic fibroma (H&E, ×90).

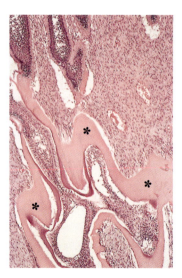

Fig 14-8 Intermediate zone characterized by the production of dentin (∗) and a few narrow areas of enamel matrix (H&E, ×90).

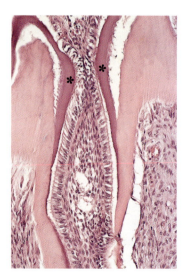

Fig 14-9 Area close to the tumor center exhibiting production of dentin. The enamel matrix (∗) is produced by pre-ameloblast-like cells (H&E, ×220).

and gelatinous. The calcified masses are a yellowish white color.

5.2 Microscopy

5.2.1 Histologic definitions

The World Health Organization (WHO)[14] defined the AFO as "a lesion similar to ameloblastic fibroma, but also showing inductive changes that lead to the formation of dentine and enamel."

The definition used by the present authors is as follows:

A hamartomatous lesion similar to the ameloblastic fibroma and fibrodentinoma, but showing further inductive changes that lead to the formation of enamel matrix in addition to dentin (dentinoid).

5.2.2 Histopathologic findings

The tissue masses of an AFO show the characteristic structure of an immature complex odontoma consisting of irregularly arranged enamel, dentinoid, cementum, and pulplike ectomesenchymal tissue (Fig 14-6). At the tumor periphery, next to the fibrous capsule, there is a zone of strands and islands of odontogenic epithelium embedded in typical cell-rich ectomesenchyme (Fig 14-7). Dentin production takes place toward the center of the lesion (Fig 14-8). The dentin may vary structurally from dentinoid to tubular dentin, as shown in Fig 14-9. Approaching the tumor center, enamel matrix is laid down by the odontogenic epithelium and may appear columnar or pre-ameloblast-like (Fig 14-9). The amount of ectomesenchyme gradually decreases as the hard tissue mass dominates the central part of the lesion. The finding of extensive pigmentation in a case of AFO in a 9-year-old Japanese girl was described by Kitano et al.[11] The authors observed an abundant deposition of melanin widely distributed in nests of odontogenic epithelium; there were also aggregations of large, rounded melanophages with large amounts of melanin similar to nevus cells in areas of the ectomesenchymal component.

5.2.3 Histochemical/immunohistochemical findings

Miyauchi et al[6] studied AFOs by immunohistochemistry using antibodies against a number of cytokeratins. Findings revealed that epithelial components showed expression of cytokeratins 8, 13, 16, 14, 18, and 19. In addition, a coexpression of these cytokeratins and vimentin were found. Sekine et al[7] studied the cell kinetics of AFOs by bromodeoxyuridine (BrdU) and proliferating cell nuclear antigen (PCNA). The results of the investigation suggested that the ectomesenchymal component was more proliferative than the epithelial component.

5.2.4 Ultrastructural findings

Using electron microscopy,[15] the epithelial cells reveal large indented nuclei with chromatin condensation in the periphery. Bundles of tonofilaments are occasionally seen in the cytoplasm. Rough endoplasmic reticulum is sparse and Golgi complexes are poorly developed. The intercellular spaces are large, showing microvilli-like projections extending into the lumina (Figs 14-10 and 14-11). A basal lamina of the epithelial cells is seen at the epithelium-ectomesenchymal interface. Adjacent to the basal lamina a rim of fine, aperiodic filaments indicating initial predentin formation may be evident. In some areas these filaments may show continuity between intracellular and extracellular filaments, suggesting a probable epithelial origin. Collagen fibers are rarely observed in this zone. Generally, the ameloblastic component is similar to that of the developing odontogenic tissue except that the ectomesenchymal cells have not developed into

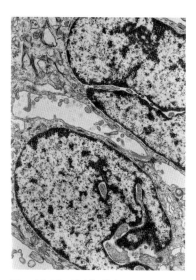

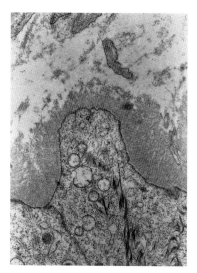

Fig 14-10 Epithelial tumor cells of an AFO revealing indented nuclei and peripheral condensation of chromatin. In the intercellular spaces microvilli-like extensions are seen projecting into the lumen. A few perinuclear tonofilaments are observed in the cytoplasm (transmission electron microscopy [TEM], ×3,500).

Fig 14-11 The epithelium-ectomesenchymal interface showing a band of aperiodic filaments adjacent to the basal lamina representing early dentinoid. Bundles of tonofilaments are noted in the cytoplasm of the epithelial tumor cells (TEM, ×10,000).

columnar odontoblasts. This finding may explain why osteodentin/dentinoid material is produced instead of tubular dentin.

6. Notes on treatment and recurrence rate

Conservative surgical enucleation is the treatment of choice for AFOs, and recurrences have not been reported. In large lesions, the removal of an associated unerupted tooth cannot always be avoided. In small lesions with minimal production of dental hard tissue, however, the associated tooth may be left in situ. The prognosis for eruption of these teeth has proved good.

References

1. Slootweg PJ, Rademakers LHPM. Immature complex odontoma: A light and electron microscopic study with reference to eosinophilic material and epithelio-mesenchymal interaction. J Oral Pathol 1983;12:103–116.

2. Hooker SP. Ameloblastic odontoma: an analysis of twenty-six cases. Oral Surg Oral Med Oral Pathol 1967;24:375–376.

3. Slootweg PJ. An analysis of the interrelationship of the mixed odontogenic tumors-ameloblastic fibroma, ameloblastic fibro-odontoma, and the odontomas. Oral Surg Oral Med Oral Pathol 1981; 51:266–276.

4. Philipsen HP, Reichart PA, Prætorius F. Mixed odontogenic tumours and odontomas. Considerations on interrelationship. Review of the literature and presentation of 134 new cases of odontomas. Oral Oncol 1997;33:86–99.

5. Baker WR, Swift JQ. Ameloblastic fibro-odontoma of the anterior maxilla—report of a case. Oral Surg Oral Med Oral Pathol 1993;76:294–297.

6. Miyauchi M, Takata T, Ogawa I, et al. Immuno-histochemical observations on a possible ameloblastic fibro-odontoma. J Oral Pathol Med 1996; 25:93–96.

7. Sekine J, Kitamura A, Ueno K, et al. Cell kinetics in mandibular ameloblastic fibro-odontoma evaluated by bromodeoxyuridine and proliferating cell nuclear antigen immunohistochemistry: Case report. Br J Oral Maxillofac Surg 1996;34:450–453.

8. Favia GF, Di Alberti L, Scarano A, Piatelli A. Ameloblastic fibro-odontoma: Report of two cases. Oral Oncol 1997;33:444–446.

9. Siegert J, Friedrich RE, Donath K, Schmelzle R. Das ameloblastische Fibroodontom. Dtsch Zahn-ärztl Z 1999; Suppl I S. 24.

10. Ozer E, Pabuccuoglu U, Gunbay U, et al. Ameloblastic fibro-odontoma of the maxilla: Case report. J Clin Pediatr Dent 1997;21:329–331.

11. Kitano M, Tsuda-Yamada S, Semba I, et al. Pigmented ameloblastic fibro-odontoma with melanophages. Oral Surg Oral Med Oral Pathol 1994; 77:271–275.

12. Lu Y, Xuan M, Takata T, et al. Odontogenic tumors. A demographic study of 759 cases in a Chinese population. Oral Surg Oral Med Oral Pathol Oral Radiol Endod 1998;86:707–714.

13. Schmidtseder R, Hausamen JE. Multiple odontogenic tumors and other anomalies. Oral Surg Oral Med Oral Pathol 1975;39:249–258.

14. Kramer IRH, Pindborg JJ, Shear M. Histologic Typing of Odontogenic Tumours. 2d ed. Berlin: Springer-Verlag, 1992.

15. Reich R, Reichart PA, Ostertag H. Ameloblastic fibro-odontome. Report of a case, with ultrastructural study. J Maxillofac Surg 1984;12:230–234.

Chapter 15

Complex Odontoma

1. Terminology

The term *odontoma* has been used as a descriptor for any tumor of odontogenic origin. However, odontomas have become known as mixed odontogenic tumors because they are composed of both epithelial and ectomesenchymal components. Both the epithelial and the ectomesenchymal tissues and their respective cells may appear normal morphologically, but they seem to have a deficit in structural arrangement. This defect has led to the opinion that odontomas are hamartomatous lesions or malformations rather than true neoplasms.

Two types of odontomas have been identified: the complex and the compound odontoma. The distinction between these two types is somewhat arbitrary, because it is based on either the appearance of well-organized toothlike structures (compound odontomas) or on a mass of disorganized odontogenic tissues (complex odontomas).

Philipsen et al[1] reviewed both types of odontomas and eight reviews, including a total of 1,040 cases, between 1976 and 1989. Due to inaccuracies in treatment data, lack of information, and presentation of pooled data, a number of published reviews were excluded; 225 cases of odontomas could be evaluated from the remaining reviews. Individual data for another 282 cases were also available. The pooled data of the reviews and the individual data are referred to in this chapter and chapter 16 as the *odontoma survey*.

In recent years several reports on larger series of odontomas have been published. MacDonald-Jankowski[2] reported on 40 cases of odontomas in a Chinese population. In 1997 Owens et al[3] published a retrospective study of 104 cases of "dental odontomas," and in 2000 Garcia-Consuegra et al[4] described data from 46 cases of odontomas in Spanish patients. A number of single case reports also have been published.[5,6] A large erupting complex odontoma,[7] peripheral odontomas,[8,9] a compound odontoma associated with a primary molar,[10] and a cystic compound odontoma[11] have all been described. Hirshberg et al[12] reported a case of an odontoma associated with a calcifying odontogenic cyst, drawing attention to this interesting association of which they reviewed 52 cases and suggested the term *odontocalcifying odontogenic cyst* (for further details, see chapter 17). The association of odontomas with Gardner's syndrome also is of diagnostic importance.[13]

2. Clinical and radiologic profile

Complex odontomas are slow-growing, expanding, and (in most cases) painless lesions. Pain and inflammation associated with

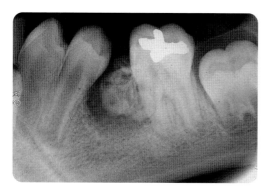

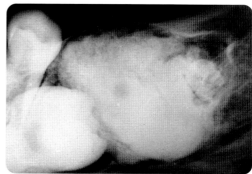

Fig 15-1 Dental radiograph showing a complex odontoma between the left mandibular second premolar and first molar. There is a radiolucent area within a radiopacity of different densities.

Fig 15-2 Periapical radiograph of a large mandibular complex odontoma. Displacement of a mandibular molar has occurred. Some complex odontomas may have a peripheral location, and are often known as erupting odontoma.

odontomas was reported in only 4% of Spanish patients.[4]

Complex odontomas are often detected on routine radiographs or diagnosed through failed eruption of a permanent tooth. The size of complex odontomas may vary from 3 to 4 cm to those that are only detectable microscopically. In a series of 46 cases of odontomas (complex and compound) from Spain,[4] the average size was 15.4 mm (range, 7 to 30 mm).

The radiologic appearance of complex odontomas depends on their developmental stage. Three stages exist based on the degree of mineralization. The first stage is characterized by radiolucency due to lack of calcification (*weiches Odontom* = soft odontoma). Partial calcification is observed in the intermediate stage, while in the third and final stage the lesion usually appears radiopaque with amorphous masses of dental hard tissue surrounded by a thin radiolucent zone (Figs 15-1 and 15-2). Resorption of neighboring teeth is rare. Unerupted teeth are associated with 10% to 44.4% of complex odontomas.[1] Patients with odontomas who experienced delayed eruption of at least

one permanent tooth totaled 74%, and in 42% of these patients, canines were involved.[4]

3. Epidemiological data

3.1 Prevalence, incidence, and relative frequency

Relative frequency of complex odontomas varies between 5% and 30%.[1] This makes the complex odontoma one of the most common odontogenic lesions, superceded in frequency only by the compound odontoma.

3.2 Age

Based on 137 cases from the odontoma survey[1] the mean age at the time of diagnosis was 19.9 years (range, 2 to 74 years). Figure 15-3 shows the age and gender distribution

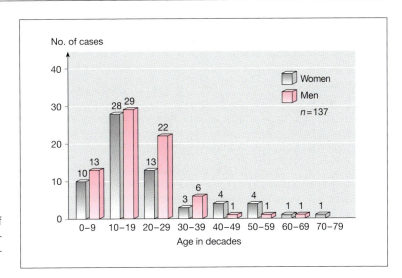

Fig 15-3 Distribution of complex odontomas according to age and gender.

at the time of diagnosis for complex odontomas in the survey; 83.9% of cases occurred before the age of 30 with a peak in the 2nd decade of life.

3.3 Gender

The male:female ratio varies from 1.5:1 to 1.6:1 to 0.8:1, according to different studies.[1] The Spanish study[4] of 46 odontomas reported a male:female ratio of 1:1.6,[4] which differs from most other reports.

3.4 Location

Although some differences exist in the literature, most authors agree that the majority of complex odontomas are located in the posterior mandible; the second most common site is the anterior maxilla.[1] Figure 15-4 shows the distribution of sites of different series of complex odontomas.[1]

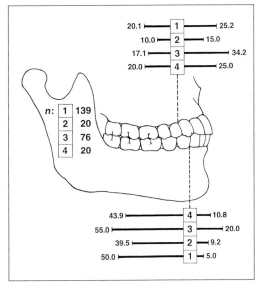

Fig 15-4 Location of complex odontomas according to the odontoma survey by Philipsen et al,[1] which evaluated four main reviews (numbers in boxes) on complex odontomas, compare with Fig 16-4.

143

4. Pathogenesis

The odontogenic origin of the complex odontoma has never been questioned. It is considered a self-limiting developmental anomaly or hamartomatous malformation characterized by nondescript masses of dental tissues. Recently, it has been suggested that odontomas tend to increase in size with the age of the patient, suggesting continuous growth.[2] This view, however, is not held by the majority of authors in this field.

The etiology of complex odontomas is unknown. Several theories have been proposed, including local trauma, infection, family history, and genetic mutation. It has also been suggested that odontomas are inherited from a mutant gene or interference, possibly postnatally with the genetic control of tooth development.[3]

Several factors may cause anomalous tissue development in odontomas. These include unsuccessful or an altered ectomesenchymal interaction in the earliest phase of dental germ development and/or alterations in the subsequent phases of the development of these tissues. It has also been assumed that alterations in the mineralization mechanisms with modifications of the mineral component in the enamel may lead to incomplete maturation.[14]

5. Pathology

5.1 Macroscopy

Cut sections of large lesions will reveal the calcified masses as a white to yellowish hard surface surrounded by a capsule of collagenous tissue.

5.2 Microscopy

5.2.1 Histologic definitions

The World Health Organization[15] (WHO) defined a complex odontoma as "a malformation in which all the dental tissues are represented, individual tissues being mainly well formed but occurring in a more or less disorderly pattern."

The definition used by the present authors is as follows:
A hamartomatous lesion in which all the dental tissues are represented, individual hard tissues being mainly well developed but occurring in a more or less disorderly pattern.

5.2.2 Histopathologic findings

Histopathologically, the complex odontoma consists primarily of a disordered mixture of dental tissues, often of spherical shape. Occasionally, the calcified masses may include tooth-like structures as in compound odontomas, indicating that the degree of morphodifferentiation varies greatly. Cementum or cementum-like structures often admixed with the dentinoid substance, small spaces with pulp tissue, enamel matrix, and epithelial remnants may be observed within the calcified/mineralized masses of dentin of different qualities. Empty spaces and clefts caused by the process of decalcification, during which mature enamel is lost, are evident. At the periphery of the lesion, islands of pulp tissue and nests and strands of odontogenic epithelium may be found (Figs 15-5 and 15-6). The enamel present in different types of odontomas is never completely mature but shows numerous mineralization and structural anomalies.

A thin, fibrous capsule and occasionally a cyst wall are seen surrounding the lesion. In 16% of complex odontomas, areas of ghost cells have been identified.[1] Some of these may present with melanin pigmentation.

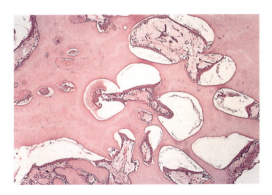

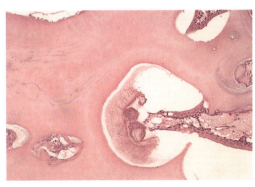

Fig 15-5 A complex odontoma showing irregularly formed dental hard structures with pulp tissue (hematoxylin-eosin [H&E], ×25).

Fig 15-6 Higher magnification of the complex odontoma shown in Fig 15-5. Enamel matrix and odontogenic epithelium are evident (H&E, ×60).

Histologic features of the complex odontoma largely depend on the developmental stage of the lesion, as do its radiologic characteristics. Therefore, it may be difficult to distinguish odontomas in the very early stages of development from ameloblastic fibromas and ameloblastic fibro-odontomas. Even after growth and mineralization have been completed, residues of the odontogenic epithelium may still be identified.

The interrelationship between the different types of odontomas and other mixed odontogenic tumors is discussed in the introduction to this section.

5.2.3 Histochemical/immunohistochemical findings

Small numbers of odontomas, including some complex odontomas, have been studied immunohistochemically. Mori et al[16] studied the expression of tenascin in a variety of odontogenic tumors. In five cases of odontomas there was a widespread stromal immunoreactivity which was, however, negative in the calcified masses. The most marked immunoreactivity was seen in the pulplike tissue adjacent to the odontoblast layer and dentinoid structures. The authors concluded that expression of tenascin in the stromal tissue of odontogenic tumors differs according to the potential of the tumor cells forming calcified structures, irrespective of the tumor cell morphology.

Papagerakis et al[17] studied late phenotypic markers of ameloblasts and odontoblasts, in particular proteins involved in biomineralization (amelogenins, keratins, collagen types III and IV, vimentin, fibronectin, osteonectin, and osteocalcin). The pattern of protein expression showed some similarities between the ameloblasts and odontoblasts in normally developing teeth and cells present in tissues of complex odontomas. The study confirmed that the differentiation of normal and tumor odontogenic cells is accompanied by the expression of some common molecules. A plausible explanation for the results (which also relates to other odontogenic tumors) could be that the odontogenic tumor epithelial cells are recapitulating genetic programs expressed during normal odontogenesis, but the tumor cells demonstrate abnormal expression patterns for these genes.

5.2.4 Ultrastructural findings

Marchetti et al[14] studied complex odontomas by scanning electron microscopy (SEM) and transmission electron microscopy (TEM). The study was performed because odontomas provide an alternative model for observing the formation of dental tissue at different stages of maturation simultaneously. Given the TEM findings, the theory that an ectomesenchymal induction failure occurs in odontomas was not confirmed. The defect seen at the beginning of the differentiated and anomalous tissue maturation may be related to later developmental events in the enamel organ.

6. Notes on treatment and recurrence rate

Conservative enucleation is recommended as the treatment of choice for complex odontomas. Special surgical considerations were described for cases of large mandibular odontomas by Blinder et al.[18] The authors suggested excision by an intraoral, lingual approach. As odontomas are often associated with unerupted, impacted teeth, the possibility of eruption after surgical removal of the odontoma should be considered. In cases without involvement of an impacted tooth, immediate surgical intervention is not always necessary considering the limited growth potential of such lesions.

Recurrences have not been reported. Although the complex odontoma seems to be self-limiting, the lesion may recur if it is incompletely removed at its early, predominantly soft tissue stage.[15]

References

1. Philipsen HP, Reichart PA, Praetorius F. Mixed odontogenic tumours and odontomas. Considerations on interrelationship. Review of the literature and presentation of 134 new cases of odontomas. Oral Oncol 1997;33:86–99.

2. MacDonald-Jankowski DS. Odontomas in a Chinese population. Dentomaxillofac Radiol 1996; 25:186–192.

3. Owens BM, Schumann NJ, Mincer HH, et al. Dental odontomas: A retrospective study of 104 cases. J Clin Pediatr Dent 1997;21:261–264.

4. Garcia-Consuegra L, Junquera LM, Albertos JM, Rodriguez O. Odontomas. A clinical-histological and retrospective epidemiological study of 46 cases. Med Oral 2000;5:367–372.

5. Owens BM, Schuman NJ, Pliske TA, Culley WL. Compound composite odontoma associated with an impacted cuspid. J Clin Pediatr Dent 1995;19:293–295.

6. Piatelli A, Perfetti G, Carraro A. Complex odontoma as a periapical and interradicular radiopacity in a primary molar. J Endod 1996;22:561–563.

7. Ragalli CC, Ferreria JL, Blasco F. Large erupting complex odontoma. Int J Oral Maxillofac Surg 2000;29:373–374.

8. Ledesma-Montes C, Perez-Bache A, Garcés-Ortíz M. Gingival compound odontoma. J Oral Maxillofac Surg 1996;25:296–297.

9. Castro GW, Houston G, Weyrauch C. Peripheral odontoma: Report of case and review of literature. J Dent Child 1994;61:209–213.

10. Piatelli M, Paolantonio M. Compound odontoma associated with a primary molar. Acta Stomatol Belg 1995;3:129–130.

11. Piatelli A, Trisi P, Romasco N. Cystic compound odontoma in an unusual pericoronal posterior location. Acta Stomatol Belg 1993;90:259–260.

12. Hirshberg A, Buchner A. Calcifying odontogenic cysts associated with odontoma: A possible separate entity (Odontocalcifying odontogenic cyst). J Oral Maxillofac Surg 1994;42:555–558.

13. Takeuchi T, Takenoshita Y, Kubo K, Iida M. Natural course of jaw lesions in patients with familial adenomatosis coli (Gardner´s syndrome). Int J Oral Maxillofac Surg 1993;22:226–230.

14. Marchetti C, Piacentini C, Menghini P, Reguzzoni M. Observations on the enamel of odontomas. Scanning Microsc1993;7:999–1007.

15. Kramer IRH, Pindborg JJ, Shear M. The Histological Typing of Odontogenic Tumours. 2d ed. Berlin: Springer-Verlag, 1992.

16. Mori M, Yamada T, Doi T, Ohmura H, Takai Y, Shrestha P. Expression of Tenascin in odontogenic tumours. Eur J Cancer B Oral Oncol 1995;31B:275– 279.

17. Papagerakis P, Peuchmaur M, Hotton D, et al. Aberrant gene expression in epithelial cells of mixed odontogenic tumors. J Dent Res 1999; 78:20–30.

18. Blinder D, Peleg M, Taicher S. Surgical considerations in cases of large mandibular angle. Int J Oral Maxillofac Surg 1993;22:163–165.

Chapter 16

Compound Odontoma

1. Terminology

The aspects of terminology for odontomas were extensively presented in Chapter 15. Information about the compound odontoma is based on the odontoma survey prepared by Philipsen et al.[1]

2. Clinical and radiologic profile

Compound odontomas are painless, benign lesions with a more limited growth potential than complex odontomas. In fact, the growth potential ends with the tooth-forming period. Since there are few clinical symptoms associated with compound odontomas, a frequent cause of discovery is the failure of a permanent tooth to erupt and/or the persistence of a deciduous tooth. The lesion is also often discovered incidentally on panoramic radiographs. Commonly, the compound odontoma is located between the apex of a root of a primary tooth and the crown of a permanent tooth, preventing the latter from erupting. The size of the lesion varies as does the number of denticles. Cases of multiple compound odontomas have been described,[2,3] prompting Mani[3] to propose the term *odontoma syndrome* for this phenome-

non. Occasionally, compound odontomas may be seen in Gardner's syndrome.[4] A case of six compound odontomas occurring in three male members of a family of seven was reported.[5] *Peripheral* compound odontomas are rare, arising extraosseously and having a tendency to exfoliate.

Radiologically, compound odontomas are characterized by a radiopaque mass of varying size which is composed of a number of toothlike structures in a disorderly pattern. The denticles are miniaturized and malformed. Persistence of one or several deciduous teeth is observed together with impaction of one or several permanent teeth. Noneruption of the normal dentition or supernumerary teeth is associated with compound odontomas in 40%[6] to 56%[7] of reported cases. The lesion is usually surrounded by a narrow, radiolucent rim corresponding to a fibrous capsule (Figs 16-1 and 16-2). The radiographic appearance is so characteristic that the diagnosis is often made solely from radiographs and macroscopic findings.

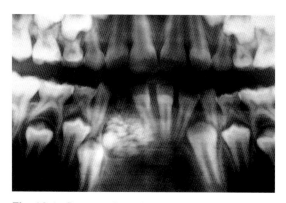

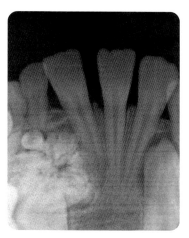

Fig 16-1 Panoramic radiograph showing a compound odontoma in the right anterior mandible. The mandibular right lateral incisor is missing and the decidous incisor persists. The mandibular right canine appears to be retained when compared with the canine on the left side.

Fig 16-2 Periapical radiograph of the region of the compound odontoma shown in Fig 16-1. The permanent right central incisor is displaced. The compound odontoma is composed of a number of denticles arranged in a disorderly pattern.

3. Epidemiological data

3.1 Prevalence, incidence, and relative frequency

The compound odontoma is the most common lesion/malformation of odontogenic origin. Its relative frequency varies between 4.2% and 73.8%.[8] Sato et al[9] recorded odontomas in 47% of their Japanese patients with benign odontogenic tumors (n=90).

3.2 Age

Based on the data of the odontoma survey by Philipsen et al[1] the mean age at the time of diagnosis was 17.2 years. Figure 16-3 shows the distribution of compound odontomas according to age and gender; 74.3% of cases were diagnosed before the age of 20 years, with a marked peak in the 2nd decade of life. The compound odontoma is clearly a lesion of childhood and adolescence.

3.3 Gender

The male:female ratio varies between 1.2:1 and 1:1, according to the odontoma survey of Philipsen et al.[1]

3.4 Location

Figure 16-4 shows the distribution of compound odontomas according to location. According to all except one of the reviews evaluated, the important finding was that the anterior maxilla is the most frequent location

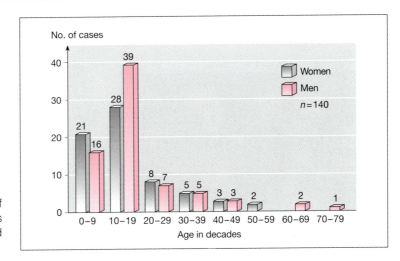

Fig 16-3 Distribution of compound odontomas according to age and gender.

for compound odontomas. When comparing compound with complex odontomas (see chapter 15), compound odontomas are more frequent in the anterior maxilla, whereas complex odontomas seem to have a predilection for the posterior mandible.[1]

4. Pathogenesis

As with the complex odontoma, the compound odontoma is of odontogenic origin. The theory that the compound odontoma develops from an ameloblastic fibroma if the latter is left untreated is questionable but still a matter of debate. The interrelationship between the different members of the mixed odontogenic tumors family are discussed in the introduction to this section.

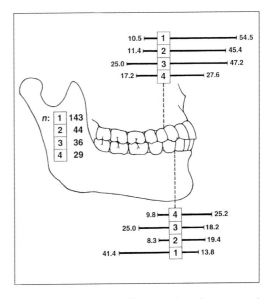

Fig 16-4 Distribution of the location of compound odontomas according to the survey prepared by Philipsen et al.[1] The numbers 1 to 4 (in square boxes) refer to four literature reviews that were used in the survey.

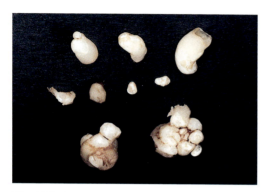

Fig 16-5 Macroscopic aspect of denticles that have been surgically removed.

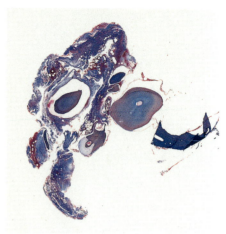

Fig 16-6 Part of a compound odontoma revealing cross sections of some of the denticles embedded in a fibrous stroma (Mallory stain, ×2.5).

5. Pathology

5.1 Macroscopy

Macroscopically, the compound odontoma is easily distinguished due to the often large numbers of toothlike structures which are removed during surgery (Fig. 16-5). The lesion is usually encapsulated.

5.2 Microscopy

5.2.1 Histologic definition

Both the World Health Organization (WHO)[10] and the present authors define the compound odontoma as follows:
A malformation in which all the dental tissues are represented in a more orderly pattern than in the complex odontoma, so that the lesion consists of many toothlike structures. Most of these structures do not morphologically resemble the teeth of the normal dentition, but in each one enamel, dentin, cementum, and pulp are arranged as in the normal tooth.

5.2.2 Histopathologic findings

Due to a higher degree of morphodifferentiation than that of the complex odontoma, compound odontomas are easily recognizable even macroscopically. Compound odontomas are usually small, but large lesions containing up to 100 denticles have been reported. Denticles are composed of enamel, dentin, cementum, and pulp tissue with a more or less regular arrangement. Morphodifferentiation and histodifferentiation of the dental hard tissues in compound odontomas have been studied in detail by Piatelli and Trisi.[11] Three percent of odontomas may contain *ghost* cells.[12]

5.2.3 Histochemical/immunohistochemical findings

Along with other odontogenic tumors, Gao et al[13] studied compound odontomas using immunohistochemistry. The aim of their study was to describe the expression and distribution of bone morphogenetic proteins (BMPs) in odontogenic tumors. BMPs, members of the transforming growth factor–beta (TGF-β) superfamily, play a role not only in bone formation, but also in epitheliomesenchymal interactions. The authors found that tumors and lesions of epithelial and/or ectomesenchymal origin, including the compound odontoma, demonstrated positive reactions while epithelial odontogenic tumors were negative. The authors concluded that BMPs may play a role in the formation of calcified tissues and the development of odontogenic tumors containing such tissues.

5.2.4 Ultrastructural findings

Not surprisingly, relatively few studies on the ultrastructure of compound odontomas have been performed. Abati et al[14] described scanning electron microscopic findings in the case of a compound odontoma.

6. Notes on treatment and recurrence rate

The treatment of compound odontomas is conservative enucleation of the lesion. Care must be taken that all denticles are removed because some may easily be overlooked. A postoperative radiograph is indicated. Unerupted neighboring teeth may be saved in those cases where the prognosis for tooth eruption is good.

References

1. Philipsen HP, Reichart PA, Prætorius F. Mixed odontogenic tumours and odontomas. Considerations on interrelationship. Review of the literature and presentation of 134 new cases of odontomas. Oral Oncol 1997;33:86–99.

2. Kaugars GE, Miller AS, Peezick B. Odontomas. Oral Surg Oral Med Oral Pathol 1989;67:172–176.

3. Mani NJ. Odontoma syndrome. Report of an unusual case with multiple multiform odontomas of both jaws. J Dent 1974;2:149–152.

4. Antoniades K, Elftheriades I, Karakasis D. The Gardner syndrome. Int J Oral Maxillofac Surg 1987;16:480–483.

5. Etnier SH, Fast TB. Complex composite odontoma. J Indianap Dist Dent Soc 1969;23:22–23.

6. Bodin I, Julin P, Thomsson M. Odontomas and their pathological sequels. Dentomaxillofac Radiol 1983;12:109–114.

7. Morning P. Impacted teeth in relation to odontomas. Int J Oral Surg 1980;9:81–91.

8. Lu Y, Xuan M, Takata T, et al. Odontogenic tumors. A demographic study of 759 cases in a Chinese population. Oral Surg Oral Med Oral Pathol Oral Radiol Endod 1998;86:707–714.

9. Sato M, Tanaka N, Sato T, Amagasa T. Oral and maxillofacial tumours in children: a review. Br J Oral Maxillofac 1997;35:92–95.

10. Kramer IRH, Pindborg JJ, Shear M. Histological Typing of Odontogenic Tumours. 2d ed. Geneva: Springer-Verlag, 1992.

11. Piatelli A, Trisi P. Morphodifferentiation and histodifferentiation of the dental hard tissues in compound odontoma: a study of undemineralized material. J Oral Pathol Med 1992;21:340–342.

12. Sedano H, Pindborg JJ. Ghost cell epithelium in odontomas. J Oral Pathol 1975;4:27–30.

13. Gao YH, Yang LJ, Yamaguchi A. Immunohistochemical demonstration of bone morphogenetic protein in odontogenic tumors. J Oral Pathol Med 1997;26:273–277.

14. Abati S, Grattini G, Carrassi A. SEM morphostructural findings in a case of compound odontoma. Dent Cadmos 1988;56:50–55.

Chapter 17

Calcifying Ghost Cell Odontogenic Cysts/Tumors (Odontogenic Ghost Cell Lesions)

1. Terminology

Ever since Gorlin et al[1,2] first identified the calcifying odontogenic cyst (COC) as a specific odontogenic lesion, controversy and confusion have existed regarding the relationship between non-neoplastic, cystic lesions and solid tumor masses that share the cellular and histomorphologic features described by the authors. No special recognition was given to solid lesions but the authors did state that the one lesion among the 15 reported cases that recurred was "a solid tumor-like mass." They also wrote, "These masses may be extensive, largely filling the cystic cavity."

The 1971 World Health Organization (WHO) classification[3] described the COC as a "non-neoplastic cystic lesion." In the 1992 edition[4] the authors replaced this phrase with "most lesions appear to be non-neoplastic." The present authors believe that the lesion has been wrongly classified as a group 1.1.2 lesion, because the stroma is not characterized by ectomesenchyme but rather by mature, collagenous connective tissue. The nature of the dentinoid material produced in COCs has not been fully clarified, but the production of this material is probably not the result of true induction (through a sequence of reciprocal epithelio-ectomesenchymal interactions) but rather as a result of a metaplastic process.

Although the COC was recognized as a distinct pathologic entity at first,[1,2] the lesion has later shown to be of extreme diversity in its clinical and histopathologic features, as well as in its biologic behavior. Because of this diversity, there has been disagreement concerning the terminology used over the past 40 years as the following list of terms clearly reveals: calcifying odontogenic cyst, Gorlin cyst, keratinizing and calcifying odontogenic cyst, atypical ameloblastoma, calcifying ghost cell odontogenic tumor, cystic calcifying odontogenic tumor, dentinogenic ghost cell tumor, calcifying odontogenic lesion, epithelial odontogenic ghost cell tumor, odontogenic ghost cell tumor, and ghost cell cyst.

Not only has confusion plagued the terminology used for this complex lesion, but a significant source of disagreement stems from the fact that there appear to be two different concepts or schools of thought when looking at the nature of COC: the monistic and the dualistic concept. Toida[5] made a comprehensive review of the attempts at classifications presented during the last 25 years and added a new dualistic classification scheme.

Although the 1992 WHO classification[4] cited the terms *dentinogenic ghost cell tumor* (DGCT, suggested by Praetorius et al[6]) and *odontogenic ghost cell tumor* (OGCT, suggested by Colmenero et al[7]), especially for the solid lesion whose neoplastic nature is apparent, the authors[4] continue to use the term *calcifying odontogenic cyst,* although this nomenclature may not be appropriate to represent a neoplastic lesion. However, if all COCs are neoplastic in nature, the term originally proposed as a substitute for COC by Fejerskov and Krogh[8]—*calcifying ghost cell odontogenic tumor* (CGCOT)—would be preferable. The cystic (non-neoplastic) and the solid (neoplastic) variants may then be called cystic CGCOT and solid CGCOT, respectively. Recent investigations[9,10] and current thinking strongly support the dualistic concept, and should this prove true, the WHO classification will have to undergo thorough revision when this lesion is reevaluated in a revised classification.

The three classifications of COC previously proposed[6,9,10] are all commonly based on the dualistic concept. However, Toida[5] raised the point that in these classifications the authors seem to have used the term *cystic* as a synonym for *non-neoplastic. Cystic* is basically a morphologic term that does not necessarily cover the term *non-neoplastic,* which is a biologic one. In other words, there may well be neoplastic lesions with a cystic histoarchitecture. To eliminate the confusion arising from the previous classifications and terminologies, Toida[5] proposed a new, simple, and basic classification based on the dualistic concept. He divided the group of COC lesions into three main groups: (*1*) the calcifying ghost cell odontogenic cyst, which should be classified with developmental odontogenic cysts; (*2*) the neoplasms, which comprise a benign and a malignant variant; and (*3*) lesions described under the first two groups and associated with odontomas, ameloblastomas, and other odontogenic lesions.

Combining these four classification attempts,[5,6,9,10] each of which contain acceptable single components, into one comprehensive and manageable classification results in the outcome shown in Table 17-1.

The suggested classification is mainly based on the proliferative activity and growth pattern of the lining cyst epithelium, as suggested by Hong et al.[10] In this context it is relevant that Takata et al[11] demonstrated that the proliferative features of the cyst lining are the main factors influencing the proliferative activity of COCs. Except for subtype 2Abβ and according to present knowledge, all lesions may occur peripherally or centrally, with the ratio between the two locations being 1:5.[9] The rest of this section provides an interpretation of this classification.

Type 1a

The non-neoplastic (simple cystic) and non-proliferative variant is lined by a nonkeratinized odontogenic epithelium of 4 to 10 cells in thickness, containing isolated or clustered ghost cells, some of which may be calcified. Juxtaepithelial dentinoid and foreign body reaction are not commonly present, but occur frequently with cholesterol granulomas and hemorrhage.

Type 1b

It was not until 1994 (Hirshberg et al[13]) that COCs associated with an odontoma (COCaO) were first reviewed in an attempt to clarify the pathogenesis of this particular variant. The authors accepted 52 cases of COCaO published in the English language literature—18 men and 34 women with a mean age of 16 years, most patients being in their 2nd decade. COCs have been reported to be associated with an odontoma in 22%[14] to 47%[15] of cases. The detailed location of the COCaOs is shown in Fig 17-1. Oral examination revealed a hard swelling in 52% of the cases. The lesion was accidentally discovered during routine radiographic examination in one fifth of cases. The radiographic

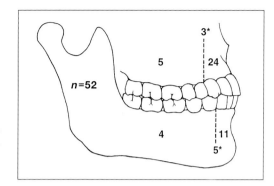

Fig 17-1 Topographic distribution of COCs associated with odontomas.[13] Numbers with asterisks indicate that these lesions occupy both the anterior and the posterior regions.

Table 17-1 Suggested classification of COCs*

1. Non-neoplastic (simple cystic) variants (CGCOC[a])
   - a. with nonproliferative epithelial lining
   - b. with nonproliferative (or proliferative) epithelial lining associated with odontomas[b]
   - c. with proliferative epithelial lining
   - d. with unicystic, plexiform ameloblastomatous proliferation of epithelial lining[c]

2. Neoplastic variants
   - A. Benign type (CGCOT[d])
     - a. cystic subtype (cystic CGCOT)
       - α) SMA ex epithelial cyst lining[e]
     - b. solid subtype (solid CGCOT)
       - α) peripheral ameloblastoma-like[f]
       - β) SMA-like[g]

   - B. Malignant type (malignant CGCOT or OGCC[h])
     - a. cystic subtype
     - b. solid subtype

---

* See Comments, page 119.
[a] Calcifying ghost cell odontogenic cyst.
[b] Also classified as compound (or complex) cystic ghost cell odontomas.
[c] Does not completely fulfill the histopathologic criteria of early ameloblastoma as suggested by Vickers and Gorlin.[12]
[d] Calcifying ghost cell odontogenic tumor.
[e] With histopathologic features of early ameloblastoma as suggested by Vickers and Gorlin.[12]
[f] Resembling a peripheral ameloblastoma (see chapter 6), hence termed peripheral epithelial odontogenic ghost cell tumor.
[g] Often called central epithelial odontogenic ghost cell tumor.
[h] Odontogenic ghost cell carcinoma (for details, see chapter 28).

appearance (*n* = 36) showed a well-defined, mixed radiolucent-radiopaque lesion in 29 cases. The radiopaque foci varied in amount from flecks to well-defined toothlike structures. In four cases, the lesion appeared radiolucent, thus demonstrating the early stages of development of the odontoma. In 20 cases (38.5%), the COCaO was associated with impacted teeth, the canine being the tooth most frequently involved.

Histomorphologic information was retrieved from 16 cases, including six cases from the authors' files. In most cases, the lesions consisted of a single large cyst, the epithelial lining of which showed a basal cell layer with hyperchromatic, polarized nuclei. Masses of "ghost" epithelial cells were present in the lining or in the fibrous tissue capsule. Elements of toothlike structures were found adjacent to the COC components either in the connective tissue capsule or in direct continuation with the epithelial cyst lining, occasionally protruding into the lumen. The components of the COC and those of the odontoma were intermingled and continuous giving the impression of a single lesion.

Hirshberg et al[13] suggested several possibilities regarding the pathogenesis of COCaOs. One was that the COC and the odontoma may represent co-incidental juxtaposition of a COC and an odontoma, because other odontogenic tumors, such as SMA, have been reported associated with COCs.[15] However, the rarity of coexistence of two separate odontogenic tumors and the relatively frequent occurrence of COCaOs make it an unlikely explanation for the pathogenesis of COCaOs. The present authors agree with this viewpoint.

A second suggestion as to the pathogenesis of COCaOs is that the odontoma develops secondarily from the lining epithelium of the COC (or CGCOC, according to Toida[5]), because the odontogenic epithelium has the potential for induction phenomena as mani-fested in odontogenic tumors belonging to group 1.1.2 in the WHO classification[4] ("odontogenic epithelium with odontogenic ectomesenchyme, with or without dental hard tissue formation"). It is, however, important to stress that there seems to be no substantial evidence that the epithelial component of the non-odontoma-producing COC (CGCOC) is supported by ectomesenchyme rather than by mature mesenchymal, fibrous connective tissue. It is therefore very unlikely that a CGCOC at some stage develops into a COCaO simply because the reciprocal epithelio-ectomesenchymal interactions responsible for a possible development of an odontoma are not operational under these conditions.

The majority of odontomas associated with a COC (CGCOC) seem to be of the compound type. When the mean age (see section 3.2 of this chapter) at the time of diagnosis of COCaO is compared to the corresponding number retrieved from a recent literature survey[16] and a similar comparison is made concerning location (Fig 17-2), the following suggestion as to the pathogenesis of COCaOs may be made. There is a remarkable similarity between the two sets of data, and the present authors interpret these findings as follows: The COCaO may be regarded as a compound odontoma (in various stages of development) in which the epithelial component—in addition to initiating the development of a compound (or more rarely a complex) odontoma—at a certain stage forms an epithelial cyst lining, eventually enveloping the odontoma. This interpretation concurs with that of Nagao et al[14] and Hong et al.[10] Because the cyst component and the odontoma are continuous with each other, it has in the past been thought that the epithelial lining of the cyst participates in the formation of the odontoma,[6,17] a concept that Hirshberg et al[13] accept. The latter authors suggested that the COCaO should be regarded as a separate entity and classified

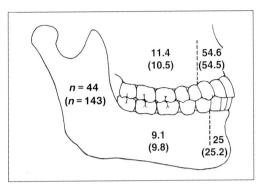

Fig 17-2 Topographic distribution (in percentages of all lesions) of COCaOs and compound odontomas (in parentheses).[16] The eight cases (see Fig 17-1) where the lesion occupied both the anterior and the posterior regions are left out. Note the remarkable similarity between the two sets of data.

as a benign mixed odontogenic tumor called odontocalcifying odontogenic cyst. This terminology seems inappropriate in that, according to the present authors' concept, this lesion is not a cyst but a compound odontoma in which an epithelial cyst has formed secondarily. The cyst lining may occasionally show some proliferative activity. Thus, it should be classified as an odontoma variant that may be called compound complex cystic ghost cell odontoma. It should be mentioned that compound (as well as complex) odontomas may contain ghost cells in as many as 11% to 18% of examined cases.[16] The feature that distinguishes the COC associated with an odontoma from an odontoma containing ghost cells is the definite formation of a cyst lined by odontogenic epithelium in the former.

Type 1c

In this subgroup the cyst lining shows proliferative activity with the formation of multiple daughter cysts in the fibrous connective tissue wall (Figs 17-3 to 17-5). Extensive ghost cell formation with a marked tendency for calcification is found in the centers of the cyst. Juxtaepithelial dentinoid is rarely seen, whereas foreign body reaction to herniated ghost cells is prominent.

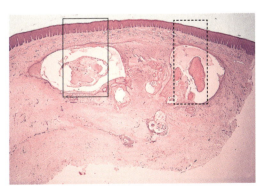

Fig 17-3 COC, type 1c, located in the gingiva with formation of multiple daughter cysts (hematoxylin-eosin [H&E], x30).

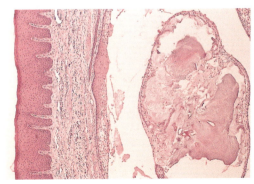

Fig 17-4 Higher magnification of the framed (solid line) area in Fig 17-3 showing clusters of ghost cells in the center of a daughter cyst (H&E, x80).

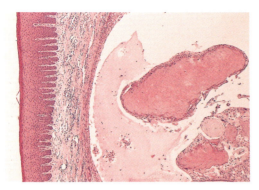

Fig 17-5 Higher magnification of the framed (broken line) area in Fig 17-3 showing a large island of ghost cells (H&E, x80).

Type 1d

This non-neoplastic, cystic subgroup is characterized by uni- or multifocal proliferative activity of the epithelial lining, resembling a plexiform unicystic ameloblastoma except for the presence of ghost cells and dystrophic calcifications within the proliferating cyst epithelium. In contrast to SMA ex COC (group 2Aaα in Table 17-1), the ghost cells and calcifications are confined to the cyst lumen. It is further differentiated from lesions in group 2Ab by its obvious cystic histoarchitecture and lack of juxtaepithelial dentinoid.

Type 2Aaα

This neoplastic variant is rare. The cyst lining shows uni- and multifocal, intramural and intraluminal proliferation of classic SMA tissue, often in a plexiform pattern with histopathologic features of early ameloblastoma according to Vickers and Gorlin.[12] The cyst lining contains a considerable number of ghost cells, whereas the transformed ameloblastomatous portion shows little or no ghost cells. Juxtaepithelial dentinoid is not present.

Type 2Abα

Lesions of this subgroup are located in the gingival soft tissue or alveolar mucosa and bear a striking resemblance to the peripheral ameloblastoma (see chapter 6) except that clusters of ghost cells are present in the central portions of the tumor cell nests and dentinoid can be found adjacent to the most peripheral cells. Multifocal downward proliferation of the oral surface epithelium is a characteristic finding, but some lesions are entirely within the lamina propria. The basal epithelial cells lack palisading of the cell nuclei. Seven of 13 cases reported by Hong et al[10] occurred in edentulous patients and 5 were seen in denture wearers. The clinical appearance of this soft tissue tumor has variously been described as exophytic and pedunculated, nodular and plaquelike with a hard, soft, or friable consistency.

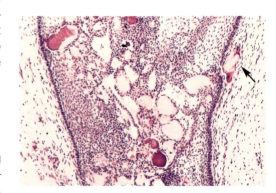

Fig 17-6 Neoplastic variant of COC (type 2Abβ) with a large island of proliferative odontogenic epithelium resembling SMA. Note the small, centrally located ghost cell clusters, some of which show calcification. A small ghost cell cluster has broken through the basement membrane of the island (*arrow*), provoking a giant cell reaction (periodic acid–Schiff, x100).

Type 2Abβ

This intraosseously located subtype is composed of nests or clusters of proliferative odontogenic epithelium resembling SMA (Fig 17-6) or occasionally adenomatoid odontogenic tumor. Ghost cells are usually encountered centrally in the epithelial islands, and juxtaepithelial dentinoid is also present. Only three cases of this lesion were included in the report by Hong et al[10] but they all lacked the ameloblastic histopathologic criteria suggested by Vickers and Gorlin.[12]

The above subclassification is, as alluded to earlier, the result of an amalgamation of four different attempts at classification[5,6,9,10] of complicated cyst/tumor variants. The classification is mainly based on pathological principles and it must be admitted that it tends to be more of an academic exercise than an attempt at finding a manageable solution to a difficult problem.

It should be mentioned that opinions differ among authors as to the need for classification of the COC (see chapter 28). Thus, Johnson et al[18] claim that "the solid variant of COC seems to represent the ultimate phase of evolution of the COC and not necessarily a separate entity. Because recurrence is uncommon (no recurrences were found among the 57 cases reported by these authors), there seems to be no clinical justification for subclassifying these lesions."

2. Clinical and radiologic profile

Because of the relatively small number of cases in the various variants and subgroups (see Table 17-1) and because the majority of published studies have not sufficiently differentiated between non-neoplastic and neo-plastic variants, deriving clinical data specific for each of the variants is difficult if not impossible at this stage. Intraosseous lesions may produce a hard bony swelling of the jaw, and peripheral lesions may appear as local gingival growths (resembling fibromas or fibrous hyperplasia). Whether centrally or peripherally located, a remarkably large number of cases have been completely symptomless, irrespective of the variant.

Radiographically, all intraosseous lesions appear as either uni- or occasionally multilocular radiolucencies (Fig 17-7). Irregular calcified bodies of varying size seen throughout the radiolucency are typical features. Larger radiopaque masses may be found in cases associated with odontomas (Figs 17-8 and 17-9). Resorption of tooth roots and root divergence has been reported,[9] and one third of intraosseous lesions were associated with one or more unerupted teeth (Fig 17-10). Extraosseous lesions may show either no radiographic alterations or a superfi-

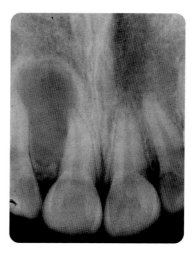

Fig 17-7 Intraoral radiograph showing a well-defined unilocular radiolucency in the maxillary right central-lateral incisor region. Histology proved this lesion to be a COC, type 1A.

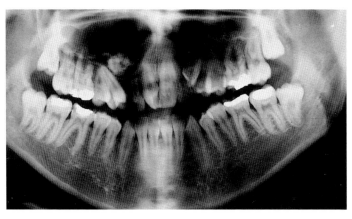

Fig 17-8 Orthopantomogram of a COC associated with an odontoma (type 1b) in the maxillary right canine–first premolar region.

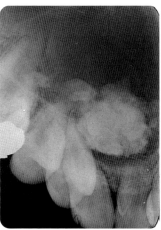

Fig 17-9 Intraoral radiograph of the tumor shown in Fig 17-8. The dislocation of the canine and first premolar caused by the presence of the odontoma is evident.

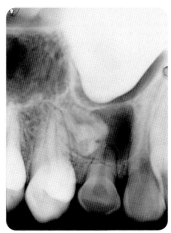

Fig 17-10 Intraoral radiograph demonstrating a COC associated with a complex odontoma. Note the persistence of the lateral incisor and impaction of the canine.

cial erosion (saucerization) of the underlying cortical bone. Erasmus et al[9] described how magnetic resonance imagery (MRI) accurately differentiates between cystic and solid variants. This method is regarded as superior to computed tomography (CT) in the evaluation of mandibular lesions because it can depict both cortical and medullary involvement. The COC, however, lacks pathognomonic clinical, radiologic, CT, and MRI features. The definitive diagnosis remains dependent on histologic evaluation.

3. Epidemiological data

3.1 Prevalence, incidence, and relative frequency

Data on prevalence and incidence are not available, irrespective of the variants of the COC. There are several sources regarding relative frequency, showing a range of 1.0% to 6.8%. All these data, however, suffer from being pooled—that is, there is no differentiation between non-neoplastic, benign neoplastic, and malignant variants of COC—and are thus of hardly any relevance. Only one report[20] has produced figures for malignant COC (odontogenic ghost cell carcinoma): 0.4% of all odontogenic tumors (of a total of 759 lesions) and 6.5% of all malignant odontogenic tumors. The authors concluded, after comparing their data with those from selected references (Chinese/African, North American, and German/Turkish), that there is a marked geographic variation in the relative frequency of several odontogenic tumors. The ameloblastomas and malignant odontogenic tumors in particular are not rare in a Chinese population.

3.2 Age

With reference to the classification suggested by the present authors, information about the age distribution of the individual COC variants and subtypes is rather sporadic or nonexistent due to the small number of cases in each variant/subtype and to the fact that available data is most often pooled. In group 1a there are, according to Hong et al,[10] two age peaks—one in the 2nd decade and one in the 8th decade, with no information about mean age. In group 1b (COCs associated with odontomas) Hong et al[10] found a sharp peak in the 2nd decade with a mean age of 14.7 years, which corresponds well with the number given by Hirshberg et al[13] (16 years), Shamaskin et al[15] (15.7 years), and Praetorius et al[6] (16.9 years), whereas the mean age reported by Ng & Siar[21] is slightly lower (13.5 years). The latter authors found a mean age of 39.5 years in the remaining non-neoplastic (cystic) variants (groups 1a, 1c, and 1d). In group 1c there is a fairly even age distribution in the 15 cases reported.[10] In group 1d, with only 10 reported cases,[10] there seem to be two minor peaks in the 2nd and 6th decades. In the neoplastic variants there are very few cases represented in Hong et al's material.[10] However, for subtypes 2Abα and 2Abβ a mean age of 62 years and 45 years, respectively, was indicated. According to Lombardi et al,[22] the neoplastic, peripheral variant showed a mean age of 59. Thus, the mean ages are, not surprisingly, higher in the neoplastic than in the non-neoplastic variants. Lastly, Shamaskin et al[15] reported a mean age of 53.8 years for peripheral variant COCs without further subclassification.

3.3 Gender

Few individual data are available. According to Hong et al,[10] the male:female ratio for non-neoplastic (cystic) COCs (not including the odontoma-associated lesions) was 1.5:1. The corresponding ratio for odontoma-associated COCs[13] was 1:1.9. Kaugars et al[23] reviewed 29 cases of peripheral COCs (with no further subclassification) from the literature and found a gender difference when comparing 10 patients younger than 40 years with 19 patients 40 years and older. Of patients younger than 40, the male:female ratio was 1:0.4, whereas for those 40 years and older the ratio was 1:2.2. Interestingly, 14 years earlier Freedman et al[24] examined 70 patients (64 cases from a literature survey and 6 cases from their own files with no further details) and arrived at almost the same numbers but in reverse order: Patients younger than 41 years exhibited a male:female ratio of 1:1.7, and patients older than 41 were 1:0.7.

3.4 Location

According to Hoffman et al,[25] 78.5% of COCs arise centrally in bone and 21.5% are observed in the gingiva. Apart from these data, specific locations related to COC variants cannot be given at present.

4. Pathogenesis

There has been universal agreement on the odontogenic origin of COCs since Gorlin et al[1,2] first suggested it. However, there has been much discussion as to the possible histopathogenesis of COCs. Shear[26] raised the question of whether those COCs that also have features of other odontogenic tumors (groups 2Aaα, 2Abα, 2Abβ) develop these secondarily, or whether the COCs are themselves secondary phenomena in preexisting odontogenic tumors. Shear[27] later answered this question himself by stating, "It is widely accepted that those COCs which have other features of odontogenic tumors develop these secondarily."

All centrally located COCs are likely to originate from reduced enamel epithelium or remnants of odontogenic epithelium.[6] Regarding the histogenesis of the peripheral, neoplastic variant (group 2Abα), two major sources of origin must be considered. Those lesions, which are located entirely within the connective tissue of the gingiva and are separated from the surface epithelium by a band of connective tissue, very likely arise from remnants of the dental lamina, whereas other lesions appear to arise from the oral surface epithelium. A similar histogenesis has

been suggested for the peripheral ameloblastoma (see chapter 6).

5. Pathology

5.1 Macroscopy

Information is not available for COCs.

5.2 Microscopy

5.2.1 Histologic definitions

According to the 1992 WHO classification,[4] the COC is "a cystic lesion in which the epithelial lining shows a well-defined basal layer of columnar cells, an overlying layer that is often many cells thick and that may resemble stellate reticulum, and masses of 'ghost' cells that may be in the epithelial cyst lining or in the fibrous capsule. The 'ghost' epithelial cells may become calcified. Dysplastic dentine may be laid down adjacent to the basal layer of the epithelium, and in some instances the cyst is associated with an area of more extensive dental hard tissue formation resembling that of a complex or a compound odontoma."

The definition used by the present authors is as follows:
Lesions in which the histopathologic features necessitate a separation into three main variants: (1) a non-neoplastic (cystic) variant with three subtypes, (2) a benign (solid) variant also with three subtypes, and (3) a malignant or carcinoma variant.

1. A lesion characterized by a simple cystic structure lined by a nonproliferative, odontogenic epithelium with a well-defined basal layer composed of 4 to 10 cell layers that may resemble stellate reticulum

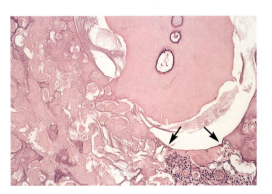

Fig 17-11 COC associated with a complex odontoma. The toothlike structure is surrounded by remnants of cyst epithelium (*arrows*) and clusters of ghost cells (H&E, x80).

and contain isolated or clustered ghost cells that may demonstrate dystrophic calcification.

In a proliferative subtype the epithelial lining shows proliferation into the surrounding fibrous capsule with the presence of multiple daughter cysts, the centers of which often show extensive ghost cell formation.

Juxtaepithelial dentinoid (osteoid) may be found in both of these COC types, in particular close to masses of ghost cells. The proliferation of the cyst lining may also show uni- or multifocal, intraluminal activity producing a netlike pattern resembling a unicystic plexiform ameloblastoma but containing isolated or clustered ghost cells and calcification.

The combined microscopic features of a COC (non-neoplastic or cystic variant) and a compound (or complex) odontoma (Fig 17-11) should be classified as a cystic ghost cell odontoma (see chapter 16) and not as a COC variant.

2. A neoplastic (solid) lesion in which the cyst lining shows both intramural and intraluminal proliferations of SMA tissue, often exhibiting a plexiform pattern. The epithelium of the cyst lining contains a large number of ghost cells in contrast to the transformed ameloblastomas epithelial portion, juxtaepithelial dentinoid is rarely, if ever, present. This neoplastic COC is known as SMA ex COC.

A subtype of the neoplastic variant is a lesion characterized by epithelial proliferations from the surface gingival epithelium into the lamina propria or proliferating epithelial islands or cords entirely located within the lamina propria and separated from the oral epithelium by a band of connective tissue. It thus bears a striking resemblance to the peripheral ameloblastoma except that ghost cells are found centrally in the epithelial tumor components and juxtaepithelial dentinoid is adjacent to the peripheral cell.

A final (rare) subtype of the neoplastic variant has histopathologic features that vary from area to area. Some portions resemble SMA-like epithelium, others show adenomatoid odontogenic tumorlike features. Both are characterized by the occurrence of ghost cells and dentinoid.

3. Malignant COCs (see chapter 28).

5.2.2 Histopathologic findings

One characteristic and distinctive histologic feature inseparably tied to the COC is the occurrence of so-called epithelial ghost cells. The nature and content of these cells have been widely discussed over the years based on histomorphologic, conventional histochemical, immunohistochemical, and ultrastructural (both transmission and scanning electron microscopy) investigations. Consequently, various theories have been proposed and recently reviewed and evaluated by Takata et al,[28] who also made extensive studies on the immunoreactivity of ghost

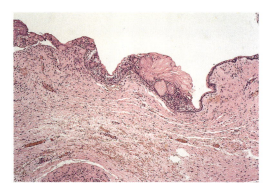

Fig 17-12 COC, type 1a, with intraepithelial ghost cells (H&E, x60).

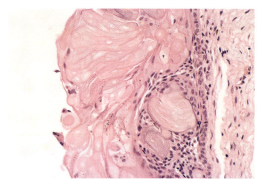

Fig 17-13 Ghost cells (shown in Fig 17-12) with the characteristic loss of nuclei. Note the early dystrophic calcification seen as fine basophilic granules or small bodies. (H&E, x120).

cells using antibodies against several enamel-related proteins.

The ghost cells, however, have been reported to occur in several other odontogenic lesions in addition to the COC such as odontomas, ameloblastic fibromas, ameloblastic fibro-odontomas, and solid/multicystic ameloblastomas.[28,29] Furthermore, ghost cells with similar histomorphologic appearance to those in odontogenic lesions are found in craniopharyngiomas and the cutaneous calcifying epithelioma of Malherbe (pilomatrixoma). The mere presence of ghost epithelial cells in a lesion does not, therefore, justify the diagnosis of COC. Ghost cells are generally described as pale, eosinophilic, balloon-shaped, elliptic epithelial cells that have lost their nuclei, leaving a faint outline of the original nuclei, hence the term *ghost* (Figs 17-12 and 17-13). Although the cell outlines are usually well defined, they may sometimes be blurred so that groups of ghost cells appeared fused. Dystrophic calcification may occur in some of the ghost cells, initially as fine basophilic granules and later as small spherical bodies. Ghost cells may break through the epithelial basement membrane (be extruded) and, when in contact with the connective tissue wall of the cyst, evoke a foreign body reaction with the formation of multinucleate giant cells.

In some variants of COC, atubular dentinoid material may be found in the cyst wall close to the epithelial lining, adjacent to epithelial proliferations, and particularly in contact with masses of ghost cells (Fig 17-14). Whether the dentinoid (or osteoid) material, some of which may become mineralized,

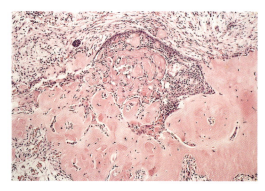

Fig 17-14 Dentinoid material found adjacent to the epithelial cyst lining which contains ghost cells. The cyst wall harbors small aggregations of inflammatory cells (H&E, x80).

should be regarded as an inflammatory (metaplastic) response to the presence of ghost cells in the cyst wall or represent a true inductive effect is still to be clarified. There is, however, a general trend in the opinions of recent authors that the former theory is favored.

Takeda et al[17] found melanin-containing cells in the epithelial islands of ameloblastomatous proliferative COCs (group 1d). Although no conclusions could be drawn as to the specific origin or pathologic significance of pigmentation in the COCs, the authors stated that the detection of melanin is not a characteristic histologic feature of this tumor. Therefore, COCs in which melanin is formed should not be considered a variant of COC as indicated by Kramer et al.[4] Takeda and coworkers[17] have described the occurrence of melanin pigment in odontogenic keratocysts, complex odontomas, ameloblastic fibro-odontomas, odontoameloblastomas, and adenomatoid odontogenic tumors. The authors noticed that all pigmented odontogenic lesions, except for odontogenic keratocysts, are associated with the formation of dental hard tissues or prominent calcification.

Ng and Siar[30] reported a case of COC (most likely group 1c) in which nests, cords, and islands of typical clear cells were found in the connective tissue wall of the cyst. The clear cells corresponded well to similar cells occurring in various odontogenic tumors (see chapters 5, 10, and 27). In a study of the occurrence of Langerhans cells in odontogenic cysts, Akhlaghi and Dourov[31] included a case of COC (no details given), where Langerhans cells were detected among the calcified ghost cells of the cyst epithelium.

5.2.3 Histochemical/immunohistochemical findings

Using methods from conventional histochemistry to immunocytochemistry, the majority of these studies have focused on the nature of the ghost cells.[28] As early as 1964,[2] Gorlin et al concluded that ghost cells in COCs, pilomatrixomas, and craniopharyngiomas represented a form of abnormal keratinization, a theory supported by many authors over the years. However, most immunohistochemical investigations on cytokeratins in the ghost cells of COCs failed to demonstrate positive staining for different kinds of keratins.[10,32–34] Takata et al[28] used a polyclonal antibody against wide-spectrum cytokeratins and found that ghost cells in COC showed only faint or no positivity, while adjacent "non-ghost" epithelial cells were obviously positive. The authors concluded that aberrant keratinization seems to make a minor contribution to the formation of ghost cells. Thus, the biologic properties of ghost cells in COCs are different from those of keratinocytes. Hong et al[10] expressed the opinion that the characteristics of ghost cells are compatible with the features of coagulative necrosis of odontogenic epithelium.

Further, Takata et al[28] showed that amelogenin was immunolocalized to ghost cells in all COC cases, irrespective of variant. In addition, enamelin, sheathlin, and enamelysin were expressed to varying degrees. Columnar and stellate reticulum cells of the epithelial cyst lining were negative for the enamel-related proteins examined as were ghost cells in pilomatrixomas (which were positive for hair keratin). The authors concluded that ghost cells in COCs contain enamel-related proteins in the cytoplasm accumulated during the process of pathologic transformation.

5.2.4 Ultrastructural findings

Fejerskov and Krogh[8] were the first to show that the ultrastructure of COC ghost cells does not reveal the so-called keratin pattern identical to that observed in epidermis and oral epithelia, the main difference being the

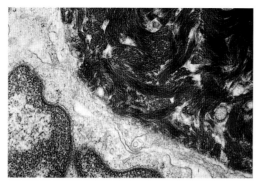

Fig 17-15 Electron micrograph showing part of an epithelial cell (lower left corner) from the cyst lining of a COC (type 1a) and an adjacent ghost cell (upper right corner). Note the coarse, thick tonofilament bundles occupying the cytoplasm of the ghost cell (TEM, x8,000).

and the squamous or papillary type, which resembles the SMA histologically and is found exclusively in adults.[37] Bernstein and Buchino[38] pointed out that the ACP often exhibits histologic features of both the COC (SMA ex COC in the nomenclature used in this chapter, and ghost cell ameloblastoma [GCA] according to Badger and Gardner[37]) and the SMA. Ghost cells are a prominent feature of both ACPs and GCAs. Based on a histopathologic comparison of 26 cases of ACPs and 3 cases of GCAs, the authors concluded that the biologic behavior of the two lesions appears to be similar and they should be considered homologous tumors.

coarse, thick tonofilament bundles in COCs as opposed to the evenly distributed, fine tonofilaments in a matrix characterizing the keratin pattern (Fig 17-15). These findings were supported by Regezi et al[29] who concluded that the ghost cells represented an aberrant or unusual form of keratin and not true keratin. Satomura et al[35] especially studied the initial calcification in COC ghost cells and found that a variety of vesicles were scattered among the tonofilament bundles. Some vesicles contained needlelike crystals which were considered initial calcification sites in ghost cells. This finding differed from previous reports where the calcification of ghost cells was found to occur in association with the bundles of tonofilaments.[8,36]

5.2.5 The relationship between adamantinomatous (ameloblastomatous) craniopharyngiomas and COCs

It is recognized that the craniopharyngioma exhibits two variants: the adamantinomatous or classic type (ACP), which is more common and occurs in the first two decades of life,

6. Notes on treatment and recurrence rate

Appropriate treatment for the non-neoplastic (cystic) variants of COC (groups 1a, 1b, 1c, and 1d) and the neoplastic variant of subtype 2Abα is believed to be conservative, surgical enucleation. For the remaining neoplastic variants (2Aaα and 2Abβ), some investigators consider their behavior and prognosis to be that of a SMA, meaning treatment must be radical. For treatment of the malignant COCs or odontogenic ghost cell carcinoma (group 2B), see chapter 28.

Recurrence of COCs is rare. According to Buchner,[9] nine cases have been reported. Since the recurrences occurred after as much as 8 years, a follow-up period of 10 years seems advisable.

References

1. Gorlin RJ, Pindborg JJ, Clausen FP, Vickers RA. The calcifying odontogenic cyst—A possible analogue of the cutaneous calcifying epithelioma of Malherbe. Oral Surg Oral Med Oral Pathol 1962; 15:1235–1243.

2. Gorlin RJ, Pindborg JJ, Redman RS, et al. The calcifying odontogenic cyst. A new entity and possible analogue of the cutaneous epithelioma of Malherbe. Cancer 1964;17:723–729.

3. Pindborg JJ, Kramer IRH. Histological Typing of Odontogenic Tumours, Jaw Cysts and Allied Lesions. Berlin: Springer-Verlag, 1971.

4. Kramer IRH, Pindborg JJ, Shear M. Histological Typing of Odontogenic Tumours. 2d ed. Berlin: Springer-Verlag, 1992.

5. Toida M. So-called calcifying odontogenic cyst: Review and discussion on the terminology and classification. J Oral Pathol Med 1998;27:49–52.

6. Praetorius F, Hjørting-Hansen E, Gorlin RJ, Vickers RA. Calcifying odontogenic cyst. Range, variations and neoplastic potential. Acta Odontol Scand 1981;39:227–240.

7. Colmenero C, Patron M, Colmenero B. Odontogenic ghost cell tumors. J Craniomaxillofac Surg 1990;18:215–218.

8. Fejerskov O, Krogh J. The calcifying ghost cell odontogenic tumor—or the calcifying odontogenic cyst. J Oral Pathol 1972;1:273–287.

9. Buchner A. The central (intraosseous) calcifying odontogenic cyst: An analysis of 215 cases. J Oral Maxillofac Surg 1991;49:330–339.

10. Hong SP, Ellis GL, Hartman KS. Calcifying odontogenic cyst. A review of ninety-two cases with reevaluation of their nature as cysts or neoplasms, the nature of ghost cells, and subclassification. Oral Surg Oral Med Oral Pathol 1991;72:56–64.

11. Takata T, Lu Y, Ogawa I, et al. Proliferative activity of calcifying odontogenic cysts as evaluated by proliferating cell nuclear antigen labeling index. Pathol Int 1998;48:877–881.

12. Vickers RA, Gorlin RJ. Ameloblastoma: Delineation of early histopathologic features of neoplasia. Cancer 1970;26:699–710.

13. Hirshberg A, Kaplan I, Buchner A. Calcifying odontogenic cyst associated with odontoma: A possible separate entity (odontocalcifying odontogenic cyst). J Oral Maxillofac Surg 1994;52: 555–558.

14. Nagao T, Nakajima T, Fukushima M, Ishiki T. Calcifying odontogenic cyst. A survey of 23 cases in the Japanese literature. J Maxillofac Surg 1983; 11:174–179.

15. Shamaskin RG, Svirsky JA, Kaugars GE. Intraosseous and extraosseous calcifying odontogenic cyst (Gorlin cyst). J Oral Maxillofac Surg 1989;47:562–565.

16. Philipsen HP, Reichart PA, Praetorius F. Mixed odontogenic tumours and odontomas. Considerations on interrelationship. Review of the literature and presentation of 134 new cases of odontomas. Oral Oncol 1997;33:86–99.

17. Takeda Y, Suzuki A, Yamamoto H. Histopathologic study of epithelial components in the connective tissue wall of unilocular type of calcifying odontogenic cyst. J Oral Pathol Med 1990;19: 108–113.

18. Johnson A, Fletcher M, Gold L, Chen S-Y. Calcifying odontogenic cyst: A clinicopathologic study of 57 cases with immunohistochemical evaluation for cytokeratin. J Oral Maxillofac Surg 1997;55: 679–683.

19. Erasmus JH, Thompson IOC, van Rensburg LJ, van der Westhuijzen AJ. Central calcifying odontogenic cyst. A review of the literature and the role of advanced imaging techniques. Dentomaxillofac Radiol 1998;27:30–35.

20. Lu Y, Xuan M, Takata T, et al. Odontogenic tumors. A demographic study of 759 cases in a Chinese population. Oral Surg Oral Med Oral Pathol Oral Radiol Endod 1998;86:707–714.

21. Ng KH, Siar CH. Morphometric analysis of epithelial components and dentinoid formation in non-neoplastic calcifying odontogenic cyst. J Nihon Univ Sch Dent 1995;37:156–165.

22. Lombardi T, Küffer R, Di Felice R, Samson J. Epithelial odontogenic ghost cell tumour of the mandibular gingiva. Oral Oncol 1999;35:439–442.

23. Kaugars CC, Kaugars GE, DeBiasi GF. Extraosseous calcifying odontogenic cyst: Report of case and review of literature. J Am Dent Assoc 1989;119:715–718.

24. Freedman PD, Lumerman H, Gee JK. Calcifying odontogenic cyst. Oral Surg Oral Med Oral Pathol 1975;40:93–106.

25. Hoffman S, Jacoway JR, Krolls SO. Intraosseous and parosteal tumors of the jaws. In: Atlas of Tumor Pathology. Washington DC: Armed Forces Institute of Pathology, 1987:30–34.

26. Shear M. Cysts of the Oral Regions. Bristol: J. Wright, 1976.

27. Shear M. Developmental odontogenic cysts. An update. J Oral Pathol Med 1994;23:1–11.

28. Takata T, Zhao M, Nikai H, et al. Ghost cells in calcifying odontogenic cyst express enamel-related proteins. Histochem J 2000;32:223–229.

29. Regezi JA, Courtney RM, Kerr DA. Keratinization in odontogenic tumors. Oral Surg Oral Med Oral Pathol 1975;39:447–455.

30. Ng KH, Siar CH. Clear cell change in a calcifying odontogenic cyst. Oral Surg Oral Med Oral Pathol 1985;60:417–419.

31. Akhlaghi E, Dourov N. Langerhans cells in odontogenic cysts. A retrospective study based on 142 cases. Bull Group Int Rech Sci Stomatol Odontol 1995;38:71–76.

32. Yamamoto Y, Hiranuma Y, Eba M, et al. Calcifying odontogenic cyst immunohistochemical detection of keratin and involucrin in cyst wall. Virchows Arch A Pathol Anat Histopathol 1988;412:189–196.

33. Kakudo K, Mushimoto K, Shirasu R, et al. Calcifying odontogenic cysts: Co-expression of intermediate filament proteins, and immunohistochemical distribution of keratins, involucrin, and filaggrin. Pathol Res Pract 1989;185:891–899.

34. Lukinmaa P-L, Leppäniemi A, Hietanen A, et al. Features of odontogenesis and expression of cytokeratins and tenascin-C in three cases of extraosseous and intraosseous calcifying odontogenic cyst. J Oral Pathol Med 1997;26:265–272.

35. Satomura K, Nakanishi H, Fujisawa K, et al. Initiation of ectopic epithelial calcification in a calcifying odontogenic cyst. J Oral Pathol Med 1999;28:330–335.

36. Chen S-Y, Miller AS. Ultrastructure of the keratinising and calcifying odontogenic cyst. Oral Surg Oral Med Oral Pathol 1975;39:769–780.

37. Badger KV, Gardner DG. The relationship of adamantinomatous craniopharyngioma to ghost cell ameloblastoma of the jaws: A histopathologic and immunohistochemical study. J Oral Pathol Med 1997;26:349–355.

38. Bernstein ML, Buchino JJ. The histologic similarity between craniopharyngioma and odontogenic lesions: A reappraisal. Oral Surg Oral Med Oral Pathol 1983;56:502–510.

Chapter 18

Odontoameloblastoma

1. Terminology

The odontoameloblastoma (OA) which is characterized as being extremely rare, was formerly known by different names such as *adamanto-odontoma, calcified mixed odontogenic tumor, soft and calcified odontoma,* and *ameloblastic odontoma.* Thoma[1] introduced the term *odontoameloblastoma* in 1970. It was considered by some to be yet another member of the odontoma group, together with the ameloblastic fibro-odontoma (AFO), until Hooker[2] showed that they are two separate tumors with different clinical behavior, though previously grouped together under the term *ameloblastic odontoma.* Hooker differentiated the ameloblastic fibro-odontoma from the ameloblastic odontoma and used the term *ameloblastic odontoma* for the more aggressive tumors composed of an SMA and a complex or compound odontoma.

In the literature, few of the reported cases satisfy the clinical and histologic criteria to substantiate the classification of odontoameloblastoma; the majority of cases reported as odontoameloblastomas appear to be examples of the less aggressive amelobastic fibro-odontoma.[3] In fact, a number of investigators in the field of odontogenic tumors still question the existence of the odontoameloblastoma. Wächter et al[4] made a critical attempt to differentiate between the OA and the AFO by means of histologic criteria

from 29 cases referred to the DÖSAK bone tumor register.* After critical revision, 18 appropriate cases were selected for evaluation. According to the 1992 World Health Organization (WHO) criteria,[5] 4 cases of OAs and 14 AFOs were classified. The authors were unable to find any significant differences between the clinical symptoms, age, radiography, and frequency of recurrences between the two entities. In addition, a decisive histologic differentiation was impossible. Therefore, the authors supported the hypothesis that there may be only one entity.

Kaugars and Zussmann[6] described a case of odontoamelobastoma in 1991 and critically reviewed the English literature of reported cases, bringing the total to 12. Acceptable cases were selected on the basis of histologic criteria in the form of published photographs or adequate descriptions and put in three categories: unequivocal ameloblastoma; connective tissue with mature, homogeneous appearance; and fragments of malformed calcified dental structures. In recent years only a few possible cases of odontoameloblastomas have been reported.[2,5,6]

*German-Austrian-Swiss register for jaw tumors, Basle, Switzerland.

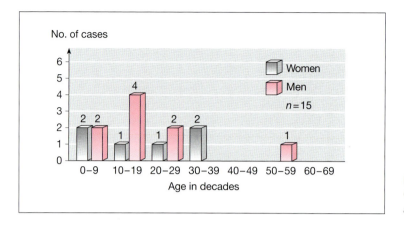

Fig 18-1 Distribution of OAs according to age and gender.[3,6–8]

2. Clinical and radiologic profile

Odontoameloblastomas have been characterized as slow, progressively growing lesions with growth characteristics similar to those of SMAs. They present as expansile, centrally destructive lesions. Symptoms include progressive swelling of the alveolar bone, dull pain, changes in occlusion, and delayed eruption of teeth.

Radiographically, the OA appears as a well-defined unilocular or multilocular radiolucency containing varying amounts of radiopaque substances. The radiopaque material may be in the form of small particles (denticles representing a compound odontomalike appearance) or of a larger centrally located mass of dental hard structures with the features of a complex odontoma (which may cause divergence of roots of the adjacent teeth).

3. Epidemiological data

3.1 Prevalence, incidence, and relative frequency

Odontoameloblastomas appear to be extremely rare and no figures on incidence, prevalence, or relative frequency are available. The situation is complicated even further by the fact that a number of cases published under the names ameloblastic odontoma or odontoameloblastoma do not meet the strict histologic criteria of this lesion and represent instead examples of the ameloblastic fibro-odontoma.

3.2 Age

Distribution of age at the time of diagnosis is shown in Fig 18-1 (n=15). The mean age of 15 cases was 18.8 years (range, 3 to 50 years).

3.3 Gender

The male:female ratio was 2:1 in the cases reviewed by Kaugars and Zussmann[6] and

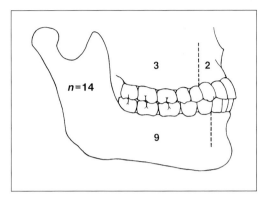

Fig 18-2 Topographic distribution of location for OAs.[4,6]

5. Pathology

5.1 Macroscopy

No detailed descriptions of the macroscopic appearance are available.

5.2 Microscopy

5.2.1 Histologic definitions

Both the 1992 WHO[5] and the present authors define the OA as follows:
A very rare neoplasm that includes odontogenic ectomesenchyme, in addition to odontogenic epithelium that resembles an ameloblastoma (SMA) in both structure and behavior. Because of the presence of the odontogenic ectomesenchyme, inductive changes take place leading to the formation of dentin and enamel in parts of the tumor.

1:3 in the four cases reported by Wächter et al.[6] Due to the small number of representative cases, no definite conclusion can be drawn for the gender distribution of OAs at present.

3.4 Location

Figure 18-2 shows the distribution of 14 cases of OAs[4,6] the majority of which is located in the posterior mandible (*n*=9).

4. Pathogenesis

The OA is clearly of odontogenic origin; however, its relationship to other odontogenic tumors—the ameloblastoma (SMA) on the one hand and the odontomas on the other—is not well understood.

5.2.2 Histopathologic findings

Microscopy reveals proliferating odontogenic epithelium in a mature connective tissue stroma, characteristic of a SMA. The epithelium is arranged in islands and rosettes with tall, columnar, peripherally palisaded epithelial cells. Reverse nuclear polarization, as seen in follicular ameloblastomas, may be found. The neoplastic odontogenic epithelium forms islands and cords between dysplastic dentinoid substances and enamel (Fig 18-3). The often large masses of dysplastic dentin and enamel are arranged in a haphazard pattern as in a complex odontoma, although rudimentary teeth (as are found in compound odontomas) also may be present. In addition, a variable amount of the characteristic cellular odontogenic ectomesenchyme is present, which gives rise to induction phenomena resulting in hard tissue formation. Wächter et al[4] who compared 4 cases of OAs with 14 cases of AFOs, found

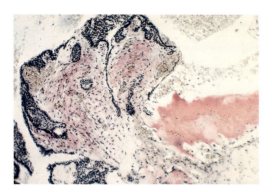

Fig 18-3   Low magnification of an odontoameloblastoma revealing odontogenic epithelial islands and cords bordering a large mass of dentinoid material (hematoxylin-eosin, ×20) (Courtesy of DÖSAK, Prof G. Jundt, Basle, Switzerland).

no decisive histologic criteria to separate these two lesions. However, it appeared that SMA-like structures were more characteristic for the odontoameloblastoma, whereas the ectomesenchymal component was more pronounced in the AFO. *Ghost cells* may be present in OAs.

5.2.3 Histochemical/immunohistochemical findings

Among a number of other mixed odontogenic tumors, Yamamoto et al[8] studied a case of OA by immunohistochemical methods. They found positive reaction of the odontogenic epithelium to KL-1 antibodies with some differences in intensity. Cells positive for proliferating nuclear cell antigen were seen more frequently in the epithelium of the OA and ameloblastic fibroma. The authors concluded that tumor cells in each odontogenic tumor possess characteristic proteins associated with proliferation potential and that ameloblastic fibromas and OAs have a higher proliferation potential than other mixed odontogenic tumors.

5.2.4 Ultrastructural findings

Studies on ultrastructural aspects of odontoameloblastomas have not been published.

6. Notes on treatment and recurrence rate

Since the OA has been considered an aggressive lesion, most authors recommend a radical treatment as applied for ameloblastomas.[3,6] In the series reviewed by Kaugars and Zussman,[6] three recurrences were noted, including one case in which the OA recurred twice. Wächter et al[4] did not record any recurrences among their cases.

Kaugars and Zussman[6] discussed the similarity of OAs with both ameloblastomas and odontomas. While the location, expansion, and recurrence rate appear to be similar to those of the SMA, the age at the time of diagnosis is more comparable to that of the complex odontoma (60% in first two decades of life; *n*=15). Wächter et al[4] considered the OA and the AFO to be one entity because of a similar biologic behavior and prognosis. Also, they considered the OA (and the AFO) to be more of a hamartomatous lesion than a true neoplasm. They recommended the performance of regular follow-up in order to detect "recurrences" early.

References

1. Thoma KH. Oral Pathology, 6th ed. St Louis: Mosby, 1970:497–499.

2. Hooker SP. Ameloblastic odontoma: An analysis of 26 cases. Oral Surg Oral Med Oral Pathol 1967;24:119–122.

3. Thompson IOC, Phillips VM, Ferreira R, Housego TH. Odontomeloblastoma: A case report. Br J Oral Maxillofac Surg 1990;28:347–349.

4. Wächter R, Remagen W, Stoll P. Kann man zwischen Odonto-Ameloblastom und ameloblastischem Fibro-Odontom unterscheiden? Dtsch Zahnärztl Z 1991;46:74–77.

5. Kramer IRH, Pindborg JJ, Shear M. Histological Typing of Odontogenic Tumours. 2d ed. Berlin: Springer-Verlag, 1992.

6. Kaugars GE, Zussmann H. Ameloblastic odontoma (odontoameloblastoma). Oral Surg Oral Med Oral Pathol 1991;77:371–373.

7. Gunbay T. Odontoameloblastoma: Report of case. J Clin Pediatr Dent 1993;18:17–20.

8. Yamamoto K, Yoneda K, Yamamoto T, et al. An immunohistochemical study of odontogenic mixed tumours. Eur J Cancer B Oral Oncol 1995, 31B:122–128.

Section Four

Benign Neoplasms and Tumor-like Lesions Showing Mesenchyme and/or Ectomesenchyme

Introduction

This section covers three different entities—odontogenic fibromas, odontogenic myxomas, and benign cementoblastomas—which are all classified in the 1992 edition of the World Health Organization (WHO) classification.[1]

However, from a histomorphologic viewpoint, neither the odontogenic fibroma nor the odontogenic myxoma contains typical cellular ectomesenchyme with few delicate connective tissue fibers as is classically seen in the ameloblastic fibroma. The connective tissue component in these two neoplasms is that of a mature, mesenchymal or mesodermal (connective tissue) type. Likewise, the benign cementoblastoma does not include a histomorphologically characteristic ectomesenchymal component, a fact the authors of the 1992 WHO classification acknowledged when they stated that "the soft tissue component consists of vascular, loose-textured fibrous tissue." In their account of the formal genesis of benign odontogenic tumors, Reichart and Ries[2] stress that from a histogenetic viewpoint, cementoblasts—together with odontoblasts—belong to the ectomesenchymally derived cells. Thus, the present authors have modified the definition of the 1992 WHO classification for the three neoplasms in this section: lesions originating from mesenchyme and/or odontogenic ectomesenchyme with or without presence of odontogenic epithelium.

Comments

Readers should note the terminology used in chapters 19, 20, and 21. During the Editorial and Consensus Conference, held in July 2003 in association with the preparation of the new WHO volume *Tumours of the Head and Neck*, the following changes in terminology were introduced for the tumors described in the aforementioned chapters of this book.

Two variants of the *odontogenic fibroma*—the simple type and the complex or WHO type—were renamed *epithelium-poor* and *epithelium-rich*, respectively. The terms *myxoma* or *myxofibroma* are unchanged. As for the benign cementoblastoma, the word "benign" has been dropped and it is now *cementoblastoma*. Because the Consensus Conference was held during the final production of this book, rewriting chapters 19, 20, and 21 to introduce the new terminology was not possible.

References

1. Kramer IRH, Pindborg, Shear M. Histological Typing of Odontogenic Tumours. 2d ed. Berlin: Springer-Verlag, 1992.

2. Reichart PA, Ries P. Considerations on the classification of odontogenic tumours. Int J Oral Surg 1983;12:323–333.

Chapter 19

Odontogenic Fibroma

1. Terminology

The odontogenic fibroma (OF) is an elusive and controversial tumor: elusive because of its rarity and controversial because of the uncertainty as to the number of distinct types that exist.[1] At present the term *odontogenic fibroma* appears to be applied to various types of lesions. It is, however, generally agreed that topographically two variants can be distinguished: an intraosseous or central type (COF) and an extraosseous or peripheral type (POF). This chapter deals only with the central variety. More information on POFs is available in Gardner,[2] Buchner et al,[3] Daley and Wysocki,[4] and Siar and Ng.[5]

According to the 1992 World Health Organization (WHO) publication,[6] the COF is derived from "odontogenic ectomesenchyme with or without included odontogenic epithelium" and is thus classified with myxomas (odontogenic myxoma, myxofibroma) and benign cementoblastomas in group 1.1.3. However, it was stressed in 1971[7] that in the absence of odontogenic epithelium, the diagnosis of odontogenic fibroma should be made "only if there is good evidence that the tumour originates from the odontogenic apparatus" (the 1992 WHO classification[6] added "with caution" to this caveat). The present authors do not agree with the WHO panel about including the odontogenic fibroma in group 1.1.3. Basically, the COF is a central (jaw) fibroma; the connective tissue is that of a mature, mesenchymal type and *not* that of the embryonic, ectomesenchymal type as exemplified by the connective tissue component of the *ameloblastic fibroma* (AFs, classification group 1.1.2). The connective tissue of COFs varies from a relatively acellular, dense, fibrous type to areas of delicate fibers interspersed with considerable amounts of ground substance (simple type) to a cellular, fibroblastic type interwoven with less cellular and often vascular areas (WHO type). The latter type also contains foci of calcified material resembling dysplastic cementum, osteoid, or dysplastic dentin.

The occurrence of odontogenic epithelium, whether by chance or as part of the pathogenesis of the lesion, varies among COFs. In the *simple type*, remnants of odontogenic epithelium are seldom numerous and they appear as inactive-looking, small, irregular islands and cords. However, odontogenic, inactive-looking epithelium is an integral component of the *WHO type*. It may be sparse but it is often conspicuous. The epithelium does *not* exhibit a central stellate reticulum or palisading of the peripheral cells, features that are characteristic of the active-looking epithelial component of the ameloblastic fibroma. These findings may support the view held by the present authors that the odontogenic epithelium in the COF does not exhibit an active-looking "induction response" because it is *not* embedded in an ectomesenchymal environment. Likewise, the calcified material found in the WHO type COF is considered to be metaplastically produced (dysplastic) cementoid/osteoid/dentinoid, and the presence of this material is not a result of true reciprocal induction phenomena.

Regarding group 1.1.3 in the WHO classification[6]—which apart from the odontogenic fibroma also includes the odontogenic myxoma (OM) or myxofibroma and the benign cementoblastoma (BC), also called cementoblastoma and true cementoma—the present authors do not see any evidence for the presence of odontogenic ectomesenchyme in the two latter entities. In fact, COFs, OMs, and BCs belong to a group of lesions characterized by mesenchymal tissue with or without odontogenic epithelium.

In 1980, Gardner[8] made an attempt to clarify the criteria by which a lesion should be diagnosed as COF. The author distinguished between three central lesions: (1) hyperplastic dental follicle, (2) simple COF, and (3) WHO type COF. The first is a well-circumscribed mass of fibrous tissue that occurs around the crown of an unerupted tooth and has a radiologic appearance similar to that of a small dentigerous (follicular) cyst. This lesion should not be considered a COF.

The second is a tumor composed of fibrous connective tissue containing scattered rests of odontogenic epithelium. Its histologic appearance is therefore quite similar to that of a dental follicle, from which it is presumably derived. The lesion is relatively acellular, the fibers are often delicate, and there is a considerable amount of ground substance yielding a fibromyxoid quality. This simple type may exhibit small islands and cords of odontogenic epithelium, but they are seldom numerous.

In contrast, the WHO type COF is a fibroblastic lesion which is interwoven with less cellular areas in which numerous small blood vessels are present. This type shows the presence of foci of calcified collagenous material resembling dysplastic cementum, osteoid (or bone), or dysplastic (atubular) dentin. As already stated, odontogenic epithelium may be sparse or conspicuous. Not everyone agrees about the desirability of distinguishing between the simple and WHO types of odontogenic fibroma. Handlers and associates[9] challenged the existence of the simple and WHO types of COF and, based on a literature review, maintained that separation of odontogenic fibromas into these two variants is inconsistent among researchers. The authors considered the two types as opposite ends of the same tumor spectrum.

It should be mentioned that neither the first[7] nor the second[6] edition of the WHO classification use the terms simple type COF or WHO type COF; both terms were proposed by Gardner[8] and have been widely accepted. Doyle et al[10] suggested the term complex odontogenic fibroma as an alternative to the WHO type. Gardner,[11] in his recent review of current knowledge concerning the COF, agreed that Doyle et al's alternative designation is probably a more suitable term and also adds the term fibroblastic odontogenic fibroma. The 1992 WHO classification only recognizes and illustrates the WHO type as a COF. The type resembling the dental follicle (simple type) is included under the subheading 1.1.3.2—myxoma (odontogenic myxoma, myxofibroma)—in the 1992 publication.

The rarity of the lesion in question became apparent when, in 1994, a study of the radiologic features of the COF,[12] including a review of articles published in the English language literature, disclosed a total of only 51 cases. The authors, however, did not distinguish between simple and WHO type cases. Due to insufficient documentation in single case reports and reports of smaller series of COFs in the literature, it is not possible to retrieve reliable data on cases of the simple type. The present authors have been able to trace and verify 15 cases of WHO type COF from a literature survey.[10,13-20]

2. Clinical and radiologic profile

The tumor is silent when small, and a painless swelling may announce its presence. A few patients may experience slight sensitivity. The growth is slow but progressive, frequently resulting in cortical expansion. Mobility of the teeth has been observed in a number of cases.

The radiographic features of the COF are not diagnostic. It is seen as a unilocular radiolucent area with well-defined borders in approximately half of cases, some of which may show a sclerotic border. The larger lesions show scalloping of the margins or multiloculation (Fig 19-1). In a few cases the occurrence of calcified material may lead to a mixed radiolucent/radiopaque appearance. Like many centrally located benign lesions of the jaws, the COF may displace teeth and cause root resorption of adjacent teeth. Lesions may be associated with the crown of an unerupted molar, premolar, or incisor (Fig 19-2).

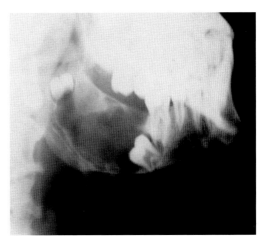

Fig 19-1 A large COF that has developed around an embedded mandibular third molar. Note the multiloculation.

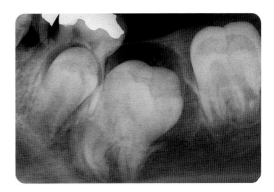

Fig 19-2 A COF in a young patient occurring around an unerupted mandibular first molar. The differential diagnosis between a COF and a dentigerous cyst cannot be made from this radiograph.

3. Epidemiological data

3.1 Prevalence, incidence, and relative frequency

No data are available concerning prevalence or incidence. A number of authors have indicated relative frequency; over the years, a wide range has been seen, from 0.7% in a Chinese population[21] to 22.8% in an unspecified American population (20,000 cases).[22] Such a range merely mirrors the lack of a uniform definition and the widespread confusion concerning the odontogenic fibroma. Regezi et al[23] did not find a single example of this tumor in a review of 706 odontogenic tumors. However, they reported two

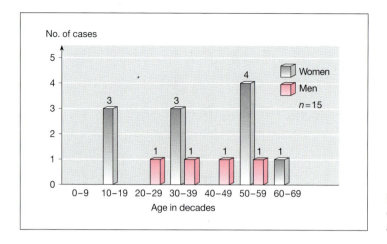

Fig 19-3 Distribution of 15 cases of WHO type COFs by age and gender.

cases of odontogenic myxoma with "3+ collagen," which may be compatible with the simple type COF.

3.2 Age

Age at the time of diagnosis ranged from 11 to 66 years (Fig 19-3). The mean age was 39.8 years.

3.3 Gender

Gender distribution showed that the male:female ratio for COF is 1:2.8 (see Fig 19-3).

3.4 Location

The sites of COF occurrence within the jaws is shown in Fig 19-4. There were considerably more cases located in the mandible than in the maxilla, giving a maxilla:mandible ratio of 1:6.5. Of the mandibular lesions, most involved the molar and premolar areas (76.9%); of the maxillary lesions, only the anterior region was affected.

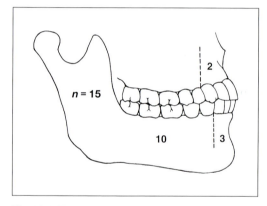

Fig 19-4 Topographic distribution within the jaws of 15 cases of WHO type COFs.

4. Pathogenesis

Some authors believe the COF to be derived from the ectomesenchymal tissue of the periodontal ligament, dental papilla, or dental follicle. It is the epithelial component of the WHO type of COF and the fact that this tumor does not occur in an extragnathic location that provide the strongest argument for this tumor being of odontogenic origin.[1] Gardner[11] stated that it is possible that the WHO type COF arises from the periodontal ligament, while the simple type is derived from the dental follicle, thus accounting for their dissimilar microscopic appearances.

The criteria for designating a central fibroma as odontogenic are still far from being defined. It may be difficult, if not impossible, to decide whether a central fibroma has arisen from the mesenchyme of the jaws rather than from the odontogenic apparatus. The presence of odontogenic epithelium embedded in the tumor tissue may be sufficient, because these structures are rarely found in nonodontogenic jaw lesions. However, some authors (WHO,[6] Gardner[8]) claim that the absence of odontogenic epithelial remnants does not preclude a central fibroma from being odontogenic. Thus, the histoarchitecture of a particular central fibroma does not prove that the lesion is nonodontogenic unless the following characteristics are found: bundles of abundant collagen fibers separated by spindle-shaped fibroblasts with elongated or ovoid nuclei[24] combined with areas of delicate collagen fibers aggregating into focal tuftlike bundles,[25] and the absence of odontogenic epithelial remnants of calcified material. If this morphologic pattern occurs in a central fibroma that has shown locally aggressive behavior, there is a considerable chance that the lesion is a nonodontogenic desmoplastic fibroma. It is, however, possible that a central desmoplastic fibroma may infiltrate or expand into an unerupted tooth and in so doing be intimately associated with its crown. This situation should not be considered evidence of odontogenic origin but must be regarded as coincidental.

The present authors agree with the idea put forward by Gardner[8] and supported by Slootweg and Müller[24] that a jaw fibroma is either a desmoplastic or an odontogenic fibroma, or as stated by the latter authors, "every jaw fibroma is odontogenic if it does not clearly demonstrate the features (stated above) of a desmoplastic fibroma."

5. Pathology

5.1 Macroscopy

The operation specimen has been described as having a gray to brownish color. Cutting through the tissue mass, the pathologist may notice calcified material.

5.2 Microscopy

5.2.1 Histologic definitions

The 1992 WHO classification[6] defines a COF as "a fibroblastic neoplasm containing varying amounts of apparently inactive odontogenic epithelium." According to the WHO panel this definition covers various types of lesions. "One resembles a thickened dental follicle both in location and in structure; tissue of this type is referred to later under the heading 'Myxoma.' Another and less common lesion is composed of a more cellular fibrous tissue, containing islands and strands of odontogenic epithelium. This second type may contain varying amounts of hard tissue resembling dysplastic cementum or bone."

The first type described in the WHO classification corresponds to the simple odontogenic fibroma. The simple type is the most collagenous variant on the histologic spectrum of myxoma, myxofibroma, and odontogenic fibroma. As pointed out by Gardner,[11] it is important to emphasize that the clinical behavior of the myxoma and the simple odontogenic fibroma are different. The sim-

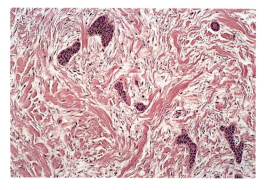

Fig 19-5 Simple type COF exhibiting thick collagen bundles with scattered, inactive-looking odontogenic epithelial remnants (hematoxylin-eosin [H&E], x80).

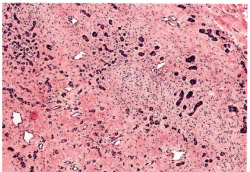

Fig 19-6 Fibroblastic COF (WHO type). The odontogenic epithelium is conspicuous. In less cellular areas there are numerous small blood vessels (H&E, x50).

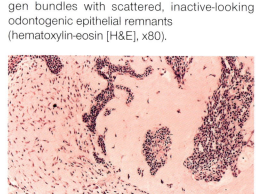

Fig 19-7 A COF (WHO type) showing a focus of calcified collagenous and cell-rich matrix with embedded inactive-looking odontogenic epithelial islands (H&E, x50).

ple odontogenic fibroma is an expansile lesion that does not infiltrate the surrounding bone, whereas the myxoma does. Consequently, from a clinical point of view, they should be considered separate entities, although they are related histogenetically. The second type of COF that is discussed by the WHO panel is identical to the odontogenic fibroma, WHO type, the term most workers appear to have accepted.

The definition used by the present authors for the simple type COF is as follows:
An expansile, noninfiltrating connective tissue lesion resembling a dental follicle. It is relatively acellular, the fibers being quite delicate, and there is a considerable amount of ground substance yielding a fibromyxoid

quality (Fig 19-5). It may exhibit inactive-looking rests of odontogenic epithelium but they are seldom numerous. Occasionally, nondescript calcifications are found.

The present authors' definition for the WHO type COF is as follows:
A benign neoplasm composed of cellular connective tissue. It often occurs in fibroblastic strands that are interwoven with less cellular areas in which numerous small blood vessels are present (Fig 19-6). Foci of calcified collagenous matrix, resembling dysplastic cementum, osteoid (or bone), or atubular dysplastic dentin often occur (Fig 19-7). Islands or strands of inactive-looking odontogenic epithelium are an integral component of this type of COF; they are usually

conspicuous. A clearly defined capsule is not encountered.

5.2.2 Histopathologic findings

Wesley et al[26] and later Watt-Smith et al[27] used electron microscopy to examine a case of WHO type COF. Watt-Smith and coworkers found that the fibroblastic cells exhibited features characteristic of both smooth muscle cells and fibroblasts. Myofibroblasts have been detected in a variety of odontogenic lesions.

5.2.2.1 The COF versus the ameloblastic fibroma

It is important to stress the histoarchitectural differences between the ameloblastic fibroma (see chapter 12) and the COF alluded to earlier. The AF is classified (by the WHO classification[6]) as a neoplasm composed of proliferating odontogenic epithelium embedded in a cellular ectomesenchymal tissue that resembles the dental papilla. The epithelial component is usually in the form of strands and islands, often consisting of a peripheral layer of cuboidal or columnar cells which may enclose a small number of cells resembling stellate reticulum. This differs considerably from the inactive-looking cell rests found in the COF. The AFs connective tissue component is embryonic looking and considerably more cellular than that seen in the COF, and there is little collagen in the form of delicate fibers.

5.2.2.2 Histologic subvariant of the simple COF

Günhan et al[28] reported an unusual example of a simple COF that exhibited numerous pleomorphic fibroblasts and an unusually large number of small calcifications. The pleomorphic fibroblasts (Fig 19-8) were similar to those that occur in the "giant cell fibroma," a soft tissue growth of the oral cavity first described by Weathers and Callihan,[29]

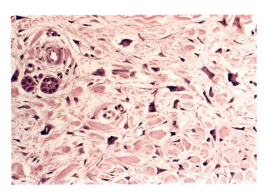

Fig 19-8 Area from a COF (WHO type) exhibiting a few inactive-looking epithelial islands and scattered pleomorphic (giant cell) fibroblasts (H&E, ×100).

and also in a number of cutaneous lesions.[30] There is no reason to suspect that the biologic behavior of this rare histologic variant differs from that of other simple COFs.

5.2.2.3 COFs (WHO type) associated with giant cell reaction

In 1992, Allen et al[20] reported three cases of WHO type COFs that were associated with a giant cell reaction similar to that seen in the central giant cell lesion (CGCL) of the jaw (see Chapter 33). A year later, Fowler et al[31] published a report in which 3 of 24 cases of COFs, exhibited an associated giant cell reaction. In one of Allen et al's cases, recurrence 14 months later displayed both the COF and the giant cell components. The nature of these unusual lesions warrants further study to clarify whether they are truly COFs that exhibit a giant cell reaction or whether the odontogenic epithelium and fibrous connective tissue are simply incidental findings associated with CGCLs.

More recently, Odell et al[32] reported on 10 lesions from 8 patients with a rare and histologically distinctive lesion composed of giant cell granuloma and fibrous tissue containing dispersed epithelial islands. It was not possible to ascertain whether this lesion was a variant of CGCL or of COF, although some of the clinical, radiologic, and histologic features were more in keeping with CGCL. The possibility that this lesion, named "hybrid CGCL and COF-like lesion of the jaws" by the authors, is a new entity cannot be ruled out.

5.2.2.4 COFs (WHO type) containing eosinophilic droplets

Two cases of WHO type COFs reported by Dunlap[1] exhibited another peculiar histologic feature. Both cases contained solitary or clustered eosinophilic hyaline droplets. The droplets were weakly positive for amyloid. A histologically identical tumor was reported as an example of atypical calcifying epithelial odontogenic tumor.[33] However, Dunlap doubted the latter diagnosis for his two cases. The origin and identity of the droplets was uncertain, but similar material has been observed in other odontogenic tumors and may be enamel matrix protein rather than amyloid.

5.2.2.5 Multiple calcifying hyperplastic dental follicles

Gardner and Radden[34] described two cases, in addition to the three previously reported, of this unusual condition. The microscopic features are those of the hyperplastic dental follicles that occur in regional odontodysplasia, although the clinical findings do not support that diagnosis. This rare condition differs in several ways from the WHO type COF—though there may be a superficial resemblance—and is, according to Gardner and Radden, sufficiently distinctive to be considered a pathologic entity.

5.2.2.6 Central granular cell odontogenic fibromas

According to the WHO classification,[6] the fibrous component of a COF may occasionally show variable numbers of cells with an acidophilic granular cytoplasm. The term

granular cell odontogenic tumor (GCOT) is sometimes applied to lesions of this type. Gardner[11] is of the opinion that the GCOT is a separate entity, although some simple COFs (but apparently not the WHO type) exhibit scattered granular cells.

6. Notes on treatment and recurrence rate

Treatment for COFs, irrespective of type, is enucleation by vigorous curettage. Long-term follow-up of a large series is not available, but the recurrence rate is considered low.

References

1. Dunlap CL. Odontogenic fibroma. Semin Diagn Pathol 1999;16:293-296.

2. Gardner DG. The peripheral odontogenic fibroma: An attempt at classification. Oral Surg Oral Med Oral Pathol 1982;54:40-48.

3. Buchner A, Ficarra G, Hansen LS. Peripheral odontogenic fibroma. Oral Surg Oral Med Oral Pathol 1987;64:432-438.

4. Daley TD, Wysocki GP. Peripheral odontogenic fibroma. Oral Surg Oral Med Oral Pathol 1994;78: 329-336.

5. Siar CH, Ng KH. Clinicopathological study of peripheral odontogenic fibromas (WHO-type) in Malaysians (1967-95). Br J Oral Maxillofac Surg 2000;38:19-22.

6. Kramer IRH, Pindborg JJ, Shear M. Histological Typing of Odontogenic Tumours. 2d ed. Berlin: Springer-Verlag, 1992.

7. Pindborg JJ, Kramer IRH. Histological Typing of Odontogenic Tumours, Jaw Cysts and Allied Lesions. Berlin: Springer-Verlag, 1971.

8. Gardner DG. The central odontogenic fibroma: An attempt at classification. Oral Surg Oral Med Oral Pathol 1980;50:425-432.

9. Handlers JP, Abrams AM, Melrose RJ, Danforth R. Central odontogenic fibroma. Clinicopathologic features of 19 cases and review of the literature. J Oral Maxillofac Surg 1991;49:46-54.

10. Doyle JL, Lamster IB, Baden E. Odontogenic fibroma of the complex (WHO) type. Report of six cases. J Oral Maxillofac Surg 1985;43:666-674.

11. Gardner DG. Central odontogenic fibroma current concepts. J Oral Pathol Med 1996;25:556-561.

12. Kaffe I, Buchner A. Radiologic feature of central odontogenic fibroma. Oral Surg Oral Med Oral Pathol 1994;78:811-818.

13. Janssen JH, Blijdorp PA. Central odontogenic fibroma. A case report. J Maxillofac Surg 1985;13:236-238.

14. Dunlap CL, Barker BF. Central odontogenic fibroma of the WHO type. Oral Surg Oral Med Oral Pathol 1984;57:390-394.

15. Schofield IDF. Central odontogenic fibroma: Report of a case. J Oral Surg 1981;39:218-220.

16. Dahl EC, Wolfson SH, Haugen JC. Central odontogenic fibroma: Review of the literature and report of cases. J Oral Surg 1981;39:120-124.

17. Mallow RD, Spatz SS, Zubrow HJ, Kline SN. Odontogenic fibroma with calcification. Oral Surg Oral Med Oral Pathol 1966;22:564-568.

18. Dixon WR, Ziskind J. Odontogenic fibroma. Oral Surg Oral Med Oral Pathol 1956;9:813-816.

19. Pincock LD, Bruce KW. Odontogenic fibroma. Oral Surg Oral Med Oral Pathol 1954;7:307-311.

20. Allen CM, Hammond HL, Stimson PG. Central odontogenic fibroma, WHO type. A report of three cases with an unusual associated giant cell reaction. Oral Surg Oral Med Oral Pathol 1992;73:62-66.

21. Lu Y, Xuan M, Takata T, et al. Odontogenic tumors. A demographic study of 759 cases in a Chinese population. Oral Surg Oral Med Oral Pathol Oral Radiol Endod 1998;86:707-714.

22. Bhaskar SN. Synopsis of Oral Pathology. 5th ed. St. Louis: CV Mosby, 1977:259.

23. Regezi JA, Kerr DA, Courtney RM. Odontogenic tumors: Analysis of 706 cases. J Oral Surg 1978;36:771-778.

24. Slootweg PJ, Müller H. Central fibroma of the jaw, odontogenic or desmoplastic. A report of five cases with reference to differential diagnosis. Oral Surg Oral Med Oral Pathol 1983;56:61-70.

25. Fisker AV, Philipsen HP. Desmoplastic fibroma of the jaw bones. Int J Oral Surg 1976;5:285-291.

26. Wesley RK, Wysocki GP, Mintz MM. The central odontogenic fibroma. Oral Surg Oral Med Oral Pathol 1975;40:235-245.

27. Watt-Smith SR, El-Labban NG, Tinkler SM. Central odontogenic fibroma. Int J Oral Maxillofac Surg 1988;17:87-91.

28. Günhan O, Gubuzer B, Gardner DG, Demiriz M, Finci R. A central odontogenic fibroma exhibiting pleomorphic fibroblasts and numerous calcifications. Br J Oral Maxillofac Surg 1991;29:42-43.

29. Weathers DR, Callihan MD. Giant-cell fibroma. Oral Surg Oral Med Oral Pathol 1974;37:374-384.

30. Houston GD. The giant cell fibroma. A review of 464 cases. Oral Surg Oral Med Oral Pathol 1982;53:582-587.

31. Fowler C, Tomich C, Brannon R, Houston G. Central odontogenic fibroma: Clinicopathologic features of 24 cases and review of the literature. Oral Surg Oral Med Oral Pathol 1993;76:587. Abstract.

32. Odell EW, Lombardi T, Barrett AW, Morgan PR, Speight PM. Hybrid central giant cell granuloma and central odontogenic fibroma-like lesions of the jaws. Histopathology 1997;30:165-171.

33. Smith RA, Hansen LS, DeDecker D. Atypical calcifying epithelial odontogenic tumor. J Am Dent Assoc 1980;100:706-709.

34. Gardner DG, Radden B. Multiple calcifying hyperplastic dental follicles. Oral Surg Oral Med Oral Pathol Oral Radiol Endod 1995;79:603-606.

Chapter 20

Odontogenic Myxoma or Myxofibroma

1. Terminology

The German pathologist Rudolph Virchow was probably the first to describe the histologic features of myxofibroma (1863), although lesions of the jaws were not particularly mentioned. In 1947, Thoma and Goldman[1] first described myxomas of the jaws. Since then the odontogenic myxoma (OM) has been a subject of continuous scientific debate. Histogenesis, pathogenesis, and particularly therapy of this benign nonencapsulated odontogenic neoplasm have been discussed avidly. In the 1992 World Health Organization (WHO) classification,[2] the term *myxoma* is used along with *odontogenic myxoma* and *myxofibroma* as alternative terms.

The odontogenic myxoma was reviewed extensively by Farman et al in 1977,[3] who evaluated 213 cases of OMs published in the international literature. Kaffe et al[4] published an analysis of the English language literature between 1965 and 1995 that included 164 cases of OMs. Smaller series of OMs—all included in the latter survey—were published by Harder,[5] Schmidseder et al,[6] Slootweg and Wittkampf,[7] and Peltola et al.[8] In 1996, Lo Muzio et al[9] reported on clinical, radiologic, immunohistochemical, and ultrastructural features of 10 cases of OMs.

2. Clinical and radiologic profile

Most OMs are first noticed as a result of a slowly increasing swelling or asymmetry of the affected jaw. Lesions are generally painless and ulceration of the overlying oral mucosa only occurs when the tumor interferes with the dental occlusion. Growth may be rapid and infiltration of neighboring soft tissue structures may occur. Most odontogenic myxomas are located intraosseously, but *peripheral variants* have been described.[6,10] Both the buccal and lingual cortical plates of the mandible may occasionally expand. Kaffe et al[4] found expansion of the jaws in 74% of patients. When the maxillary sinus is involved, the OM often fills the entire antrum. In severe cases, nasal obstruction or exophthalmos may be the leading symptoms. Displacement of tooth roots has been registered in 74% of patients and root resorption in 9.5%.[4] Association with unerupted teeth was only seen in 5% of OM cases reviewed. There appears to be no specific predilection of OM for any ethnic group.[4]

The radiologic appearance of odontogenic myxomas is variable, although the majority are characterized by a multilocular radiolucency with a "soap bubble" or honeycomb appearance (Figs 20-1 to 20-3). Kaffe et al[4] extensively reviewed the radiologic features of OM, finding a multilocular appearance in 53 cases (55%) and a unilocular appearance in 34 cases (36%). Nine cas-

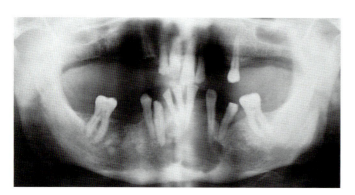

Fig 20-1 Panoramic radiograph showing a multilocular lesion in the anterior mandible. Several of the anterior teeth are severely displaced.

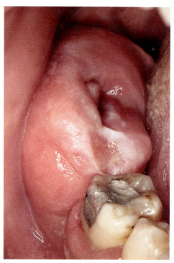

Fig 20-2 Soft tissue mass overlying the posterior right mandibular alveolar process (see Fig 20-3).

es (9%) were considered nonloculated. Correlation between size and locularity revealed that most of the unilocular lesions (85%) were smaller than 4 cm, with a mean size of 2.8 cm. In contrast, 74% of the multilocular lesions were larger than 4 cm, with a mean size of 5.7 cm. These authors also gave a detailed account of the characteristics of the radiologic borders of OMs. In 77 cases (80%), OMs were characterized as radiolucent lesions. Twelve lesions (12.5%) were mixed and seven revealed radiopacities (7.5%). Radiopaque lesions occurred in the maxilla with the tumors extending into the maxillary sinuses.

The significance of computed tomography (CT) and magnetic resonance imaging (MRI) for the diagnosis of OMs was discussed by Kawai et al.[11] Magnetic resonance imaging revealed a well-defined, well-enhanced lesion with homogeneous signal intensity on every pulse sequence. The lesion showed intermediate signal intensity on the T1- and T2-weighted images. The authors compared these findings with those for soft tissue myxomas and found discrepancies for T1- and T2-weighted signals. A similar study,[12] however, found correspondence between the MRI findings for both OMs and soft tissue myxomas. Since OMs may present with a variety of radiologic features, including poor definition on plain radiographs, imaging techniques such as CT and MRI have become indispensible for reliable diagnoses.

3. Epidemiological data

3.1 Prevalence, incidence, and relative frequency

The odontogenic myxoma is a rare neoplasm and rates for prevalence and incidence are not available. Regezi et al[13] found 3.1% of

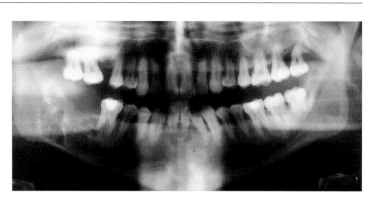

Fig 20-3 Panoramic radiograph of the lesion shown in Fig 20-2. A multilocular radiolucency is seen involving the right angle of the mandible and part of the mandibular ramus.

641 cases of odontogenic tumors were OMs. In a recent study of 759 odontogenic tumors in a Chinese population, Lu et al[14] found OMs represented 8.4%. The relative frequency for various geographic regions varied from 1.3% to 13.8%. Adekeye et al[15] stated that the absolute incidence of OMs in their geographic region (Nigeria) could not be assessed; however, they estimated the OM frequency to be between 1% and 3% among fibro-osseous lesions.

3.2 Age

Age and gender distribution of 164 cases of odontogenic myxomas are shown in Fig 20-4.[4] Age at the time of diagnosis ranged from 1 to 73 years, with a mean of 30 years; 75% of cases were detected between the 2nd and 4th decades. These figures are comparable to those of Farman et al,[3] who differentiated between maxillary and mandibular OMs as to gender and age. The mean age at the time of diagnosis of maxillary OMs in men was 29.2 years (mandibular OMs, 25.8 years) and in women 35.3 years (mandibular OMs, 29.3 years). Harder[5] held the view that the OM only rarely occurs before the age of 10.

3.3 Gender

In the analysis of Kaffe et al,[4] the male:female ratio was 1:1.6. Farman et al[3] differentiated their material further into maxillary and mandibular OMs by gender: 42.6% of maxillary OMs occurred in men (mandibular OMs, 44.4%) and 57.4% occurred in women (mandibular OMs, 55.6%).

3.4 Location

Topographic distribution of odontogenic myxomas ($n = 125$) is shown in Fig 20-5.[4] Mandibular OMs accounted for 66.4%, with 33.6% in the maxilla. Whereas 65.1% of mandibular cases were located in the molar and premolar areas, 73.8% were seen in the same areas of the maxilla.

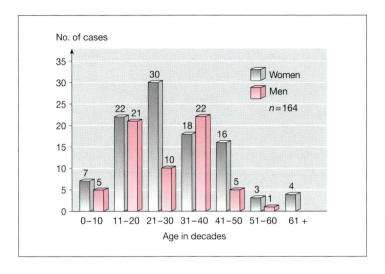

Fig 20-4 Distribution of OM cases according to age and gender.[4]

4. Pathogenesis

The pathogenesis of odontogenic myxomas has been discussed extensively during the last two decades, and it has been argued that the designation of the OM as an odontogenic tumor is uncertain. According to Lucas,[16] the classification of the OM as an odontogenic tumor has been justified by its frequent occurrence in adolescence; its association with missing or unerupted teeth; and the sporadic presence of odontogenic epithelium within the neoplastic, myxomatous tissue. Adekeye et al,[15] however, expressed the view that the frequency and significance of these features may have been overstated. The authors supposed that the rarity of OMs in any extragnathic bone could be the only firm reason for suggesting an odontogenic origin.

While some analogy between the appearance of the epithelial and/or ectomesenchymal/mesenchymal components and a phase of normal odontogenesis is apparent in most odontogenic tumors, such an analogy seems open to several interpretations in OMs.[15] The OM seems to behave differently from myxomatous tumors of the long bones, which recur more often and may transform into malignancies.[5]

A comparatively wide spectrum of cells of origin has been proposed for the OM since it was first described. Adekeye et al[15] reviewed the different arguments for individual tissues that have been considered as possible sources of OMs. The dental papilla, dental follicle, and periodontal tissues have been implicated as possible "germ centers" of OMs. However, there are a number of arguments against these possiblities. Adekeye et al.[15] proposed that no strong evidence for an odontogenic origin could be found except that the OM may represent a degenerative form of odontogenic fibroma. These authors postulated that the intraosseous neurofibroma, showing extensive myxomatous changes, would have a number of features in common with the so-called OM.

Only in recent years have ultrastructural and, in particular, immunohistochemical studies shed more light on the possible origin of OMs. In an attempt to characterize the extracellular matrix of OMs, Schmidt-Westhausen et al[17] found no resemblance between the matrix in OMs and that found in normal tooth development. Lombardi et al[18] also did not find similar staining patterns for vimentin and S-100 protein in OMs compared to dental follicle, dental papilla, and periodontal ligament cells, suggesting a nonodontogenic origin for the tumor. Other studies suggested that cells in OMs are of myofibroblastic origin[19] or that OMs are of dual fibroblastic-histiocytic origin.[20]

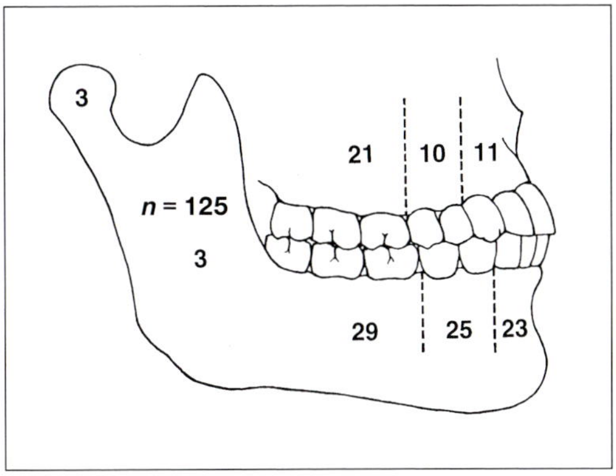

5. Pathology

5.1 Macroscopy

The cut sections of OM specimens characteristically reveal a white-gray color in the mucoid substance, which will stick to an instrument when touched.

5.2 Microscopy

5.2.1 Histologic definition

Both the 1992 WHO[2] and the present authors use the following definition for an odontogenic myxoma:
A locally invasive neoplasm consisting of rounded and angular cells lying in an abundant mucoid stroma.

5.2.2 Histopathologic findings

Odontogenic myxomas are locally aggressive, nonencapsulated, nonmetastasizing neoplasms that infiltrate bone marrow spaces. Histopathologically, the OM is characterized by loose, abundant mucoid stroma that contains rounded, spindle-shaped, or angular cells. Cellular and nuclear polymorphism is rare, as is mitotic activity. Usually tumor cells are evenly spaced within a fine fibrillar mucinous matrix. The stroma may be relatively avascular or may exhibit delicate

Fig 20-5 Topographic distribution of location of 125 cases of OMs.[4]

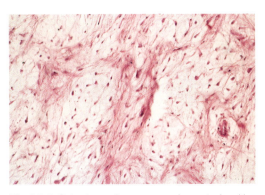

Fig 20-6 Odontogenic myxoma characterized by abundant mucoid stroma that contains spindle-shaped or angular cells. The amount of collagen is moderate (hematoxylin-eosin [H&E], x80).

capillaries. In cases of myxofibroma, the amount of collagen in the mucoid stroma is more prominent. The fibrils have been shown by silver impregnation to be reticulin.[3] Inflammatory infiltration is rarely seen (Fig 20-6). Remnants of odontogenic epithelium have occasionally been noted; sometimes they are surrounded by a narrow zone of hyalinization. The myxomatous component of OMs (Fig 20-7) has been compared to primitive mesenchyme which is found throughout the body. It has also been com-

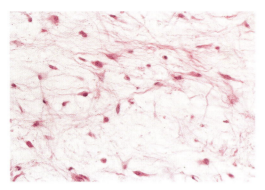

Fig 20-7 Higher magnification of the tumor shown in Fig 20-6 showing the mucoid ground substance with little collagen in the form of delicate fibrils. The cells are rounded, spindle shaped, or angular (H&E, x120).

pared to the dental papilla and the dental follicle.

From the differential diagnostic point of view, the histopathologic appearance of the OM should not be confused with that of the thickened follicle of a tooth with delayed eruption. Histopathologically, thickened follicles are characterized by a non-neoplastic, myxoid, basophilic ground substance and commonly by islands of odontogenic epithelium. Odontogenic myxomas may also be confused with myxomatous degeneration as observed in fast-growing neoplasms, particularly fibrosarcomas, chondrosarcomas, and liposarcomas.

5.2.3 Histochemical/immunohistochemical findings

Farman et al[3] reviewed histochemical findings in OMs. The ground substance of OMs has been shown to consist of about 80% hyaluronic acid and 20% chondroitin sulphate. Tumor cells appear to be relatively inactive with low levels of oxidative enzymes. Tumor cells also show slight alkaline phosphatase activity. The myxoid intercellular ma-

trix stains positively with Alcian blue, but periodic acid–Schiff staining may be negative.

Takahashi et al[20] studied OMs immunohistochemically using a number of antibodies (S-100 protein, vimentin, transferrin, ferritin, alpha-1-antichymotrypsin, alpha-1-antitrypsin neuron-specific enolase, CK1, and others). Staining patterns of spindle, stellate, and hyaline cells suggested a dual fibroblastic-histiocytic origin.

In 1992, Lombardi et al[18] published a study in which they compared the staining patterns of OMs and human tooth germs using antibodies against S-100 protein and vimentin. Whereas odontogenic myxomas were positive for S-100 protein and vimentin, normal developmental odontogenic structures were positive for only S-100 protein. Given their findings together with biochemical results from previous studies on glycosaminoglycans, the authors suggested that these data contradict an odontogenic origin for OMs. Moshiri et al,[19] who did a similar study using S-100 protein, vimentin, and actin, could not find a positive staining reaction for S-100 in OMs. They suggested that the OM tumor cells might be myofibroblastic. Lombardi et al[21] published a 1995 study on immunohistochemical findings (S-100, alpha-smooth muscle actin, and cytokeratin 19) comparing OMs and soft tissue myxomas. A minority of OMs (3 in 7) were positive for S-100; soft tissue myxomas, normal and enlarged dental follicles, and intramuscular myxomas were S-100 negative. Due to the staining patterns, the authors had some difficulty in distinguishing between OMs and myxoid nerve sheath tumors. In another study,[22] however, the authors were able to distinguish nerve sheath myxomas from other oral myxomas using neural antigens as immunohistochemical markers.

Recently, Jaeger et al[23] studied a novel cell line (Mix 1) of OM that retained the morphologic characteristics of the OM cells and matrix. The cell line was characterized as a well-differentiated fibroblast able to synthesize different proteins (type I collagen, fibronectin, tenascin) of the tumor matrix. Myofibroblastic differentiation was not found in this study.

In summary, OM tumor cells are mesenchymal and express vimentin; occasional positivity to S-100 protein and muscle-specific actin is found. The matrix exhibits different proteins, mostly type I and type VI collagen, tenascin, fibronectin, and proteoglycans; OM tumor cells have been characterized as secretory.[23]

5.2.4 Ultrastructural findings

An extensive study on the ultrastructure of OMs was published by Goldblatt in 1976.[24] Two basic types of tumor cells were described: secretory and nonsecretory. The secretory cell type was considered the principal tumor cell and resembled fibroblasts. However, ultrastructural findings indicated an abortive collagen fibrillogenesis. In addition, prominent secretory activity resulting in an excessive production of acid-mucopolysaccharide matrix was noted. Goldblatt suggested the term *myxoblast* for the tumor cells in the OM. The OM tumor cells showed many commonalities with fibroblasts of the dental papilla, dental pulp, and odontogenic fibroma, a finding which would be compatible with an odontogenic origin. However, ultrastructural features were also similar to cells of the umbilical cord. Therefore, Goldblatt concluded that origin from primitive nonodontogenic mesenchyme cannot be completely ruled out by transmission electron microscopy (TEM) studies alone.

Lo Muzio et al[9] studied OMs by immunohistochemistry and TEM. Results indicated the tumor cells had a myofibroblastic origin. Using TEM, Jaeger at al[23] found an OM tumor cell population that consisted mostly of one type of cell resembling a fibroblast. Tu-

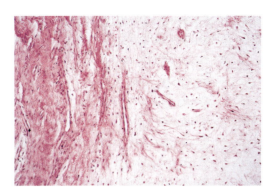

Fig 20-8 Odontogenic myxoma with an area of prominent collagen component (myxofibroma). Note the delicate blood vessels in the stroma (H&E, x60).

mor cells were spindle shaped with cell processes. Nuclei were indented with moderate margination of condensed heterochromatin. The cytoplasm was rich in intermediate filaments and variable amounts of organelles. Cells presented a prominent Golgi apparatus, dilated endoplasmic reticulum, and free ribosomes. Banded collagen fibrils in the stroma were found in close contact with the cells.

6. Notes on treatment and recurrence rate

While generally considered a slow-growing neoplasm, odontogenic myxomas may be infiltrative and aggressive with high recurrence rates. Due to poor follow-up and lack of reports, a precise analysis of recurrence rates is still missing. However, recurrence rates have been reported with an average of 25% (range, 10% to 33%).[25] Treatment has varied from local excision, currettage, or enucleation to radical resection. Recurrence is considered to be directly related to the type of therapy, with conservative surgery resulting in a higher number of recurrences. For smaller OMs, the treatment of choice is currettage because a tumor-free border may be confirmed more easily. Frozen sections, particularly in larger OMs, has been recommended for adequate control of the borders. Radical surgery is necessary when borders are poorly defined. Maxillary OMs must undergo radical resection. As is often the case, "recurrence" of OMs may, in a number of cases, be due to incomplete removal of the tumor rather than to true recurrence. Radiotherapy, electrocautery and chemotherapy have occasionally been used, but these therapies seem to be ineffective, though only a few studies on this problem have been published. Several reports on surgical and prosthetic reconstruction have been published.[26-28]

References

1. Thoma KH, Goldman HM. Central myxoma of the jaw. J Oral Surg Orthod 1947;33:532.

2. Kramer IRH, Pindborg JJ, Shear M. Histologic Typing of Odontogenic Tumours. 2d ed. Berlin: Springer-Verlag, 1992.

3. Farman AG, Nortjé CHF, Grotepass FW, et al. Myxofibroma of the jaws. Brit J Oral Surg 1977; 15:3-18.

4. Kaffe I, Naor H, Buchner A. Clinical and radiological features of odontogenic myxoma of the jaws. Dentomaxillofac Radiol 1997;26:299-303.

5. Harder F. Myxomas of the jaws. Int J Oral Surg 1978;7:148-155.

6. Schmidseder R, Groddeck A, Scheunemann H. Diagnostic and therapeutic problems of myxomas (myxofibromas) of the jaws. J Maxillofac Surg 1978;6:281-286.

7. Slootweg PJ, Wittkampf RM. Myxoma of the jaws. An analysis of 15 cases. J Maxillofac Surg 1986;14:46-52.

8. Peltola J, Magnusson B, Happonen R-P, Borrman H. Odontogenic myxoma—a radiographic study of 21 tumours. Br J Oral Maxillofac Surg 1994; 32:298-302.

9. Lo Muzio LL, Nocini PF, Favia G, et al. Odontogenic myxoma of the jaws. A clinical, radiologic, immunohistochemical, and ultrastructural study. Oral Surg Oral Med Oral Pathol Oral Radiol Endod 1996;82:426-433.

10. Tahsinoğlu M, Cöloğu S, Kuralay T. Myxoma of the gingiva: A case report. Br J Oral Surg 1975; 13:95-97.

11. Kawai T, Murakami S, Nishyama H, et al. Diagnostic imaging for a case of maxillary myxoma with a review of the magnetic resonance images of myxoid lesions. Oral Surg Oral Med Oral Pathol Oral Radiol Endod 1977;84:449-454.

12. Sumi Y, Miyaishi O, Ito K, Ueda M. Magnetic resonance imaging of myxoma in the mandible: A case report. Oral Surg Oral Med Oral Pathol Oral Radiol Endod 2000;90:671-676.

13. Regezi J, Kerr DA, Courtney RM, Arbor A. Odontogenic tumors: Analysis of 706 cases. J Oral Surg 1978;36:771-778.

14. Lu Y, Xuan M, Takata T, et al. Odontogenic tumors. A demographic study of 759 cases in a Chinese population. Oral Surg Oral Med Oral Pathol Oral Radiol Endod 1998;86:707-714.

15. Adekeye EO, Avery BS, Williams HK, Edwards MB. Advanced central myxoma of the jaws in Nigeria. Clinical features, treatment and pathogenesis. J Oral Surg 1984;13:177-186.

16. Lucas RB. Pathology of Tumours of the Oral Tissues. 2nd ed. London and Edinburgh: Churchill Livingstone, 1972:156-163.

17. Schmidt-Westhausen AM, Becker J, Schuppan D, Burkhardt A, Reichart PA. Odontogenic myxoma—characterization of the extracellular matrix (ECM) of the tumour stroma. Eur J Cancer B Oral Oncol 1994;30B:377-380.

18. Lombardi T, Samson J, Bernard J-P, et al. Comparative immunohistochemical analysis between jaw myxoma and mesenchymal cells of tooth germ. Pathol Res Pract 1992;188:141-144.

19. Moshiri S, Oda D, Worthington P, Myall R. Odontogenic myxoma: Histochemical and ultrastructural study. J Oral Pathol Med 1992;21:401-403.

20. Takahashi H, Fujita S, Okabe H. Immunohistochemical investigation in odontogenic myxoma. J Oral Pathol Med 1991;20:114-119.

21. Lombardi T, Locks C, Samson J, Odell EW. S100, α-smooth muscle actin and cytokeratin 19 immunohistochemistry in odontogenic and soft tissue myxomas. J Clin Pathol 1995;48:759-762.

22. Green TL, Leighty SM, Walters R. Immunohisto-chemical evaluation of oral myxoid lesions. Oral Surg Oral Med Oral Pathol 1992;73:469–471.

23. Jaeger M, Santos J, Domingues M, et al. A novel cell line that retains the morphological character-istics of the cells and matrix of odontogenic myx-oma. J Oral Pathol Med 2000;29:129–138.

24. Goldblatt LI. Ultrastructural study of an odonto-genic myxoma. Oral Surg 1976;42:206–220.

25. Barker BF. Odontogenic myxoma. Semin Diagn Pathol 1999;4:297–301.

26. Arcuri MR, Tabor M, Fergason H. Treatment of odontogenic myxoma of the mandible with bone graft and dental implant supported fixed partial denture: a clinical report. J Prosthet Dent 1994;72:230–232.

27. Arcuri MR, Tabor MW, Fergason HW, Haganman C. Odontogenic myxoma of the maxillary sinus: A clinical report. J Prosthet Dent 1993;70:111–113.

28. Chiodo AA, Strumas N, Gilbert RW, Birt BD. Man-agement of odontogenic myxoma of the maxilla. Otolaryngol Head Neck Surg 1977:573–576.

Chapter 21

Benign Cementoblastoma

1. Terminology

The benign cementoblastoma (BC) or true cementoma was first described by Norberg in 1930.[1] It is a rare benign odontogenic tumor of ectomesenchymal origin. It is considered to be the only true neoplasm of cemental origin and is characterized by the proliferation of cellular cementum. Ulmansky et al[2] reviewed the international literature on BC and found 66 bona fide cases of this neoplasm in addition to five of their own (n = 71). Additional cases of BCs have been reported by MacDonald-Jankowski and Wu[3] (n = 4), Slootweg[4] (n = 3), Jelic et al[5] (n = 15), Biggs and Benenati[6] (n = 1), Mogi et al[7] 1996 (n = 1), and Piatelli et al[8] 1997 (n = 1). In 1999, El-Mofty[9] published a short review on BCs and cemento-ossifying fibromas.

2. Clinical and radiologic profile

The benign cementoblastoma, intimately associated with a tooth root, generally presents as a slow-growing, unilateral swelling with expansion of the affected bone. Ulmansky et al[2] recorded swelling and expansion in 70% of their cases. In contrast to most other benign odontogenic tumors, BCs are associated with pain and occasionally with pares-thesia. In the survey published by Ulmansky et al,[2] 61% of the patients had a history of pain. Of 15 cases of BCs reported by Jelic et al,[5] 9 were symptomatic and patients complained of pain. The type of pain is usually characterized as a toothache arising in the pulp. A vitality test of teeth involved in the process is generally positive. A BC may resorb roots and even invade root canals.[2] In rare cases it may involve unerupted teeth.[8]

Radiographically, benign cementoblastomas have a characteristic, almost pathognomonic appearance (Figs 21-1 and 21-2). The lesion appears as a radiopaque, often round mass, fused with one or several roots of the associated tooth, thus obliterating the radiopaque details of the root(s). The opacity is surrounded by a thin, well-defined radiolucent border. This type of appearance was evident in 93.8% of the cases reviewed by Ulmansky et al.[2] The size of lesions reported by Jelic et al[5] (n = 11) varied between 0.5 cm and 5 cm, with an average of 1.36 cm if the 5-cm lesion was excluded. The authors stressed that the spectrum of a BC's radiographic appearance depends on its degree of mineralization. Thus, early-stage BCs generally appear more radiolucent. In such cases differential diagnoses should include periapical inflammatory lesions, focal (periapical) cemento-osseous dysplasia, central giant cell lesions, odontogenic myxomas, or solid/multicystic ameloblastomas. Mature, more calcified BC lesions may mimic ce-

199

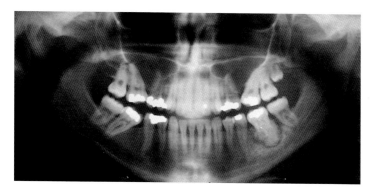

Fig 21-1 Panoramic radiograph showing a benign cementoblastoma at the root of the mandibular left first molar. The central radiopaque mass is surrounded by a radiolucent zone characteristic of BCs.

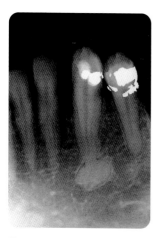

Fig 21-2 Periapical dental radiograph showing a benign cementoblastoma at the apex of the root of the mandibular left canine. There is only a fine radiolucent rim around the periapical radiopaque lesion.

mento-
ossifying fibromas, osteoblastomas, odontomas, calcifying ghost cell cysts, or calcifying epithelial odontogenic tumors. Computed tomography or magnetic resonance imaging are usually not necessary for diagnostic purposes.

3. Epidemiological data

3.1 Prevalence, incidence, and relative frequency

Since the benign cementoblastoma is a rare neoplasm, few epidemiological data are available. Benign cementoblastomas make up between 0.2% and 6.2% of odontogenic tumors.[10]

3.2 Age

The distribution of benign cementoblastomas by age and gender for cases published in references 2 to 9 (n = 93) is shown in Fig 21-3. At the time of diagnosis, the patient's age may range from the 1st to the 7th decade. However, 46.2% of BCs are diagnosed before the age of 20 years and 71% before age of 30.

3.3 Gender

Gender distribution varied among different smaller series of benign cementoblastomas. The male:female ratio of the 93 cases already mentioned[2-9] was 1:1.2.

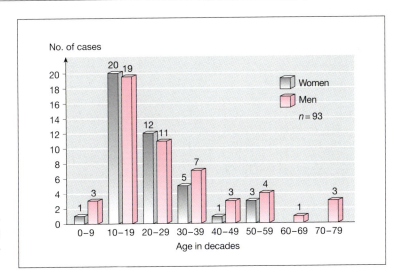

Fig 21-3 Age and gender distribution of 93 cases of benign cementoblastomas.

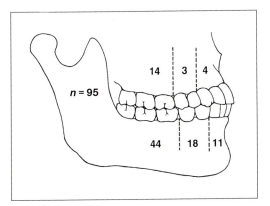

Fig 21-4 Topographic distribution of 95 cases of benign cementoblastomas according to permanent tooth groups.[2-9] One additional case not shown involved the roots of a deciduous molar.

3.4 Location

Locations of BCs according to tooth groups involved are shown in Fig 21-4 (n = 95). The mandibular permanent molars and premolars are most commonly involved, with 66% of cases occurring in these regions. El-Mofty[9] mentioned in his review that the mandibular first molar and premolars may be affected in 75% of cases. The maxillary molars and premolars are the second most affected regions. Deciduous teeth are rarely affected. Several teeth may be involved, and bilateral lesions have been reported.

4. Pathogenesis

Little is known about the pathogenesis of benign cementoblastomas. They are odontogenic tumors and are derived from ectomesenchymal cells of the periodontium, including cementoblasts. The benign cementoblastoma is thought to evolve in three stages. The first stage is characterized by periapical osteolysis, followed by a cementoblastic stage, and then an inactive stage of maturation and calcification. The BC is considered a neoplasm with unlimited growth potential. Its etiology is unknown, and trauma does not seem to play a role.

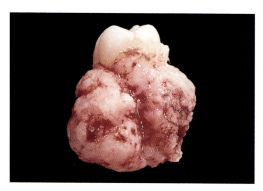

Fig 21-5 Macroscopic view of the surgical specimen shown in Fig 21-1. The lesion is large and extends up to the cementoenamel junction of the tooth.

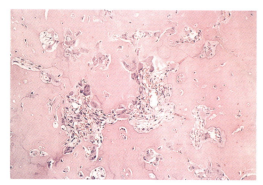

Fig 21-6 Sheets of cementum-like hard tissue with some reversal lines as seen in Paget disease. Small areas of connective vascular tissue are interspersed between the cementum-like masses (hematoxylin-eosin [H&E], x50).

5. Pathology

5.1 Macroscopy

Macroscopically, the benign cementoblastoma appears as a mineralized mass which is fused to the root(s) of a tooth, in most cases involving the apical third (Fig 21-5).

5.2 Microscopy

5.2.1 Histologic definition

Both the 1992 World Health Organization (WHO) classification[11] and the present authors define the BC as follows:
A neoplasm characterized by the formation of sheets of cementum-like tissue which contains a large number of reversal lines and is unmineralized at the periphery of the mass or in the more active growth area.

5.2.2 Histopathologic findings

The numerous basophilic reversal lines are similar to those observed in Paget disease (Figs 21-6 and 21-7). Cemental trabeculae are rimmed with plump, active cemento-

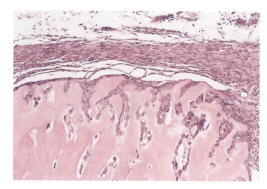

Fig 21-7 The periphery of the lesion shown in Fig 21-6. A capsule-like condensation of fibrous connective tissue with an abundance of active-looking cementoblasts is seen (H&E, x70).

blasts. Fibrous tissue with dilated vessels and multinucleated clastic giant cells may be observed between the calcified bands. At the periphery of the mineralized mass, proliferation of cementoblasts and cementoclasts is evident. It has been stressed that in many instances it is difficult to differentiate these cells from osteoblasts, and they may exhibit pleomorphism. Increased mitotic activity has not been reported. The peripheral unmineralized border of the BC corresponds to the radiolucent zone seen in radiographs. Often a correct diagnosis can be made after correlating the histopathologic, clinical, and radiologic features.

Since in many cases the cementum produced in the BC is indistinguishable from bone, it may be misinterpreted as a cementifying/ossifying fibroma, a benign osteoblastoma, an osteoid osteoma, or fibrous dysplasia. Cases in which osteocementumlike material is formed make the diagnosis particularly difficult, especially when differentiating a BC from an osteoblastoma which has a tendency to recur. Slootweg[4] compared cases of BCs and osteoblastomas and concluded that from a histologic view the two lesions cannot be separated. The diagnosis of BC is made easier when the lesion is fused to the root of a tooth. Chronic focal sclerosing osteitis has also been considered as a differential diagnosis histopathologically. Finally, according to some authors, BCs may be mistaken for osteosarcomas.

5.2.3 *Histochemical/immunohistochemical findings*

No histochemical or immunohistochemical studies of BCs have been published to date.

5.2.4 *Ultrastructural findings*

No ultrastructural studies of BCs have been published to date.

6. Notes on treatment and recurrence rate

The recommended treatment of choice is early surgical removal due to the BC's capacity for persistent growth, expansion, and involvement of adjacent structures. The growth rate has been estimated to be approximately 0.5 cm per year. The tumor is readily enucleated and does not recur. "Recurrence" is usually the result of incomplete removal. The affected tooth has been removed with the tumor in almost all reported cases. Biggs and Benenati,[6] however, described a case in which the tumor was surgically separated from the involved molar.

References

1. Norberg O. Zur Kenntnis der dysodontogenetischen Geschwülste der Kieferknochen. Wschr Zahnheilkd 1930;46:321–355.

2. Ulmansky M, Hjørting-Hansen E, Praetorius F, Haque MF. Benign cementoblastoma. A review and five new cases. Oral Surg Oral Med Oral Pathol 1994;77:48–55.

3. MacDonald-Jankowski DS, Wu PC. Cementoblastoma in Hong Kong Chinese. A report of four cases. Oral Surg Oral Med Oral Pathol 1992; 73:760–764.

4. Slootweg PJ. Cementoblastoma and osteoblastoma: A comparison of histologic features. J Oral Pathol Med 1992;21:385–389.

5. Jelic JS, Loftus M, Miller AS, Cleveland D. Benign cementoblastoma: Report of an unusual case and analysis of 14 additional cases. J Oral Maxillofac Surg 1993;51:1033–1037.

6. Biggs JT, Benenati FW. A case report. Surgically treating a benign cementoblastoma while retaining the involved tooth. J Am Dent Assoc 1995; 126:1288–1290.

7. Mogi K, Belal E, Kano A, Otake K. Benign cementoblastoma. Case report. Aust Dent J 1996; 41:9–11.

8. Piatelli A, Di Alberti L, Scarano A, Piatelli M. Benign cementoblastoma associated with an unerupted third molar. Oral Oncol 1998,34:229–231.

9. El-Mofty S. Cemento-ossifying fibroma and benign cementoblastoma. Semin Diagn Pathol 1999;16:302–307.

10. Lu Y, Xuan M, Takata T, et al. Odontogenic tumors. A demographic study of 759 cases in a Chinese population. Oral Surg Oral Med Oral Pathol Oral Radiol Endod 1998;86:707–714.

11. Kramer IRH, Pindborg JJ, Shear M. Histologic Typing of Odontogenic Tumors. 2d ed. Berlin: Springer-Verlag, 1992.

Section Five

Malignant Epithelial Odontogenic Neoplasms

Introduction to Odontogenic Carcinomas

During the past 20 years considerable confusion has existed about the definition and classification of malignant odontogenic carcinomas, in particular the definition of the primary intraosseous squamous cell carcinoma (PISC, or sometimes PIOC) and its variants, as well as the differentiation between malignant ameloblastomas and ameloblastic carcinomas. The nosology of malignant neoplasms derived from odontogenic epithelium has therefore varied considerably. In 1982, Elzay[1] proposed a modification of the first World Health Organization (WHO) classification which appeared in 1971[2] and suggested a classification of primary (de novo) PISC and PISC arising ex ameloblastoma in addition to distinguishing between a well-differentiated variant (malignant ameloblastoma, type A) and a poorly differentiated variant (ameloblastic carcinoma, type B).

In 1984, Slootweg and Müller[3] suggested the following subclassification of PISC:

Type 1   Primary intraosseous carcinoma ex odontogenic cyst
Type 2   A. Malignant ameloblastoma
         B. Ameloblastic carcinoma, arising de novo, ex ameloblastoma, or ex odontogenic cyst
Type 3   Primary intraosseous carcinoma arising de novo
         A. Nonkeratinizing
         B. Keratinizing

The authors also discussed some of the problems associated with the definition and classification of odontogenic carcinomas. They pointed out that there is lack of histologic delineation, as demonstrated by the fact that tumors consisting exclusively of conventional well-differentiated ameloblastoma in the primary tumor and in metastases have been classified as malignant ameloblastomas. Further, classification is complicated by the fact that some PISCs may reveal areas that are histologically similar to malignant ameloblastomas (that is they have *no* morphologic features of malignancy). Therefore, it is possibile that the same lesion may have been classified as a malignant ameloblastoma (exhibiting morphologic features of classic ameloblastomas) or as a PISC in the absence of metastasis. In addition, matters have been complicated by the use of the term malignant ameloblastoma for cases showing ameloblastomatous foci with a more anaplastic component and exhibiting a more locally destructive pattern in comparison to conventional ameloblastomas.

Waldron and Mustoe[4] suggested a revised classification of the primary intraosseous carcinomas. In 1999, Eversole[5] revised the classification of malignant epithelial odontogenic neoplasms based on more recent publications.

In this classification Eversole introduces an entry under the name of *malignant (metastasizing) ameloblastoma.* This tumor is not included in the 1992 WHO classification,[6] which uses the term *malignant ameloblastoma* as the equivalent of Eversole's ameloblastic carcinoma.

The present authors consider Eversole's classification to be the most appropriate one until more detailed information on pathogenesis, biologic profile and behavior becomes evident. Thus, the Eversole classification forms the basis of the following chapters on malignant epithelial odontogenic neoplasms with the changes in classification and terminology agreed upon during the Editorial and Consensus Conference in Lyon (IARC/WHO) in July 2003 in association with the preparation of the new WHO volume "Tumours of the Head and Neck". To fully appreciate these changes with special emphasis on the interpretation of chapters 22 to 26 of the present book, the reader is strongly advised to consult the WHO volume on "Tumours of the Head and Neck", chapter 6.

References

1. Elzay RP. Primary intraosseous carcinoma of the jaws: Review an update of odontogenic carcinomas. Oral Surg Oral Med Oral Pathol 1982;54: 299–303.

2. Pindborg JJ, Kramer IRH. Histologic Typing of Odontogenic Tumours, Jaw Cysts and Allied Lesions. Berlin: Springer-Verlag, 1971.

3. Slootweg PJ, Müller H. Malignant ameloblastoma or ameloblastic carcinoma. Oral Surg Oral Med Oral Pathol 1984;57:168–176.

4. Waldron CA, Mustoe TA. Primary intraosseous carcinoma of the mandible with possible origin in an odontogenic cyst. Oral Surg Oral Med Oral Pathol 1989;67:716–724

5. Eversole LR. Malignant epithelial odontogenic tumours. Semin Diagn Pathol 1999;16:317–324

6. Kramer IRH, Pindborg JJ, Shear M. Histological Typing of Odontogenic Tumours. 2d ed. Berlin: Springer-Verlag, 1992.

Chapter 22

Metastasizing, Malignant Ameloblastoma

1. Terminology

The solid/multicystic ameloblastoma (SMA) of the mandible and maxilla is an epithelial odontogenic tumor, the biologic profile of which has recently been reviewed by Reichart et al.[1] The relative frequency of ameloblastomas varies between 11% and 92%.[1] Only 0.02% to 0.7% of general pathology biopsies are ameloblastomas. Ameloblastomas are generally considered benign, although they are locally invasive and have a high recurrence rate depending on the type of initial surgical treatment.[1] As such, they share a number of features with the basal cell carcinoma of skin, both in biologic behavior and histopathologic features. In rare cases, an ameloblastoma may undergo malignant transformation (becoming an ameloblastic carcinoma; see chapter 23). Like basal cell carcinomas of skin, SMAs may—in rare instances—metastasize. Emura[2] was probably the first to describe metastasis to local lymph nodes.

Vorzimer and Perla[3] mentioned metastasis of ameloblastoma to the lung for the first time in 1932. Other reviews of metastasis have been published by Laughlin,[4] Ueda et al,[5] Ameerally et al,[6] and Henderson et al.[7] Malignant behavior is present in about 2% of SMAs.[8]

2. Clinical and radiologic profile

Generally, ameloblastomas that may metastasize do not have any specific clinical features. In their review, Reichart et al[1] found swelling, pain, delayed tooth eruption, ulceration, and tooth mobility to be the most common symptoms (see chapter 5). There are, however, a number of factors that appear to contribute to a potential metastatic spread, including duration of the neoplasm, extent and size of the initial tumor, initial type of surgery (conservative versus radical therapy), multiple recurrences and respective surgical interventions, and use of radiation or chemotherapy. An analysis of the cases reviewed by Ameerally et al[6] revealed that 8 cases (33%) had evidence of metastasis within 6 years of diagnosis, a shorter period from initial tumor to metastatic disease than the 10 years and 4 months reported by Ueda et al.[5] Also, repeated surgical intervention was not always a prominent feature in the history of metastasizing, malignant ameloblastoma (MA). Seven patients (29%) had only two courses of surgery, and in nine there was no evidence of the primary tumor at the time metastasis occurred, indicating that uncontrolled local disease is not always a prerequisite for distant spread.[6]

The most common site of metastasis is the lung. From the analysis of Ameerally et al,[6] it appeared that 75% of the cases evaluated had lung metastasis, including hilar lymph nodes; 25% involved bones, including skull, vertebrae, and femur; 18% cervical lymph nodes; 11% liver; 10% brain; and 3.5%, other nodes, spleen, and kidney. Henderson et al[7] recently reviewed 41 cases of MAs with metastasis to the lung. For this specific location, the time from diagnosis to the detection of metastasis ranged from 3 months to 31 years, with a median disease-free interval of 9 to 12 years. Pulmonary metastases are most commonly found bilaterally and with multiple nodules.[7] Lung metastatic disease may sometimes manifest clinically as subacute respiratory obstruction or dyspnea,[6] but in the majority of cases thorax radiography (computed tomography, magnetic resonance imagery) will reveal only metastases. Submandibular or cervical lymph nodes may be palpated or diagnosed by sonographic techniques. Duffey et al[9] analyzed cases of MAs with metastasis to cervical lymph nodes, and retrieving nine cases from the literature and adding one of their own. The time from first presentation to the detection of metastases was a mean of 11.7 years ($n = 7$) with a range of 2 to 24 years. Five of nine patients had additional distant metastases.

In rare cases, the metastatic ameloblastoma may be associated with hypercalcemia.[10] In the case report by Harada et al,[10] it was elevated to 12.8 mg/d, the inorganic phosphate level was 2.2 mg/d, and the alkaline phosphate level was 170 U. The humoral hypercalcemia is considered to be the result of osteolytic factors such as a transforming growth factor or parathyroid-like substance. Substances secreted by the metastatic ameloblastoma have also been considered.[10]

Radiologically, MAs cannot be distinguished from their nonmetastasizing counterparts. Since metastasis often occurs only after one to several local recurrences of the tumor, radiographic interpretation of the primary site becomes more and more difficult. Computed tomography (CT) and magnetic resonance imagery (MRI) are needed for adequate diagnosis in such cases.

3. Epidemiological data

3.1 Prevalence, incidence, and relative frequency

Malignant ameloblastomas are rare, and only about 65 cases have been described in the literature, the majority (75%) of which developed pulmonary metastasis. Compared to ameloblastic carcinomas, however, they seem to be more common (see chapter 23). Due to its rarity, no details on prevalence, incidence, or relative frequency for the MA have been published to date.

3.2 Age

The mean age of 65 cases of MAs—based on 43 cases reviewed by Laughlin,[4] 7 cases by Ueda et al,[5] 11 cases by Ameerally et al,[6] and single cases reported by Duffey et al,[9] Sugiyama et al,[11] Weir et al,[12] and Witterick et al[13]—was 34.4 years with a range of 5 to 74 years. Figure 22-1 shows the age distribution of MAs in this sample.

3.3 Gender

The female:male ratio for the same sample ($n = 65$) was 1:1.2 (see Fig 22-1).

3.4 Location

Of 43 cases reviewed by Laughlin,[4] 38 were located in the mandible and 5 in the maxilla (7.6:1). Henderson et al[7] reviewed cases of

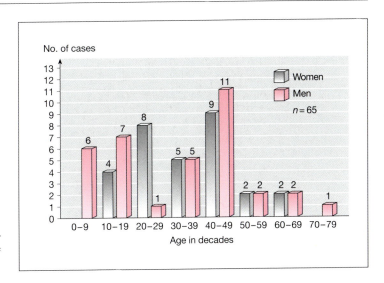

Fig 22-1 Age and gender distribution for 65 cases of MAs.

MAs with pulmonary metastasis only (n = 41) and found a mandible:maxilla ratio of 4.1:1.

4. Pathogenesis

The origin of metastasizing malignant ameloblastoma is likely to be the same as that of nonmetastasizing ameloblastoma. However, the precise mechanism by which slow-growing, cytologically nonmalignant ameloblastomas spread to distant locations and how such behavior can be predicted in the presence of histologic benignity has been the subject of considerable debate. Metastasis of the ameloblastoma is usually preceded by local recurrences of the tumor, which has been treated by surgery, radiation, or chemotherapy.[8] Curettage, the surgical procedure most commonly used in treating the primary tumor until 20 to 30 years ago, was followed by recurrences in up to 90% of mandibular and 100% of maxillary ameloblastomas.[4] Because metastasis of ameloblastomas is preceded by local recurrences, the spread of the tumor could result from either increasingly malignant behavior stimulated by multiple recurrences of the tumor itself or implantation of the tumor into lymphatic or blood vessels by repeated surgical interventions. Eisenberg[14] discussed the development of metastasis in cases of MAs and concluded that surgical transplantation of tumor cells is unlikely; the vast majority of these cells are destroyed by natural defense mechanisms, and the remaining cells would fail to thrive and attain sufficient size or biochemical capability to survive and attain deleterious effects. In this context, it is noteworthy that most MA cases have occurred only after a delay of more than 10 years after the initial treatment, somewhat disqualifying the theory of metastasis due to surgical transplantation.[7]

Generally, metastasis is defined as the active or passive dissemination of neoplastic disease from the site of origin to a distant site or organ in the host. When the MA is being considered, three routes of spread are commonly suggested: hematogenous, lymphatic, or aspiration.[7] Cases of MAs with pulmonary metastasis are generally considered to be of hematogenous spread. The fact that lung metastasis of MAs is most often found bilaterally and with multiple nodules lends support to the idea of a hematogenous spread. This is also supported by the fact that diffusely scattered tumor foci are often found bilaterally, and clusters of tumor cells are commonly observed in the surrounding blood vessels.

Lymphatic spread of malignant tumor cells is generally a well-accepted route of metastasis. Eisenberg,[14] however, questioned this mode of spread for MAs. She considered it very unlikely that a lymph node metastasis could reside in an indolent or dormant state from the time of initial therapy to clinical presentation of lymph node involvement, which in the case that she discussed was 17 years. Eisenberg proposed that in some cases the lymph node tumor may represent neoplasia occurring in conjunction with the phenomenon of heterotopia. This theory would imply that odontogenic epithelium may become trapped in lymphoid tissue during embryogenesis and later undergoes benign neoplastic transformation to an ameloblastoma in situ. This would also imply that the process was multifocal from the beginning, so that the jaw tumor and the tumor in the lymph node bore no direct relationship to one another. Such a hypothesis would (in some cases of lymph node involvement of MAs) account for why, after long periods of time, a single (metastatic) lesion arose distant from the primary tumor location but within its general anatomic region. As such, the presence of an ameloblastoma in a lymph node may not be based on lymphatic or hematogenous spread but may represent another (ectopic) primary lesion. More cases of MAs have to be studied to better understand the pathogenetic and pathologic processes of the SMA and its capability to metastasize.

5. Pathology

5.1 Macroscopy

No detailed descriptions on the gross pathology of resected specimens of malignant ameloblastomas have been published in the literature. However, it may be assumed that the macroscopy of MAs does not differ from that of conventional ameloblastomas.

Cranin et al[15] described a massive *granular cell ameloblastoma* with metastasis. The cut surface of the resected specimen revealed the tumor to be partially solid and partially cystic.

5.2 Microscopy

5.2.1 Histologic definitions

The 1992 World Health Organization (WHO) classification[16] used the term *malignant ameloblastoma* to describe a tumor that today would qualify as an ameloblastic carcinoma. The MA was neither defined nor commented on in the WHO classification.

The definition used by the present authors is as follows:
A neoplasm in which both the primary and metastatic growths are characterized histologically by benign, innocuous-appearing SMA tissue components that lack any features of malignancy.

5.2.2 Histopathologic findings

Although a variety of histologic ameloblastoma subtypes are known, in MA cases, plexiform histopathologic types prevail, with 80% of metastatic lesions being either mixed or of the pure plexiform type (see chapter 5). Despite the fact that most MAs are of the plexiform type (Figs 22-2 and 22-3), it is not possible to predict metastatic potential. Further, instances of metastasis have arisen from sol-

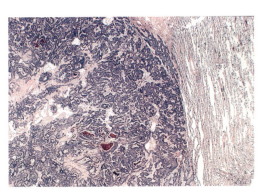

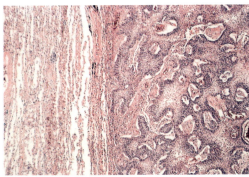

Fig 22-2 Metastasizing/malignant ameloblastoma of predominantly plexiform type. The tumor is that of a SMA in a fibrous stroma (hematoxylin-eosin [H&E], x60). (Courtesy of Professor J.J. Sciubba, Baltimore, MD.)

Fig 22-3 Malignant ameloblastoma (lung metastasis) from the same patient shown in Fig 22-2. Note how clearly the classic appearance of a benign ameloblastoma is retained (H&E, x60). (Courtesy of Professor J.J. Sciubba, Baltimore, MD.)

id invasive variants of ameloblastomas rather than from the unicystic type. In very rare cases the MA may be associated with fibrosarcoma (malignant mixed tumor).[17]

Ueda et al[5] studied the tumor doubling time of three metastatic nodules of MA. In this case, volume doubling time was constant among individual nodules from 129 days to 201 days. The semilog graph revealed a relatively parallel slope of tumor growth, indicating that the nodules were slow growing. It has been stated that patients with a tumor doubling time of 45 days or less had a significantly reduced survival expectancy after surgical treatment of metastasis of the lung.

5.2.3 Histochemical/immunohistochemical findings

The malignant ameloblastoma has not been studied by immunohistochemistry.

5.2.4 Ultrastructural findings

Studies on the ultrastructure of malignant ameloblastomas have not been published in the English literature.

6. Notes on treatment and recurrence rate

Adequate initial surgical treatment of the primary neoplasm plays the most important role in the prevention of postoperative metastasis. Radical resection with primary reconstruction of mandibular ameloblastomas has become the most accepted therapeutic concept.

Several modalities for the treatment of pulmonary metastasis of MAs have been used, but little has been published on these methods. The most common treatment of choice is surgery, although radiation and chemotherapy also have been described. Current strategies support the use of chemotherapy and radiation for palliative therapy and an aggressive surgical approach for treatable lesions.[7] Surgical treatment consists of local excision or lobectomy. Computed tomography—guided fine-needle aspiration or biopsy techniques may be used in preoperative histologic/cytologic diagnosis. Multiple metastases may only be removed if sufficient pulmonary reserve is maintained.

Radiation therapy has shown high recurrence rates.[7] Laughlin[4] recommended radiation only for inoperable metastatic lesions. Eliasson et al[18] discussed the limitations of chemotherapy in detail. Chemotherapy has been shown to have a palliative effect and may in some cases reduce the size of the tumor, but based on their review of MAs and lung metastasis, Henderson et al[7] could not see a role for chemotherapy as a primary treatment of MAs.

The median disease-free interval between initial presentation and the occurrence of metastasis of MA was 9 years in the review by Laughlin.[4] Of the 43 patients he studied, 19 (44.2%) were known to have died of the tumor and/or metastasis. The time from initial diagnosis to the detection of pulmonary metastasis ranged from 3 months to 31 years, with a median disease-free period of 9 to 12 years. The median survival time after treatment of the primary tumor ranged from 11 to 14 years. After the diagnosis of metastasis, median survival ranged from 3 months to 5 years.[7] The longest survival time recorded after the appearance of metastatic disease was 25 years.[8]

As with many other malignant odontogenic neoplasms, knowledge and experience is still limited in cases of malignant ameloblastomas. Therefore, Henderson et al[7] recommended continued reporting of such cases to fully understand the mechanism and optimal treatment methods for MAs.

References

1. Reichart PA, Philipsen HP, Sonner S. Ameloblastoma: Biological profile of 3677 cases. Eur J Cancer B Oral Oncol 1995;31B:86–99.

2. Emura M. A case of metastatic ameloblastoma. Jpn J Surg 1923;24:760–764.

3. Vorzimer J, Perla D. An instance of adamantinoma of the jaw with metastasis of the right lung. Am J Pathol 1932;8:445–453.

4. Laughlin EH. Metastasizing ameloblastoma. Cancer 1989;64:776–780.

5. Ueda M, Kaneda T, Imaizumi M, Abe T. Mandibular ameloblastoma with metastasis to the lungs and lymph nodes: A case report and review of the literature. J Oral Maxillofac Surg 1989;47:623–628.

6. Ameerally P, McGurk M, Shaheen O. Atypical ameloblastoma: Report of 3 cases and review of the literature. Br J Oral Maxillofac Surg 1996;34:235–239.

7. Henderson J, Sonnet JR, Schlesinger C, Ord RA. Pulmonary metastasis of ameloblastoma: Case report and review of the literature. Oral Surg Oral Med Oral Pathol 1999;88:170–176.

8. Houston G, Davenport W, Keaton W, Harris St. Malignant (metastatic) ameloblastoma. Report of a case. J Oral Maxillofac Surg 1993;51:1152–1155.

9. Duffey DC, Bailet JW, Newman A. Ameloblastoma of the mandible with cervical lymph node metastasis. Am J Otolaryngol 1995;16:66–73.

10. Harada K, Kayano T, Nagura H, Enomoto S. Ameloblastoma with metastasis to the lung and associated hypercalcemia. J Oral Maxillofac Surg 1989;47:1083–1087.

11. Sugiyama M, Ogawa I, Katayama K, Ishikawa T. Simultaneous metastatic ameloblastoma and thyroid carcinoma in the cervical region: Report of a case. J Oral Maxillofac Surg 1999;57:1255–1258.

12. Weir M, Centeno BA, Szyfelbein WM. Cytological features of malignant metastatic ameloblastoma: A case report and differential diagnosis. Diagn Cytopathol 1998;18:125–130.

13. Witterick IJ, Parikh S, Mancer K, Gullane PJ. Malignant ameloblastoma. Am J Otolaryngol 1996;17:122–126.

14. Eisenberg E. Malignant (metastatic) ameloblastoma: Report of a case. J Oral Maxillofac Surg 1983;51:1156–1157.

15. Cranin AN, Bennett J, Solomon M, Quarcoo S. Massive granular cell ameloblastoma with metastasis: Report of a case. J Oral Maxillofac Surg 1987;45:800–804.

16. Eversole LR. Malignant epithelial odontogenic tumors. Semin Diagn Pathol 1999;16:317–324.

17. Tanaka T, Ohkubo T, Jujitsuka H, et al. Malignant mixed tumor (malignant ameloblastoma and fibrosarcoma) of the maxilla. Arch Pathol Lab Med 1991;115:84–87.

18. Eliasson MAH, Roy MJ, Tenholder CMF. Diagnosis and treatment of metastatic ameloblastoma. Metastatic ameloblastoma. South Med J 1998; 82:1165–1168.

Chapter 23

Ameloblastic Carcinoma (Primary, Secondary [Dedifferentiated] Intraosseous; Secondary [Dedifferentiated] Extraosseous)

1. Terminology

Carcinomas derived from ameloblastomas have been classified a number of ways, including *malignant ameloblastoma, ameloblastic carcinoma, metastatic ameloblastoma,* and *primary intra-alveolar epidermoid carcinoma.*[1] The term *ameloblastic carcinoma* (AC) was introduced by Shafer in 1974.[2] The World Health Organization (WHO) classifications of 1971[3] and 1992[4] do not include this term in the section on odontogenic carcinomas.

In 1987, Corio et al[1] reported eight cases of ACs from the U.S. Armed Forces Institute of Pathology (Washington DC). These authors classified ameloblastic carcinomas as "any ameloblastoma in which there is histologic evidence of malignancy in the primary or the recurrent tumor, regardless of whether it has metastasized." The ameloblastic carcinoma is currently defined as a malignant epithelial odontogenic tumor that histologically has retained the features of ameloblastic differentiation, yet also exhibits cytologic features of malignancy.[5] Primary and secondary (dedifferentiated) intra- and extraosseous AC variants have been described in the literature.

In 1991 Nagai et al[6] reviewed the literature on ameloblastic carcinomas and found 46 cases, but features of individual cases were not shown. Lolachi et al[7] reported on 34 cases of ACs from the English language literature and one of their own. Small series of ACs were reported by Lau et al[8] (two cases) and Infante-Cossio et al[9] (three cases). Single case reports were published by Slootweg and Müller,[10] Andersen and Bang,[11] Lee et al,[12] Bruce and Jackson,[13] Ingram et al,[14] and Simko et al.[15] Recently, Cox et al[16] described a case of ameloblastic carcinoma with malignancy-associated hypercalcemia; a peripheral AC was reported by McClatchey et al[17]; and Kao et al[18] described the case of an odontogenic carcinoma with distant metastasis which, according to the histology, could probably also represent an AC.

2. Clinical and radiologic profile

Common clinical signs and symptoms of ameloblastic carcinomas include swelling, pain, trismus, and dysphonia.[5] Rapid growth of the tumor is another important clinical finding. Mental nerve paresthesia may also occur.[7] In cases of maxillary ACs the most frequent clinical complaint is a mass in the cheek, but other clinical findings such as pain, anesthesia of the infraorbital nerve, and a fistula in the palate have also been noted.

In rare cases[16] an AC may occur with malignancy-associated hypercalcemia. Hypercalcemia is considered a metabolic complication of malignancy and is divided into two

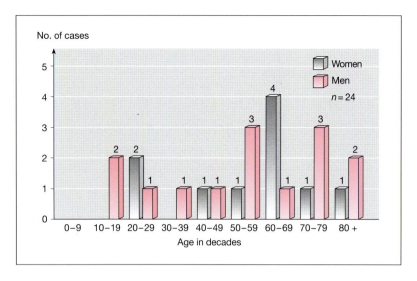

Fig 23-1 Age and gender distribution of 24 cases of ameloblastic carcinomas.

variants: humoral hypercalcemia of malignancy and local osteolytic hypercalcemia. Not more than four cases of MAHC-associated ACs have been reported.[16]

Principally, ameloblastic carcinomas may arise de novo, ex ameloblastoma, or ex odontogenic cyst. Most ACs are thought to have arisen de novo, with a few cases of malignant transformation of ameloblastomas being apparent. Such was the case described by Cox et al[16] in which multiple recurrences of a mandibular ameloblastoma occurred with the eventual development of an ameloblastic carcinoma in the same site as the previously diagnosed ameloblastoma. Ameloblastic carcinomas have been reported to metastasize to the lungs and to distant sites; however, in other cases with extended follow-up, metastasis has not been observed, regardless of the malignant histopathology.[1]

Radiologically, ameloblastic carcinomas may resemble SMAs, but in most cases they present as ill-defined radiolucencies. Foci of radiopacities, probably due to dystrophic calcification, have also been observed. Often lesions present with perforation of the cortical bone and may extend into the neighboring soft tissue; pathologic fractures may occur.[17] Axial and coronal CT scans may reveal cortical thinning, perforations, and soft tissue invasion.

3. Epidemiological data

3.1 Prevalence, incidence, and relative frequency

Cases of ameloblastic carcinomas are rare and no details on prevalence, incidence, or relative fequency are presently available. Compared to the metastasizing, malignant ameloblastoma, however, the AC seems to be more common (2:1).[6]

3.2 Age

The age distribution of 24 cases of ACs[1,6-18] is shown in Fig. 23-1. Ameloblastic carcinomas mainly affect the elderly, but the age range is 15 to 84 years.

3.3 Gender

The male:female ratio of 24 AC cases[1,6-18] was 1.4:1 (see Fig 23-1).

3.4 Location

The topographic distribution of 24 cases of AC[1,6-18] is shown in Fig 23-2; the majority of cases were found in the mandible.

4. Pathogenesis

The pathogenesis of ameloblastic carcinomas is not clear. They may originate ex ameloblastoma or ex odontogenic cyst, and both central (intraosseous) and peripheral (extraosseous) variants have been described. An ameloblastic carcinoma originating from the gingival or alveolar mucosa epithelium is very rare. *Peripheral* ACs may arise de novo and as dedifferentiated ACs from preexisting benign peripheral ameloblastomas.

Histomorphogenetically, two different AC entities may be recognized. One is characterized by lesions that initially demonstrate the morphology of a SMA but *dedifferentiate* over time. Dedifferentiation may occur spontaneously or be related to surgical procedures that become necessary due to recurrences of the primary tumor or therapeutic radiation. The second entity comprises those ACs that have *malignant cytologic features* de novo. Among the cases of ACs reviewed by Slootweg and Müller,[10] there were two cases in which the metastasis exhibited a less differentiated pattern than the primary tumor. In nine cases, the primary tumor and metastasis exhibited dedifferentiation. In 14 cases, the primary ameloblastoma had undergone anaplastic transformation but metastatic disease was not present or, if present, was not histologically proven.

5. Pathology

5.1 Macroscopy

Few descriptions of the macroscopic aspects of ACs have been published. Cox et al[16] described a large AC specimen measuring 17 x 16 x 13 cm and weighing 1,875 g. The internal portion of the tumor was tan-yellow with a necrotic and friable appearance; several large cystic spaces were noted within the necrotic area. In another case,[7] the cut surface of the tumor was gray-white and smooth with a central cystic area.

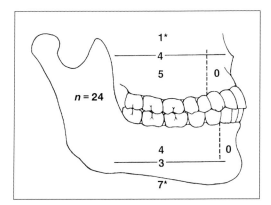

Fig 23-2 Topographic distribution of 24 cases of ameloblastic carcinoma. Asterisk indicates that no specific location was given.

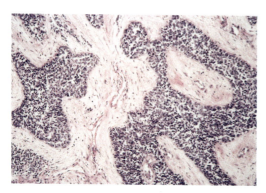

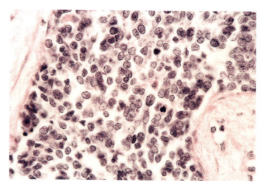

Fig 23-3 Islands and cords of highly cellular odontogenic (ameloblastomatous) epithelium in a mature fibrous stroma. Peripheral palisading is not obvious (hematoxylin-eosin [H&E], x80). (Courtesy of DÖSAK, Professor G. Jundt, Basle, Switzerland.)

Fig 23-4 A higher magnification of the AC in Fig 23-3. Nuclear enlargement and hyperchromatism of the ameloblastomatous component are evident (H&E, x160).

5.2 Microscopy

5.2.1 Histologic definitions

The WHO classification of 1992[4] did not use the term *ameloblastic carcinoma*. However, the authors described this entity under the name *malignant ameloblastoma*, thus causing considerable confusion (see chapter 22).

The definition used by the present authors is as follows:

A neoplasm in which the histologic pattern of a SMA has been retained in the primary growth in the jaws and/or in any metastasic growth, yet also exhibits cytologic features of malignancy.

5.2.2 Histopathologic findings

The AC is composed of islands and cords of ameloblastomatous odontogenic epithelium in an infiltrative pattern within a stroma of mature fibrous tissue (Fig 23-3). The epithelium may reveal a single outer layer of ameloblastic cells of columnar to cuboidal shape which exhibit a tendency for palisading and reverse nuclear polarization; peripheral palisading and polarization are not always clearly evident. The stellate reticulum within epithelial islands is often condensed and hypercellular, presenting a less orderly pattern. The characteristic differentiating features are nuclear enlargement with granular stippled nucleoplasm, nuclear hyperchromatism, mild pleomorphism, an increased nuclear cytoplasmic ratio, and increased mitotic activity with abnormal forms of mitoses (Fig 23-4). Mitotic figures may attain a count of 2 to 5 per high-power field.[5] In some cases, individual cell keratinization and keratin pearl formation may be seen. Necrosis and dystrophic calcifications also may be observed in some of the epithelial islands, histologic features not usually characteristic for ameloblastomas. Different histologic patterns may be noted within the malignant component: highly differentiated squamous cells or a more basaloid, poorly differentiated variety.[1] The connective tissue is usually composed of mature collagen fibers with occasional inflammatory cells, hemorrhage, and/or hemosiderin pigment.

In rare cases, ameloblastic carcinomas may reveal *clear cell* differentiation. These tumors demonstrate tumor islands with peripheral palisading of columnar or cuboidal cells with reversed nuclear polarity. Prominent clear cells may be observed within follicular epithelial islands. The clear cell component may be misinterpreted as a salivary gland clear cell adenocarcinoma, a mucoepidermoid carcinoma, or a metastatic neoplasm. Although only a few cases of the clear cell variant of AC have been described, they seem to have an aggressive clinical course.

Bruce and Jackson[13] have drawn attention to the difficulty in differentiating between the histologic appearance of the primary intraosseous squamous cell carcinoma and the AC. In this context, Corio et al[1] stated that "Although the primary intra-alveolar carcinoma (PISC) and the ameloblastic carcinoma exhibit some clinical differences, their histological features are similar enough to suggest a histogenetic relationship. It is possible then that the primary intra-alveolar carcinoma (PISC) may represent simply a less differentiated, usually non-keratinizing form of ameloblastic carcinoma, both lesions being derived from odontogenic epithelial remnants."

In a few cases, fine-needle aspiration cytology has been applied for the initial diagnosis of AC.[14]

5.2.3 Histochemical/immunohistochemical findings

Systematic histochemical or immunohistochemical studies have not been performed with tissues derived from ameloblastic carcinomas. Lau et al[8] studied their two cases for the presence of cytokeratins and showed that the ameloblastomatous areas of the ACs reacted strongly with antibodies directed against cytokeratins CAM 5.2 and AE1 and AE3; the basaloid and spindle cells were

negative for these markers, as well as for vimentin, desmin, actin, and factor VIII. The entire tumor was negative for carcinoembryonic antigen (CEA).

Mueller et al[19] studied the DNA ploidy of ameloblastomas (SMAs) and ameloblastic carcinomas. Of the primary SMAs, 14 (82%) were diploid; 3 of 5 recurrent ameloblastomas were diploid. No significant differences in ploidy between primary and recurrent ameloblastomas or among plexiform, follicular, or acanthomatous ameloblastoma variants were demonstrated. Of five ACs, four were aneuploid; ploidy did not correlate significantly with the incidence of metastasis. Aneuploidy seems to be more common than ploidy in ACs and may be regarded as a strong predictor for malignant potential.

5.2.4 Ultrastructural findings

Ultrastructural studies on ameloblastic carcinomas have not been published to date.

6. Notes on treatment and recurrence rate

The rarity and unusual biologic behavior of ACs make it difficult to develop effective treatment protocols. However, the clinical course of these tumors is aggressive with extensive local destruction. The treatment of choice is radical surgery with neck dissection.[13] Some authors have recommended preoperative irradiation to decrease tumor size, but this seems to be of only limited value.[11] The resistance of ACs to radiotherapy has been described, but the significance of chemotherapy as a form of treatment is not clear.[13]

Local recurrences and metastasis to the neck and lung seem to be common,[13] and questions as to the modes of metastasis of ACs have been raised. Aspiration of malignant cells into the lung, hematogenous spread, and spread via lymphatics have all been proposed. Three of seven cases reported by Corio et al[1] had recurrences within 1 year. Patients with ACs in whom both the primary tumor and metastasis revealed dedifferentiation died within 2 years after metastasis.[10] Patients with maxillary ACs seem to have an even more serious prognosis.[12]

Survival of patients with ACs has to be evaluated over a long period of time due to the possibility of recurrence and the appearance of local and distant metastasis.

References

1. Corio RL, Goldblatt LI, Edwards PA, Hartmann KS. Ameloblastic carcinoma: A clinicopathologic study and assessment of eight cases. Oral Surg Oral Med Oral Pathol 1987;64:570–576.

2. Shafer WG, Hine MK, Levy BM. A Textbook of Oral Pathology. 3rd ed. Philadelphia: WB Saunders, 1974:254.

3. Pindborg JJ, Kramer IRH. Histologic Typing of Odontogenic Tumors, Jaw Cysts, and Allied Lesions. Berlin: Springer-Verlag, 1971.

4. Kramer IRH, Pindborg JJ, Shear M. Histological Typing of Odontogenic Tumours. 2d ed. Berlin: Springer-Verlag, 1992.

5. Eversole LR. Malignant epithelial odontogenic tumors. Semin Diagn Pathol 1999;16:317–324.

6. Nagai N, Takeshita N, Nagatsuka H, et al. Ameloblastic carcinoma: Case report and review. J Oral Pathol Med 1991;20:460–463.

7. Lolachi CM, Shashi K, Madan MD, Jacobs JR. Ameloblastic carcinoma of the maxilla. J Laryngol Otol 1995;109:1019–1022.

8. Lau S, Tideman H. Ameloblastic carcinoma of the jaws. A report of two cases. Oral Surg Oral Med Oral Pathol Oral Radiol Endod 1998;85:78–81.

9. Infante-Cossio P, Hernandez-Guisado JM, Fernandez-Machin P, et al. Ameloblastic carcinoma of the maxilla: A report of 3 cases. J Oral Maxillofac Surg 1998;26:159–162.

10. Slootweg PJ, Müller H. Malignant ameloblastoma or ameloblastic carcinoma. Oral Surg Oral Med Oral Pathol 1984;57:168–176.

11. Andersen E, Bang G. Ameloblastic carcinoma of the maxilla. J Maxillofac Surg 1986;14:338–340.

12. Lee L, Maxymiw WG, Wood RE. Ameloblastic carcinoma of the maxilla metastatic to the mandible. Case report. J Craniomaxillofac Surg 1990;18:247–250.

13. Bruce RA, Jackson IT. Ameloblastic carcinoma. Report of an aggressive case and review of the literature. J Craniomaxillofac Surg 1991;19:267–271.

14. Ingram EA, Evans ML, Zitsch RP. Fine-needle aspiration cytology of ameloblastic carcinoma of the maxilla: A rare tumor. Diagn Cytopathol 1996;14:249–252.

15. Simko EJ, Brannon RB, Eibling DE. Ameloblastic carcinoma of the mandible. Case report. Head Neck 1998;20:654–659.

16. Cox DP, Muller S, Carlson GW, Murray D. Ameloblastic carcinoma ex ameloblastoma of the mandible with malignancy-associated hypercalcemia. Oral Surg Oral Med Oral Pathol Oral Radiol Endod 2000;90:716–722.

17. McClatchey KD, Sullivan MJ, Paugh DR. Peripheral ameloblastic carcinoma: A case report of a rare neoplasm. J Otolaryngol 1989;18:109–111.

18. Kao SY, Pong BY, Li WY, et al. Maxillary odontogenic carcinoma with distant metastasis to axillary skin, brain, and lung: Case report. Int J Oral Maxillofac Surg 1995;24:229–232.

19. Mueller S, DeRose PB, Cohen C. DNA ploidy of ameloblastoma and ameloblastic carcinoma of the jaws. Analysis by image and flow cytometry. Arch Pathol Lab Med 1993;117:1126–1131.

Chapter 24

Primary Intraosseous Squamous Cell Carcinoma (Solid)

1. Terminology

According to Morrison and Deeley,[1] the central squamous cell carcinoma of the jaw was first described by Loos in 1913. In 1948, Willis[2] suggested the term *intra-alveolar epidermoid carcinoma*, and Shear[3] later revised this to *primary intra-alveolar epidermoid carcinoma*. Pindborg et al[4] suggested the term *primary intraosseous carcinoma*, which was accepted by the World Health Organization (WHO) classification of 1992.[5]

Primary intraosseous squamous cell carcinoma (PISC or PIOC) must be differentiated from other odontogenic carcinomas, such as malignant ameloblastomas and carcinomas arising from odontogenic cysts. Squamous cell carcinomas (SCCs) involving the jaw as an infiltration from the gingiva, alveolar ridge, floor of the mouth, or maxillary sinus or via metastases have to be excluded.

The primary intraosseous squamous cell carcinoma has been described, often incorrectly, under a variety of names, which include *primary epithelial tumor of the jaw, carcinoma of the jaw, central epidermoid carcinoma of the jaw, intra-alveolar carcinoma, intra-alveolar epidermoid carcinoma, central squamous cell carcinoma of the jaw, primary odontogenic carcinoma of the jaw, intramandibular carcinoma, central mandibular carcinoma, primary intra-alveolar epidermoid carcinoma*, and *primary intra-alveolar squamous cell carcinoma*.[6]

Primary intraosseous squamous cell carcinomas are rare. Elzay[6] reviewed the literature in 1982 and found 12 cases. Ohtake et al[7] published a series of 28 cases of central carcinomas in 1989 without clearly separating solid PISCs from cystogenic PISCs. Suei et al[8] reviewed the literature on PISCs in 1994, describing 39 cases from 24 publications; however, details of individual cases were not shown.[8] The most recent and comprehensive review of PISCs is that of Thomas et al,[9] who included one case of their own for a total of 29 cases. The cases described by Bridgeman et al[10] in 1996, Kaffe et al[11] in 1998, and Ide et al[12] in 1999 were not included in the cases reviewed by Thomas and coworkers. The latter case[9] is of interest because it was suggested that the tumor may have originated from reduced enamel epithelium.

2. Clinical and radiologic profile

Persistent symptoms like postextraction pain, toothache, periodontal disease, or pericoronitis were the presenting complaints reported by Thomas et al.[9] The diagnosis of PISC was delayed, mainly because the dental problems were given top priority and the underlying disease was missed. Other symp-

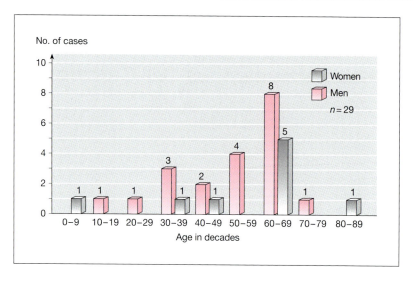

Fig 24-1 Age distribution of 29 cases of PISCs.[9]

toms were swelling, pain, and sensory disturbances. Since persistent pain and swelling of the jaw seem to be important presenting symptoms of PISCs, this diagnosis has to be considered in all cases where initial dental treatment has failed. The diagnosis of PISC is difficult, and an infectious etiology may often (wrongly) be considered. Once the histologic diagnosis of PISC has been made, metastatic disease has to be ruled out. Principally, the investigation of the primary tumor should include a chest radiograph to exclude lung metastasis.

The radiographic features of PISC were reviewed by Kaffe et al.[11] Osteolytic bone changes are characteristic. The margins of PISC lesions are poorly defined, diffuse, and irregular in most cases.

3. Epidemiological data

3.1 Prevalence, incidence, and relative frequency

Primary intraosseous squamous cell carcinomas of the jaw arising de novo are more rare than cystogenic PISCs (see chapter 26). Thomas et al[9] reviewed the English language literature in 2000 and found 29 acceptable cases. While there may be a few more cases hidden away in the international literature, the PISC still appears to be an extremely rare odontogenic lesion. Rates of prevalence, incidence, and relative frequency are not currently available.

3.2 Age

Primary intraosseous squamous cell carcinomas commonly occur in elderly patients. According to the review of Thomas et al,[9] the mean age of patients with PISCs ($n = 29$) was 53 years with a range of 4 to 81 years. Figure 24-1 shows the age distribution of these cases.

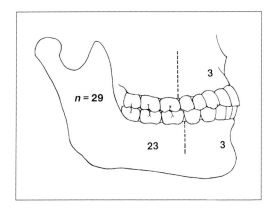

Fig 24-2 Topographic distribution of 29 cases of PISC.[9]

3.3 Gender

Of 29 cases of PISCs,[9] 20 were men and 9 women; the male:female ratio is 2.2:1. The male predominance is in agreement with previous reviews.[6,11]

3.4 Location

The distribution of PISCs according to location is shown in Fig 24-2. The majority of 29 cases were located in the posterior mandible. Six cases occurred in the midlines of the maxilla and mandible, three in each jaw.

4. Pathogenesis

The etiology and pathogenesis of PISCs are unknown. However, the cells of origin are odontogenic epithelial cells consisting of the reduced enamel epithelium, the rests of Malassez in the periodontal ligament and in the alveolar bone subsequent to tooth loss, and remnants of the dental lamina in the gingiva. Eversole[13] suggested that future studies should focus on disturbances in cell cycling, proto-oncogene expression, and tumor suppressor gene mutations to gain a better understanding of the pathogenesis of malignancy. To study the pathogenesis of PISCs, however, is particularly difficult because of their rarity.

5. Pathology

5.1 Macroscopy

Details on the macroscopic appearance of PISCs have not been published.

5.2 Microscopy

5.2.1 Histologic definition

Both the 1992 WHO classification[5] and the present authors define the PISC as follows: A squamous cell carcinoma arising within the jaw, having no initial connection with the oral mucosa, and presumably developing from residues of odontogenic epithelium.

5.2.2 Histopathologic findings

Some of the reported cases of PISCs have revealed histologic features of squamous cell carcinomas which were indistinguishable from SCCs of the oral mucosa. In such cases, a definitive diagnosis may be impossible without reliable clinical and radiographic data. Primary intraosseous squamous cell carcinomas may reveal a distinct odontogenic pattern with basal-type cells forming alveoli or arranged in a plexiform pattern with palisading of the peripheral cells. The nuclei of these cells are often oriented away from

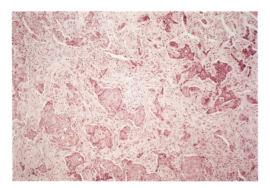

Fig 24-3 Primary intraosseous squamous cell carcinoma exhibiting irregular islands of well-differentiated SCC (hematoxylin-eosin, x40). (Courtesy of DÖSAK, Professor G. Jundt, Basle, Switzerland.)

the basement membrane. Squamous metaplasia and keratinization, as observed in acanthomatous ameloblastomas, may be seen. In a few cases, foci of central necrosis or degeneration within the epithelial islands have been observed. Since the histologic characteristics of PISCs are not pathognomonic, a diagnosis can be made only if there is no evidence of the tumor arising from either the oral mucosa or from an odontogenic cyst. Serial section of the main specimen has been recommended to exclude other origins of SCCs. Further, PISC has to be differentiated from metastatic tumors and from primary intraosseous mucoepidermoid carcinomas (Fig 24-3).

5.2.3 Histochemical/immunohistochemical findings

No detailed histochemical or immunohistochemical studies of PISCs have been published.

5.2.4 Ultrastructural findings

Ruskin et al[14] published electron micrographs of PISCs with their two case reports. The histologic diagnosis of well-differentiated SCC was supported by ultrastructural findings. The squamous epithelial cells revealed prominent desmosomal connections and large irregular nuclei with prominent nucleoli.

6. Notes on treatment and recurrence rate

Of the 29 cases evaluated by Thomas et al,[9] 14 were treated with surgery as the primary modality. Seven patients received combination therapies (surgery and radiotherapy, surgery and chemotherapy, etc). Out of 14 patients treated surgically, 11 underwent hemimandibulectomy in conjunction with a radical or modified radical neck dissection. Ten (34.5%) of 29 patients had lymph node metastasis.

Radical surgery is accepted as the primary mode of therapy for PISCs. Involvement of the lymph nodes requires block resection combined with the excision of the primary tumor.

The prognosis for patients with PISCs is difficult to determine because of the small number of reported cases, the different treatment modalities, and the variable follow-up time (from 5 to 60 months in the review by Thomas et al[9]). The 5-year survival rate of patients with PISCs has been reported as between 30% and 40%.[3] Of the 12 patients evaluated by Elzay,[6] 40% had a 2-year survival. To et al[15] stated that involvement of the lymph nodes did not affect the prognosis, as is the case for oral SCCs. In addition, it was noted that patients with a delayed diagnosis seem to have a poor prognosis.

References

1. Morrison R, Deeley TJ. Intra alveolar carcinoma of the jaw: Treatment by supervoltage radiotherapy. Br J Radiol 1964;35:321–326.

2. Willis RA. Pathology of tumors. London: CV Mosby, 1948:310–316.

3. Shear M. Primary intra-alveolar epidermoid carcinoma of the jaw. J Pathol 1969;97:645–651.

4. Pindborg JJ, Kramer IRH. Histologic Typing of Odontogenic Tumours, Jaw Cysts and Allied Lesions. Berlin: Springer-Verlag, 1971.

5. Kramer IRH, Pindborg JJ, Shear M. Histological Typing of Odontogenic Tumours. 2d ed. Berlin: Springer-Verlag, 1992.

6. Elzay RP. Primary intraosseous carcinoma of the jaws. Review and update of odontogenic carcinomas. Oral Surg Oral Med Oral Pathol 1982;54:299–303.

7. Ohtake K, Yokobayashi Y, Shingaki S, et al. Central carcinoma of the jaw. A survey of 28 cases in the Japanese literature. J Craniomaxillofac Surg 1989;17:155–161.

8. Suei Y, Tanimoto K, Taguchi A, Wada T. Primary intraosseous carcinoma: Review of the literature and diagnostic criteria. J Oral Maxillofac Surg 1994;52:580–583.

9. Thomas G, Sreelatha KT, Balan A, Ambika K. Primary intraosseous carcinoma of the mandible—a case report and review of the literature. Eur J Surg Oncol 2000;26:82–86.

10. Bridgeman A, Wiesenfeld D, Buchanan M, et al. A primary intraosseous carcinoma of the anterior maxilla. Report of a new case. Int J Oral Maxillofac Surg 1996;25:279–281.

11. Kaffe I, Ardekian L, Peled M, et al. Radiological features of primary intraosseous carcinoma of the jaw. Analysis of the literature and report of a new case. Dentomaxillofac Radiol 1998;27:209–214.

12. Ide F, Shimoyama IF, Horie N, Kaneko T. Primary intraosseous carcinoma of the mandible with probable origin from reduced enamel epithelium. J Oral Pathol Med 1999;28:420–422.

13. Eversole LR. Malignant epithelial odontogenic tumors. Semin Diagn Pathol 1999;16:317–324.

14. Ruskin JD, Cohen DM, Davis LF. Primary intraosseous carcinoma: Report of two cases. J Oral Maxillofac Surg 1988;46:425–432.

15. To EHW, Brown JS, Avery BS, Ward-Booth RP. Primary intraosseous carcinoma of the jaw. Three new cases and a review of the literature. Br J Oral Maxillofac Surg 1991;29:19–25.

Primary Intraosseous Squamous Cell Carcinoma Derived from Odontogenic Cysts

1. Terminology

In rare cases, primary intraosseous squamous cell carcinomas (PISCs) may arise from the epithelial lining of odontogenic cysts. Either nonkeratinizing or odontogenic keratocysts now termed *keratinizing cystic odontogenic tumor* (KCOT) (see chapter 26) may be the origin of PISCs. The total number of reported cases of PISCs ex odontogenic cysts is difficult to determine because diagnostic criteria have been missing. The fact that a number of cases have been published as possible or probable cases of PISCs ex odontogenic cysts is a clear indication that it is sometimes difficult to prove conclusively that a PISC has developed from the lining of a cyst.[1,2] Eversole et al[3] critically reviewed the literature on PISCs ex odontogenic cysts and accepted 36 cases, of which 33 were excluded because of insufficient data. In 1989, Waldron and Mustoe[2] added another 13 cases that had been published since 1973 and added their own probable case. Schwimmer et al[4] summarized the clinical data of 56 previously reported cases in addition to a case of their own. As early as 1975, Gardner[5] stated that to establish that the malignancy was primary in the cyst, one must demonstrate the transition of the epithelial lining of the cyst to carcinoma in situ and to invasive carcinoma. Recently, Berens et al[6] published a case of PISC ex odontogenic cyst. In their accompanying literature review, the authors found 31 well-documented cases in which transition between the normal cyst epithelium and the squamous cell carcinoma was demonstrated histologically.

2. Clinical and radiologic profile

Clinical symptoms are nonspecific and include pain and swelling. Cases in which the mandible is affected may involve expansion of the cortical plates. Cervical lymphadenopathy has also been reported. Paresthesia or anesthesia is uncommon but may occur after local invasion of the inferior alveolar nerve.

Radiologically, PISCs ex odontogenic cysts are nonspecific and are characterized by a radiolucency surrounded by a relatively well-defined radiopaque border (Figs 25-1 and 25-2).

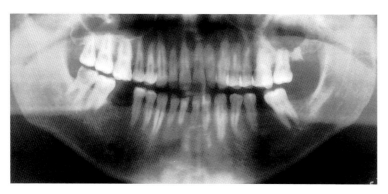

Fig 25-1 Panoramic radiograph of a 40-year-old man with a well-defined cystic lesion in the left maxilla. A tentative diagnosis of radicular (residual) cyst was made. The patient did not return for treatment.

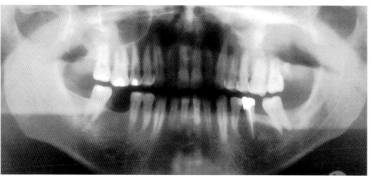

Fig 25-2 Panoramic radiograph of the same lesion shown in Fig 25-1 after 2 years. The border of the enlarged radiolucent lesion was ill defined. Histopathology revealed a PISC ex odontogenic cyst.

3. Epidemiological data

3.1 Prevalence, incidence, and relative frequency

The PISC ex odontogenic cyst is rare. Incidence has been estimated at 0.31% to 3%.[7] Other estimates say that one case per million population may occur.[8]

3.2 Age

The median age of 56 reported cases[4] was 57 years, with a range of 4 to 90 years; 5.4% occurred in the first two decades, 25.0% in the 3rd to 5th decades, and 69.9% in the 6th to 8th decades. Data for a detailed age distribution are not readily available.

3.3 Gender

Of 51 cases of PISC ex odontogenic cysts, 33.9% were women and 66.1% were men with a male:female ratio of 1:1.8.[4]

3.4 Location

Of 56 cases of PISC ex odontogenic cysts,[4] 42 (80.3%) cases were located in the mandible and 14 (19.7%) in the maxilla. The ratio of mandibular to maxillary lesions was 3:1. In the review by Berens et al,[6] 19 cases were located in the mandible and 9, including their own case, were maxillary lesions (mandible:maxilla ratio, 2:1).

4. Pathogenesis

The pathogenesis and etiology of PISC ex odontogenic cysts is unknown. Long-standing chronic inflammatory changes have been proposed as possible predisposing factors of malignant transformation of the epithelial lining of the cyst, but this cannot be substantiated. Some reports have emphasized that keratinization of the cyst epithelium may be associated with a higher risk of transformation[4] (see chapter 26).

5. Pathology

5.1 Macroscopy

Detailed reports on the macroscopic appearance of PISC ex odontogenic cysts have not been published. The cystic nature of the lesions, however, is evident in all cases.

5.2 Microscopy

5.2.1 Histologic definition

No particular definition for PISC ex odontogenic cyst has been published by the World Health Organization (1992). However, the basic criterion for the diagnosis of this type of lesion is that the transition between normal cyst epithelium and squamous cell carcinoma has to be demonstrated histologically. Thus, the present authors use the following definition:
A squamous cell carcinoma arising from the epithelial lining of an odontogenic cyst.

5.2.2 Histopathologic findings

Primary squamous cell carcinomas may arise from a variety of cysts. Schwimmer et al[4] reviewed 56 cysts associated with PISC ex odontogenic cyst and found the majority (37.5%) of cysts to be of the inflammatory residual type, 17.8% were keratinized residual cysts, 19.7% were follicular cysts, and 17.8% were apical or lateral radicular cysts. The remaining 7.2% of the cysts were not classified. Eversole[9] doubted that the lateral periodontal cyst was place of origin for PISCs.

Dysplastic changes of the stratified squamous epithelium are common and include pleomorphism, increased mitotic activity, dropping off of bulbous rete ridges, hyperchromatism, and cellular crowding. Secondary squamous epithelial changes such as pseudoepitheliomatous hyperplasia, acanthosis, and hyperkeratosis also may be observed (Figs 25-3 to 25-7). Foci of invasion of the cyst epithelium may be evident in early cases of PISCs. In advanced cases, solid tumor islands may invade the fibrous cyst wall and alveolar bone. Most carcinomas arising from cyst epithelium are well or mod-

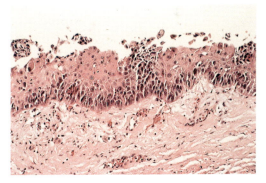

Fig 25-3 Nonkeratinizing odontogenic cyst (residual type) with carcinoma in situ of the epithelial lining. Only a slight inflammatory reaction is seen in the connective tissue wall (hematoxylineosin (H&E], x80). (Courtesy of Professor J.J. Sciubba, Baltimore, MD.)

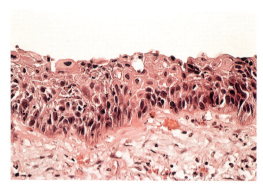

Fig 25-4 Higher magnification of a different area of the cyst lining shown in Fig 25-3. Notice severe epithelial dysplasia with nuclear hyperchromatism, cellular polymorphism, and loss of intercellular cohesion. The basal membrane is still intact (H&E, x120). (Courtesy of Professor J.J. Sciubba, Baltimore, MD.)

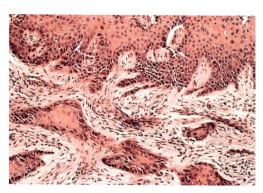

Fig 25-5 Epithelial lining of a nonkeratinized cyst exhibiting infiltrative squamous cell carcinoma arising from cyst epithelium (H&E, x80). (Courtesy of Professor J.J. Sciubba, Baltimore, MD.)

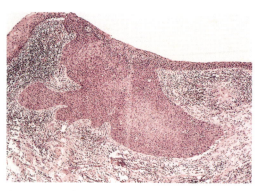

Fig 25-6 Squamous cell carcinoma arising from the reduced enamel epithelium of a retained tooth (H&E, x60). (Courtesy of Professor P.J. Slootweg, Utrecht, The Netherlands.)

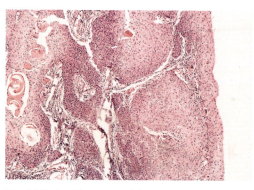

Fig 25-7 Another area of the same lesion shown in Fig 25-6. The well-differentiated squamous cell carcinoma is evident (H&E, x80).

erately well differentiated.[9] The fibrous capsule of the cyst may be thickened as a result of chronic inflammation. When histologically evaluating an odontogenic cyst for the occurrence of primary malignancy, other possibilities—such as the invasion of the cyst lining from an adjacent primary or metastatic carcinoma and cystic degenerative changes that have occurred in a primary or metastatic carcinoma—must be excluded.

5.2.3 Histochemical/immunohistochemical findings

Primary intraosseous squamous cell carcinomas arising from nonkeratinizing odontogenic cysts have rarely been studied with special staining methods. Recently, McDonald et al[10] found a squamous cell carcinoma ex odontogenic cyst to be p53 positive.

5.2.4 Ultrastructural findings

No studies on the ultrastructure of PISC ex odontogenic cysts have been published in the English language literature.

6. Notes on treatment and recurrence rate

Since odontogenic cysts with PISC cannot be differentiated clinically and radiographically from conventional cysts, most of them are enucleated at first-stage surgery. After the histopathologic diagnosis has been established the treatment of choice for the PISC ex odontogenic cyst is radical surgery. Treatment has varied, however, depending on the degree of invasion noted at biopsy and the presence or absence of lymph node metastasis. Larger lesions require mandibulectomy, maxillectomy, or partial resection of the affected jaw with lymph node dissection to radical neck dissection.

The 2-year survival rate of patients with PISC ex odontogenic cysts varies among different studies[6] from 53% to 80%. Figures on recurrence rates have not been indicated in the majority of reported cases.

References

1. Hampl PF, Harrigan WF. Squamous cell carcinoma arising from an odontogenic cyst: Report of case. J Oral Surg 1973;31:359–362.

2. Waldron C, Mustoe TA. Primary intraosseous carcinoma of the mandible with probable origin in an odontogenic cyst. Oral Surg Oral Med Oral Pathol 1989;67:716–724.

3. Eversole LR, Sabes WR, Rovin S. Aggressive growth and neoplastic potential of odontogenic cysts. Cancer 1975;35:270–281.

4. Schwimmer AM, Aydin F, Morrison SN. Squamous cell carcinoma arising in residual odontogenic cyst. Report of a case and review of literature. Oral Surg Oral Med Oral Pathol 1991;72:218–221.

5. Gardner AF. A survey of odontogenic cysts and their relationship to squamous cell carcinoma. J Can Dent Assoc 1975;3:161–167.

6. Berens A, Kramer JF, Kuettner C, et al. Entstehung eines Plattenepithelkarzinoms auf dem Boden einer odontogenen Zyste. Mund Kiefer Gesichtschir 2000;4:330–334.

7. Fanibunda K, Soames JV. Malignant and premalignant change in odontogenic cysts. J Oral Maxillofac Surg 1995;53:1469–1472.

8. Otten J-E, Joos U, Schilli W. Karzinomentstehung auf dem Boden des zystenbildenden odontogenen Epithels. Dtsch Zahnärztl Z 1985;40:544–547.

9. McDonald AR, Progrel A, Carson J, Regezi J. p53-positive squamous cell carcinoma originating from an odontogenic cyst. J Oral Maxillofac Surg 1996;54:216–218.

Primary Intraosseous Squamous Cell Carcinoma Derived from Keratinizing Cystic Odontogenic Tumor

1. Terminology

Primary intraosseous squamous cell carcinomas (PISCs) ex keratinizing cystic odontogenic tumors (KCOTs) are very rare when compared to PISCs arising from other odontogenic (nonkeratinizing) jaw cysts (see chapter 25). Before 1992, only 6 cases of PISCs arising from KCOTs had been described.[1] Additional cases were published by Yoshida et al,[2] Dabbs et al,[3] Hennis et al,[4] and Foley et al.[5] Cases of squamous cell carcinomas (SCCs) arising from KCOTs in patients with Gorlin syndrome have been described by Ramsden and Barrett[6] as well as Moos and Rennie.[7] Herbener et al[8] reported a case of juxtaposed KCOT and squamous cell carcinoma. Although some morphologic similarities between the KCOT and the tumor were observed, definitive evidence of a common origin was not demonstrable.

To qualify as a PISC, there must be no initial connection with the oral mucosa, overlying skin, or antral or nasal mucosa. The possibility that the PISC represents a metastasis from a distant primary tumor must be ruled out by physical and radiographic (computed tomography and magnetic resonance imagery) examination, and the subsequent clinical course. As with the PISC ex odontogenic cyst, the only criterion that proves that a squamous cell carcinoma has arisen from a KCOT is the demonstration of direct transition from the normal epithelial lining to invasive carcinoma.

2. Clinical and radiologic profile

Since there seem to be less than a dozen acceptable cases of PISCs ex odontogenic keratocysts in the English language literature, specific clinical and radiographic criteria of these tumors are still unclear and may not be very different from those of PISCs ex odontogenic cysts (see chapter 25) (Figs 26-1 to 26-3).

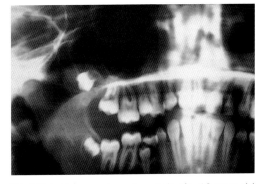

Fig 26-1 Panoramic radiograph of a 13-year-old boy with a displaced maxillary right third molar. The borders of the floor of the maxillary sinus are indistinct. (Courtesy of Professor W. Wagner, Mainz, Germany.)

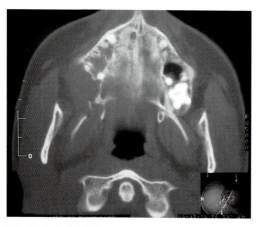

Fig 26-2 Axial CT scan (same as Fig 26-1) showing destruction of the right posterior maxilla. (Courtesy of Professor W. Wagner, Mainz, Germany.)

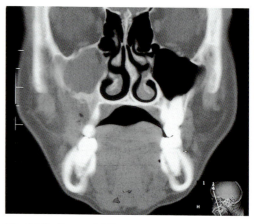

Fig 26-3 Coronal CT scan showing destruction of the right maxillary sinus with a homogeneous radiopaque mass filling the entire sinus. (Courtesy of Professor W. Wagner, Mainz, Germany.)

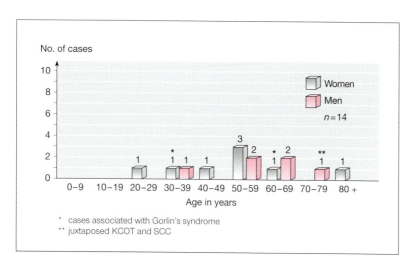

* cases associated with Gorlin's syndrome
** juxtaposed KCOT and SCC

Fig 26-4 Age distribution of 14 cases of PISC ex KCOTs.

3. Epidemiological data

3.1 Prevalence, incidence, and relative frequency

Since the number of well-documented cases of PISCs ex KCOTs is extremely small, no figures on prevalence, incidence, or relative frequency are available.

3.2 Age

Figure 26-4 shows the distribution of 14 cases of PISC ex KCOTs. Although the sample is small, cases tend to involve mainly elderly patients.

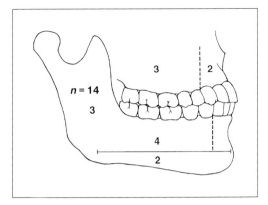

Fig 26-5 Topographic distribution of 14 cases of PISC ex KCOTs.

3.3 Gender

The male:female ratio of tumors in 14 patients was 1.3:1. These are our own (non-published) data prepared for this book.

3.4 Location

Figure 26-5 shows the topographic distribution of 14 cases. Two cases involved the entire mandible.

4. Pathogenesis

Although the epithelium of the KCOT seems to have a higher mitotic activity than that of other odontogenic cysts, there is little evidence that the KCOT is associated with malignant change more often than any other type of odontogenic cyst. In fact, the potential for malignant transformation in KCOTs seems to be quite low. Browne and Gouch[9]

suggested that keratin metaplasia, followed by epithelial hyperplasia and development of epithelial dysplasia of cyst epithelia, were the significant events in the development of SCCs in odontogenic cysts. It was also suggested that cyst linings that reveal keratinization were at greater risk for development of SCCs. Furthermore, while there are several well-documented cases in which a KCOT and an SCC are juxtaposed,[8] it was not possible to determine whether these represent malignant transformation within the cyst or collision of two pathogenetically distinct entities. As with PISC in odontogenic cysts, there is a relative dearth of pathogenetic information for PISC ex odontogenic keratocysts. The same (unknown) factors that lead to transformation of cyst epithelium in nonkeratinizing cysts may also be relevant for KCOTs.

5. Pathology

5.1 Macroscopy

No detailed descriptions of the macroscopic aspects of PISC ex KCOTs have been published.

5.2 Microscopy

5.2.1 Histologic definitions

No specific definition of PISC ex KCOTs was proposed by the World Health Organization (WHO) classification of 1992,[10] although the odontogenic keratocyst—as it was known until now—as an entity was defined as "a cyst arising in the tooth-bearing areas of the jaws, or posterior to the mandibular third molar, and characterized by a thin fibrous capsule and a lining of keratinised stratified epithelium usually about five to eight cells in thickness and generally without rete ridges."

The definition of PISC ex KCOT used by the present authors is as follows: "A squamous cell carcinoma arising from the epithelial lining of a keratinizing cystic odontogenic tumor."

5.2.2 Histopathologic findings

In order to confirm a histologic diagnosis of PISC ex KCOT, the histologic criteria of the KCOT and the transition of the normal cyst epithelium of KCOT to SCC have to be demonstrated. The PISC ex KCOT may develop from parakeratinized or orthokeratinized cyst epithelium. Minic[1] claimed to have described the first case of PISC ex KCOT from orthokeratinized cyst epitheli-

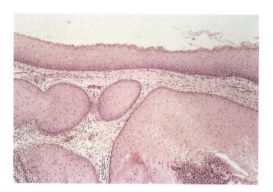

Fig 26-6 KCOT with infiltrating large islands of well-differentiated squamous cell carcinomas (same patient shown in Figs 26-1 to 26-3) (hematoxylin-eosin [H&E], x50).

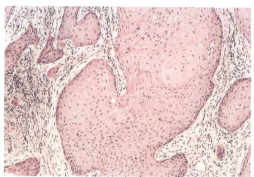

Fig 26-7 Higher magnification of the tumor in Fig 26-6 showing infiltrating large and small, predominantly well-differentiated squamous cell carcinoma islands (H&E, x80).

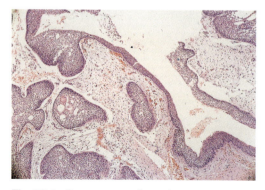

Fig 26-8 Squamous cell carcinoma ex KCOT. The transition zone between the cyst lining of the KCOT and several islands of the SCC is clear (H&E, x25). (Courtesy of Professor P.J. Slootweg, Utrecht, The Netherlands.)

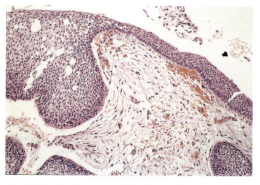

Fig 26-9 Higher magnification of the transitional zone revealing squamous cell carcinomas that have arisen from the cyst lining of the KCOT (H&E, x60). (Courtesy of Professor P.J. Slootweg, Utrecht, The Netherlands.)

um.[1] Epithelial dysplasia of varying degrees are often found. Histopathologic features of cystogenic SCCs parallel the progressive changes from dysplasia to SCC that typically occur in precancerous lesions of the oral mucosa.[11] It is of further interest that metastasis to cervical and submandibular lymph nodes occurs in up to 50% of reported cases of PISC ex odontogenic cysts; indeed, an enlarged lymph node may be the initial presenting sign of a cystogenic SCC (Figs 26-6 to 26-9).

5.2.3 Histochemical/immunohistochemical findings

No histochemical or immunohistochemical studies have been published on the PISC ex KCOT. However, High et al[12] examined the DNA content of a KCOT and the subsequent SCC. Using flow cytometry, they were able to show a prominent, abnormal DNA stemline in the KCOT, which was also present in the subsequent SCC.

5.2.4 Ultrastructural findings

Herbener et al[8] studied the ultrastructure of a KCOT and a juxtaposed SCC. At the ultrastructural level, some of the cells observed in both the KCOT and the SCC had a remarkable resemblance to ameloblasts of developing teeth and ameloblast-like cells of ameloblastoma. The authors saw some indications of a possible relationship between the KCOT and SCC, but their observations were not sufficient to support a conclusion of a shared origin.

6. Notes on treatment and recurrence rate

The treatment of choice for the PISC ex KCOT is radical surgery with neck dissection of lymph nodes. Due to the small number of cases of PISC ex KCOTs, no relevant information on recurrence rate, frequency of metastasis, or prognosis are available. Long-term follow-up, as with patients with oral cancer, is mandatory.

References

1. Minic AJ. Primary intraosseous squamous cell carcinoma arising in a mandibular keratocyst. Int J Oral Maxillofac Surg 199;21:163–165.

2. Yoshida H, Onizawa K, Yusa H. Squamous cell carcinoma arising in association with an orthokeratinized odontogenic keratocyst. Report of a case. J Oral Maxillofac Surg 1996;54:647–651.

3. Dabbs DJ, Schweitzer RJ, Schweitzer LE, Mantz F. Squamous cell carcinoma arising in recurrent odontogenic keratocyst: Case report and literature review. Head Neck 1994;16:375–378.

4. Hennis HL, Stewart WC, Neville B, O'Connor KF, Apple DJ. Carcinoma arising in an odontogenic keratocyst with orbital invasion. Doc Ophthalmol 1991;77:73–79.

5. Foley WL, Terry BC, Jacoway JR. Malignant transformation of an odontogenic keratocyst: Report of a case. J Oral Maxillofac Surg 1991;49:768–771.

6. Ramsden RT, Barrett A. Gorlin's syndrome. J Laryngol Otol 1975;89:615–629.

7. Moos KF, Rennie JS. Squamous cell carcinoma arising in a mandibular keratocyst in a patient with Gorlin's syndrome. Br J Oral Maxillofac Surg 1987;25:280–284.

8. Herbener GH, Gould AR, Neal DC, Farman AG. An electron and optical microscopic study of juxtaposed odontogenic keratocyst and carcinoma. Oral Surg Oral Med Oral Pathol 1991;71:322–328.

9. Browne RM, Gough NG. Malignant change in the epithelial lining of odontogenic cysts. Cancer 1972;29:1199–1207.

10. Kramer IRH, Pindborg JJ, Shear M. Histologic Typing of Odontogenic Tumors. 2d ed. Berlin: Springer-Verlag, 1992.

11. Eversole LR, Sabes WR, Rovin S. Aggressive growth and neoplastic potential of odontogenic cysts. Cancer 1975;35:270–281.

12. High AS, Quirke P, Hume WJ. DNA-ploidy studies in a keratocyst undergoing subsequent malignant transformation. J Oral Pathol 1987;16: 135–138.

Chapter 27

Clear Cell Odontogenic Carcinoma

1. Terminology

In 1985, two groups of research workers (Hansen et al[1] and Waldron et al[2]) described a total of five cases of an aggressive, intrabony neoplasm of putative odontogenic origin. All cases were characterized by a bimorphic cell population consisting of polygonal cells and clear cells. The presence of clear cells in various odontogenic tumors should not be surprising because the dental lamina is thought to be a common origin, and the remnants of these odontogenic cell rests are reported to contain clear cells as one of their components.[3]

In the three cases published by Hansen et al,[1] there were no local or distant metastatic foci. The authors were therefore unable to say whether this tumor had the potential to metastasize. However, they stated that the locally destructive effect seen in their patients suggested, at the very least, that the tumor was locally aggressive and coined the name *clear cell odontogenic tumor* (CCOT) for this lesion.

Waldron and coworkers[2] reported two cases that demonstrated a biphasic histologic pattern with areas resembling follicular ameloblastoma, although with atypical features and containing areas with a conspicuous clear cell epithelial component. One of the patients had multiple recurrences with extension into the infratemporal fossa, retro-orbital region, and base of the skull, as well as regional lymph node metastasis. The patient died of the disease after 15 years. The authors labeled these cases clear cell ameloblastoma (CCA) and concluded that the two lesions should properly be considered malignant (clear cell) ameloblastomas (MCCAs). In a later personal communication with Gardner[4] Waldron suggested that the CCOT and the MCCA may be part of a histopathologic spectrum and not separate entities.

In 1995, Eversole et al[5] analyzed 17 cases of CCOTs and MCCAs (8 cases from the literature and 9 cases from their own files, including an evaluation of the long-term follow-up of the 3 cases initially reported by Hansen et al[1]) and concluded that CCOTs exhibit metastatic potential and should be referred to as clear cell odontogenic carcinomas (CCOCs), as was suggested by Bang et al[6] in 1989. It seems that even prior to 1985, at least two cases of what today is known as CCOC were diagnosed. These cases were not reported in the literature but were referred to by Bang et al[6]; the first (mandibular midline lesion in a 52-year-old woman) was seen by Dr Lou Hansen in 1979 and at that time was diagnosed as an "atypical epithelial odontogenic tumor" since it did not fit into any known histologic pattern. The second case (a 65-year-old man with a mandibular lesion) was presented at an international slide seminar in 1981 by Drs Rick and Shear.

Based on the histologic findings and the tumor's clinical behavior, Dr Rick chose to designate the lesion a clear cell odontogenic carcinoma.

Odontogenic tumors containing a significant number of clear cells are rare. They are represented by the clear cell variant of the calcifying epithelial odontogenic tumor (CC-CEOT, see chapter 10), the clear cell ameloblastoma (CCA/MCCA), and the clear cell odontogenic carcinoma. A relationship, if any, between the latter two entities is an interesting and controversial issue, and it has yet to be fully elucidated. Piattelli et al[7] was the first to theorize that the CCOC is a distinct and separate entity and not a clear cell variant of the ameloblastoma (MCCA). In the review by Eversole et al,[5] however, the authors evaluated only the pooled data regarding CCOCs and MCCAs without differentiating between the two.

The present authors analyzed the total number of available cases of CCOCs and CCAs/MCCAs at the end of 2000, and it seemed that on the basis of demographic, clinical, and histologic features, the tumors could be divided into 26 cases of CCOCs[1,5,7-18] and 9 cases of CCAs/MCCAs.[19-25] It must be stressed that the available data are still too few to allow definitive conclusions as to whether the lesions are separate entities.

2. Clinical and radiologic profile

The most common presenting sign of both CCOCs and CCAs/MCCAs is jaw enlargement. Sensory deficit, which is often encountered in metastatic carcinomas of the mandible (as with the hypernephroma), is a rare feature. Some patients may complain of mild pain or a dull ache in the affected area and mobility of the teeth is often present. In edentulous patients, a poorly fitting denture may be an early sign of tumor presence. The CCOC occurs as a central tumor in either jaw, whereas the CCA/MCCA may in extremely rare cases be located in the gingival soft tissues (peripheral variant described by Ng and Siar[21]).

Radiographically, the CCOC appears as a poorly delineated uni- or multilocular radiolucent lesion that occurs with prominent bone destruction. Divergence of roots with or without root resorption is common. Nair et al[18] found that in its initial stages the CCOT may resemble early periodontitis that fails to resolve in spite of periodontal therapy. The CCA/MCCA has the same radiographic appearance as that of its benign counterpart, the solid/multicystic ameloblastoma.

3. Epidemiological data

3.1 Prevalence, incidence, and relative frequency

In a demographic study of 759 cases of odontogenic tumors in a Chinese population, Lu et al[26] found that the relative frequency of CCOTs was 0.3%. This is the only data available as yet.

3.2 Age

The mean age at time of diagnosis for CCOCs ($n = 26$) was 56.7 years with a range of 17 to 89 years. The mean age for women was slightly higher (57.6 years) than that for men (55.3 years) (Fig 27-1). The mean age for CCAs/MCCAs was 44.6 years with a range of 14 to 71 years; with 45.7 years for women and 44.0 years for men. This seems

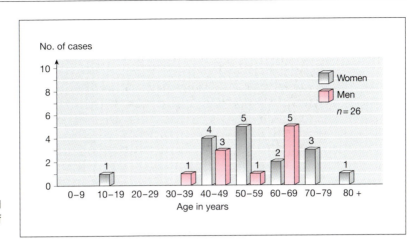

Fig 27-1 Age and gender distribution of CCOCs.

to indicate a difference in mean age between the two tumor forms, with the CCA/MCCA approaching the mean age for the SMA (37.4 years).[27]

3.3 Gender

The male:female distribution for CCOCs was 1:1.6 (see Fig 27-1) and 1:2 for CCAs/MC-CAs.

3.4 Location

The maxillary:mandibular ratio for 21 cases of CCOCs was 1:7.7 (Fig 27-2). In other words, the tumor is almost eight times more common in the mandible than in the maxilla. The ratio for CCAs/MCCAs was 1:3.5. Thus, both tumor forms have a clear predilection for the mandible. Cases in which the exact location within the jaw has been registered show that the posterior region of the mandible is a more common site for CCOCs (90%), whereas the CCA/MCCA so far seems evenly distributed between anterior and posterior regions. In one of the cases reported by Waldron et al,[2] the MCCA was associated with

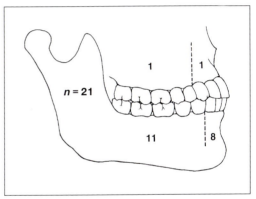

Fig 27-2 Topographic distribution of CCOCs.

an impacted third molar. Cases of CCOCs associated with an unerupted tooth have not been reported so far.

241

4. Pathogenesis

Based on ultrastructural and histochemical findings, Eversole et al[28] concluded that the CCOT is a primary, nonglandular epithelial neoplasm of odontogenic origin, a view shared by Fan et al.[8] The absence of similar tumors in any other part of the body supports the supposition of primary odontogenic origin. The CCOT, according to the 1992 World Health Organization (WHO) classification,[29] probably arises from residues or derivatives of the dental lamina or from rests of Malassez.

With regard to the CCA/MCCA, there is hardly any doubt that this tumor is of odontogenic origin. Regardless of their location, these tumors characteristically exhibit features of a classic follicular SMA in which clear cells have replaced the stellate reticulum.[2,22]

5. Pathology

5.1 Macroscopy

Macroscopic features of CCOCs or CCAs/MCCAs are rarely described. Hansen et al[1] found that sections of surgical specimens of CCOT disclosed a homogenous, pinkish-gray or white, solid (often glistening) tumor with no necrotic areas.

5.2 Microscopy

5.2.1 Histologic definitions

When the 1992 WHO classification[29] was written, the malignant potentiality of the CCOT/CCOC had not yet been realized, so the CCOC was not considered in that edition. The CCOT was defined as "a benign but lo-

cally invasive neoplasm originating from odontogenic epithelium and characterized by sheets and islands of uniform, vacuolated and clear cells."

The definition used by the present authors for CCOC is as follows:

A malignant neoplasm capable of locally destructive growth and both nodal and distant metastasis. Two histologic variants are identifiable. The most common does not resemble the SMA: the islands of cells are biphasic; contain both clear cells and more hyperchromatic-appearing polygonal cells; and exhibit cytoplasmic eosinophilia that fails to show any squamous, glandular, or ameloblastic features (Fig 27-3). Occasionally, these two cell populations coexist in a tumor nest, creating a "glomeruloid" appearance. The islands are separated by zones of a mature, fibrous, and partly hyalinized connective tissue stroma. There is no encapsulation and tumor cells invade medullary bone. Cellular pleomorphism and mitotic activity are rarely seen, but are generally within the population of polygonal cells when present. The second histologic variant

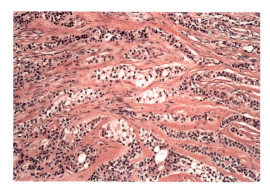

Fig 27-3 CCOC showing no ameloblastomatous features. The strand of tumor tissue contains a mixed population of clear cells and hyperchromatic, polygonal cells traversed by septae of dense fibrous stroma (hematoxylin-eosin [H&E], x150).

of CCOC has islands that are almost exclusively of the clear cell phenotype.

A definition of the CCA/MCCA was not contained in the 1992 WHO classification.[29] The present authors use the following definition:

A malignant neoplasm showing areas consistent with a diagnosis of a follicular ameloblastoma in which varying numbers of tumor islands show peripheral palisading of cuboidal and cylindrical cells with reversed nuclear polarity (directed away from the basal lamina). A prominent clear cell component is present within the follicular nests replacing the stellate reticulum (Fig 27-4). The stroma is composed of dense, fibrous connective tissue with hyalinized areas.

The CCOC was considered an entity in Eversole's 1999 classification of odontogenic carcinomas.[30] Eversole distinguished between three histopathologic patterns, of which the first two corresponded to the present authors' definition. Eversole's third pattern corresponded to what the present authors call clear cell ameloblastoma/malignant clear cell ameloblastoma. Thus, the

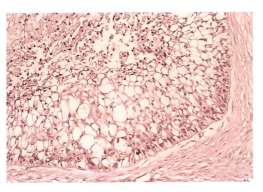

Fig 27-4 CCA/MCCA follicular (SMA-like) tumor island with peripheral palisading of cuboidal and columnar cells that have reversed nuclear polarity. The stellate reticulum has been replaced by clear cells (H&E, x150).

present authors believe that the CCOC and the CCA/MCCA constitute separate tumors. Future studies of larger numbers of these two tumors may reveal whether they should be viewed as entities or variants of a biologic and histopathologic spectrum.

5.2.2 Histopathologic findings

The diagnosis of CCOC is based on histopathologic findings as outlined in the preceding section. Tumors with clear cells impose serious problems for differential diagnosis since clear cell tumors in the head and neck region can originate from a number of sources, including salivary glands (clear cell mucoepidermoid carcinomas, clear cell acinic cell carcinomas, clear cell oncocytomas, and epithelio-myoepithelial carcinomas, to name a few), other odontogenic tumors (such as the clear cell variant of CEOT), and metastatic renal clear cell carcinomas (hypernephromas). Clear cell nests or islands may be a prominent feature in developmental lateral periodontal cysts and in the gingival cyst of the adult.[3] The problem of differential diagnosis of clear cell tumors of the head and neck was reviewed by Eversole[31] and Maiorano et al.[32]

Several authors have noticed the occurrence of hyalinized or partly hyalinized stroma in both CCOCs[6,14] and CCAs/MCCAs.[19,20] Miyauchi et al[15] and Kumamoto et al[17] found eosinophilic hyaline deposits (reminiscent of amyloid-like globules in calcifying epithelial odontogenic tumors) formed in direct contact with the epithelial nests in their reported cases of CCOCs. However, these deposits did not stain with Congo red. The authors suggested it is possible that the CCOC is capable of epithelioectomesenchymal induction, a view the present authors do not support.

The pathologist will probably find the diagnosis of CCA/MCCA less difficult than that of CCOC. Histologically, typical SMA-like (follicular) structures with palisading of the peripheral cylindric cells and reversed nuclear polarity, combined with central areas of clear cells where a stellate reticulum would be expected, are characteristic features. This clear cell differentiation in a SMA was first noticed by Waldron et al.[2] Both the primary and metastatic foci are characterized histologically by benign, innocuous-appearing tumor islands, which lack any features of malignancy.[30] This is in contrast to the malignant epithelial odontogenic tumor, in Eversole's classification[30] called ameloblastic carcinoma, that histologically retains the features of ameloblastic differentiation yet also exhibits cytologic features of malignancy.

5.2.3 Histochemical/immunohistochemical findings

Histochemically, clear cells in both CCOCs and CCAs/MCCAs show identical reactions. Studying fresh-frozen tumor sections, Eversole et al[28] found that the cytoplasm in clear tumor cells of CCOTs (CCOCs) exhibits prominent diastase-digested PAS-positive granules. Both formalin-fixed and fresh-frozen sections failed to disclose cytoplasmic alcianophilia. These findings were confirmed by Miyauchi et al.[15] Further, Eversole et al[28] found that enzyme histochemical reactions disclosed diffuse granular positivity for acid phosphates, nonspecific esterase, and NADH diaphorase, but the cells were negative for alkaline phosphatase.

Immunohistochemically, several authors have examined tumor tissue from CCOCs[8,12,15,17] and CCAs/MCCAs.[20] However, the immunohistochemical features of CCOCs are still unclear. Most authors agree that tumor cells stain diffusely and intensely positive for CK 19, epithelial membrane antigen (EMA), and filaggrin but are negative for S-100 protein, glial fibrillary acidic protein, involucrin, vimentin, and smooth muscle actin.

Muramatsu et al[12] found that the foci of some cells were S-100 protein positive and suggested that these might be Langerhans cells. Eversole et al[5] reported to have found moderately intense positivity for S-100 protein and cytokeratin, more so in the polygonal cells than in the clear cells. De Aguiar et al[20] found positivity for only cytokeratins 14 and 13 in their case of CCA/MCCA. Cytokeratin 14 is one of the major cytokeratins of neoplastic cells in SMAs.[33]

5.2.4 Ultrastructural findings

Eversole et al[28] gave ultrastructural descriptions of tissue samples from a case (at the time diagnosed as CCOT) reported by Hansen et al.[1] They found the presence of abundant glycogen rosettes in the cytoplasm of the clear cells. No well-developed Golgi apparatus, free tonofilaments, or secretory granules were observed, supporting the theory of a nonglandular epithelial origin. Annulate lamellae were frequently present in the cytoplasm, as were lysosomes. Many cells had centrioles or microtubule organizing centers adjacent to the nuclei. Desmosomes linked adjacent tumor cells. The plasma membranes were often convoluted, with interdigitating microvilli. These findings were generally confirmed by Fan et al[8] and Miyauchi et al.[15] However, Fan et al[8] did not find conspicuous cytoplasmic glycogen; rather the cytoplasm was characterized by sparse organelles. Maiorano et al[32] pointed out that clear cells most often result from fixation artifacts and glycogen storage; in some instances they may be a reflection of peculiar functional states of the tumor cell or may result from a lack of organelles. Guilbert et al,[23] who examined the ultrastructure of a CCA/MCCA, found the cytoplasm of the clear cells to be rich in glycogen and lysosomes.

In 1994, Milchgrub et al[34] described a unique salivary gland tumor which they called hyalinizing clear cell carcinoma (HCCC). This tumor, most frequently occurring in women in minor salivary glands (particularly at the base of the tongue or palate) is composed of nests or solid sheets of uniformly clear cells and others with weakly eosinophilic cytoplasm. The clear cells have a polyhedral appearance, round nuclei, inconspicuous nucleoli, and no nuclear atypia. The cytoplasm is filled with PAS-positive, diastase-sensitive glycogen granules but is devoid of mucin.

Immunohistochemistry shows the expression of epithelial markers—cytokeratin, EMA, and occasionally carcinoembryonic antigen (CEA)—but an absence of myoepithelial determinants—S-100 protein, actin, and vimentin. Clusters of tumor cells in HCCCs are separated by broad bands of PAS-positive, hyalinized fibrous stroma that may undergo myxoid or hyaline degeneration. The stroma may hence resemble amyloid but it is negative for Congo red. Although capable of lymph node metastasis, the HCCC appears to behave in a less aggressive fashion than other malignant clear cell tumors of the salivary glands. Occurrences of this tumor in intraosseous jaw locations was recently reported by Berho and Huvos[35] in two women, 66 and 53 years of age. One tumor arose in the mandible, the other in the maxilla. The authors were aware of the close resemblance between HCCCs and CCOCs (CCOTs) and did not believe that their cases satisfied the histologic criteria for CCOCs. Both cases reported showed an overgrowth of a heavily hyalinized stroma (not illustrated in the article). The authors further claimed that the characteristic peripheral arrangement of the polyhedral cells seen in CCOCs were not found in their HCCCs. Lastly, they found the immunohistochemical profiles of their cases to be more in keeping with the one described for HCCCs than for that of CCOCs. Both patients exhibited good health 14 and 17 months, respectively, after diag-

nosis with no evidence of metastasis or recurrence.

The present authors do not support the interpretation of Berho and Huvos's findings. The demographic data of their cases exactly match those of CCOC cases. The histologic criteria as well as the immunohistochemical profiles of the HCCCs also fit those of CCOCs. The disagreement with Berho and Huvos's view may be explained by the fact that they only referred to 5 out of the 15 reports on CCOCs available at the time of their report. It should be added that recurrence and metastatic disease may occur more than 5 years after initial diagnosis,[30] so follow-up periods of 14 and 17 months do not rule out metastatic potential.

6. Notes on treatment and recurrence rate

The reason for the change in nomenclature—from CCOT to CCOC—is to be found in the continued follow-up of the three cases initially reported by Hansen et al[1] and reviewed by Eversole et al[5] 10 years later. One of the three patients, a 74-year-old woman with an anterior maxillary tumor, developed widespread local extension and regional lymph node and pulmonary metastasis. Death occurred 7 years after the initial diagnosis. In a second case involving the anterior mandible of a 41-year-old woman, multiple recurrences with regional and distant metastasis resulted in death 15 years after the initial diagnosis. In both these cases, the original diagnosis did not allude to malignancy and the primary treatment consisted only of curettage. Cases with a favorable outcome were usually treated by radical resection at the time of initial surgery, whereas some of the cases that involved multiple recurrences, metastasis, and death were initially treated by local enucleation and curettage.

Of the nine reported cases of CCAs/MC-CAs, only two did not show recurrence—one peripheral variant with a 5-year follow-up[21] and one case of a 14-year-old boy followed for 15 years.[22] The remaining cases showed multiple recurrences with and without lymph node metastasis.[21,22]

Thus, early aggressive surgery is clearly the therapy of choice and a close follow-up for several years is mandatory.

References

1. Hansen LS, Eversole LR, Green TL, Powell NB. Clear cell odontogenic tumor—a new histologic variant with aggressive potential. Head Neck Surg 1985;8:115–123.

2. Waldron CA, Small IA, Silverman H. Clear cell ameloblastoma—an odontogenic carcinoma. J Oral Maxillofac Surg 1985;43:707–717.

3. Wysocki GP, Brannon RB, Colonel L, et al. Histogenesis of the lateral periodontal cyst and the gingival cyst of the adult. Oral Surg Oral Med Oral Pathol 1980;50:327–334.

4. Gardner DG. Some current concepts on the pathology of ameloblastomas. Oral Surg Oral Med Oral Pathol Oral Radiol Endod 1996;82:660–669.

5. Eversole LR, Duffey DC, Powell NB. Clear cell odontogenic carcinoma. A clinicopathologic analysis. Arch Otolaryngol Head Neck Surg 1995;121:685–689.

6. Bang G, Koppang HS, Gilhuus-Moe O, et al. Clear cell odontogenic carcinoma: Report of three cases with pulmonary and lymph node metastases. J Oral Pathol Med 1989;18:113–118.

7. Piattelli A, Sesenna E, Trisit P. Clear cell odontogenic carcinoma. Report of a case with lymph node and pulmonary metastases. Eur J Cancer B Oral Oncol 1994;30B:278–280.

8. Fan J, Kubota E, Imamura H, et al. Clear cell odontogenic carcinoma. A case report with massive invasion of neighboring organs and lymph node metastasis. Oral Surg Oral Med Oral Pathol 1992;74:768–775.

9. Milles M, Doyle JL, Mesa M, Raz S. Clear cell odontogenic carcinoma with lymph node metastasis. Oral Surg Oral Med Oral Pathol 1993;76:82–89.

10. Nikai H, Miyauchi M, Ljuin N. A case of clear cell odontogenic tumor. Tr Soc Pathol Jpn 1993;82: 127. Abstract.

11. Sadeghi EM, Levin S. Clear cell odontogenic carcinoma of the mandible: Report of a case. J Oral Maxillofac Surg 1995;53:613–616.

12. Muramatsu T, Hashimoto S, Innoue T, et al. Clear cell odontogenic carcinoma in the mandible: Histochemical and immunohistochemical observations with review of the literature. J Oral Pathol Med 1996;25:516–521.

13. Vesper M, Wilck T, Donath K, Schmelzle R. Helzelliges odontogenes Karzinom in Verbindung mit einem Plattenepithelkarzinom. Fallbericht und Literaturübersicht. Mund Kiefer Gesichtschir 1998;2:270–274.

14. Yamamoto H, Inui M, Mori A, Tagawa T. Clear cell odontogenic carcinoma. A case report and literature review of odontogenic tumours with clear cells. Oral Surg Oral Med Oral Pathol Oral Radiol Endod 1998;86:86–89.

15. Miyauchi M, Ogawa I, Takata T, et al. Clear cell odontogenic tumour: A case with induction of dentin-like structures. J Oral Pathol Med 1998; 27:220–224.

16. Kumamoto H, Kawamura H, Ooya K. Clear cell odontogenic tumor in the mandible: Report of a case with an immunohistochemical study of epithelial cell markers. Pathol Int 1998;48:618–622.

17. Kumamoto H, Yamazaki S, Sato A, et al. Clear cell odontogenic tumor in the mandible: Report of a case with duct-like appearances and dentinoid induction. J Oral Pathol Med 2000;29:43–47.

18. Nair MK, Burkes EJ, Chai-U-Dom O. Radiographic manifestation of clear cell odontogenic tumor. Oral Surg Oral Med Oral Pathol Oral Radiol Endod 2000;89:250–254.

19. Mari A, Escutia E, Carrera M, Pericot J. Clear cell ameloblastoma or odontogenic carcinoma. A case report. J Craniomaxillofac Surg 1995;23: 387–390.

20. de Aguiar MCF, Gomez RS, Silva EC, de Araujo VC. Clear-cell ameloblastoma (clear-cell odontogenic carcinoma). Report of a case. Oral Surg Oral Med Oral Pathol Oral Radiol Endod 1996;81: 79–83.

21. Ng KH, Siar CH. Peripheral ameloblastoma with clear cell differentiation. Oral Surg Oral Med Oral Pathol 1990;70:210–213.

22. Müller H, Slootweg P. Clear cell differentiation in an ameloblastoma. J Maxillofac Surg 1986;14:158–160.

23. Guilbert F, Auriol M, Chomette G. Une forme rare d'épithelioma primitif de la mandibule: Le carcinome odontogénique à cellules claires. Etude clinique et morphologique. Rev Stomatol Chir Maxillofac 1991;92:277–280.

24. Odukoya O, Arole O. Clear-cell ameloblastoma of the mandible (a case report). Int J Oral Maxillofac Surg 1992;21:358–359.

25. Duffey DC, Bailet JW, Newman A. Ameloblastoma of the mandible with cervical lymph node metastasis. Am J Otolaryngol 1995;16:66–73.

26. Lu Y, Xuan M, Takata T, et al. Odontogenic tumors. A demographic study of 759 cases in a Chinese population. Oral Surg Oral Med Oral Pathol Oral Radiol Endod 1998;86:707–714.

27. Reichart PA, Philipsen HP, Sonner S. Ameloblastoma: Biological profile of 3677 cases. Eur J Cancer B Oral Oncol 1995;31B:86–99.

28. Eversole LR, Belton CM, Hansen LS. Clear cell odontogenic tumor: Histochemical and ultrastructural features. J Oral Pathol 1985;14:603–614.

29. Kramer IRH, Pindborg JJ, Shear M. Histological Typing of Odontogenic Tumours. 2d ed. Berlin: Springer-Verlag, 1992.

30. Eversole LR. Malignant epithelial odontogenic tumors. Semin Diagn Pathol 1999;16:317–324.

31. Eversole LR. On the differential diagnosis of clear cell tumours of the head and neck. Eur J Cancer B Oral Oncol 1993;29B:173–179.

32. Maiorano E, Altini M, Favia G. Clear cell tumors of the salivary glands, jaws, and oral mucosa. Semin Diagn Pathol 1997;14:203–212.

33. Vigneswaran N, Whitaker SB, Budnick SD, et al. Expression patterns of epithelial differentiation antigens and lectin-binding sites in ameloblastomas: A comparison with basal cell carcinomas. Hum Pathol 1993;24:49–57.

34. Milchgrub S, Gnepp DR, Vuitch F, et al. Hyalinizing clear cell carcinoma of salivary gland. Am J Surg Pathol 1994;18:74–82.

35. Berho M, Huvos AG. Central hyalinizing clear cell carcinoma of the mandible and the maxilla. A clinicopathologic study of two cases with an analysis of the literature. Hum Pathol 1999;30:101–105.

Chapter 28

Ghost Cell Odontogenic Carcinoma

1. Terminology

A malignant counterpart of the odontogenic lesion formerly known as the calcifying odontogenic cyst (COC) (see chapter 17) is extremely rare, with only 17 cases having been reported in the English language literature as of 2000. The first case was illustrated in a photomicrograph in the 1971 World Health Organization (WHO) classification[1] of odontogenic tumors, but no clinical information was provided. The first well-documented case of a malignancy arising in a COC was reported by Ikemura et al in 1985.[2] They described the simultaneous occurrence of a malignant epithelial tumor and typical COC in the maxilla of a 48-year-old woman who eventually died of intracranial extension of the tumor 20 months following diagnosis. Since then, case reports have described such tumors in a variety of ways, including malignant COC, odontogenic ghost cell carcinoma (OGCC), carcinoma arising in a COC, aggressive epithelial ghost cell odontogenic tumor, dentinogenic ghost cell ameloblastoma, and malignant calcifying ghost cell odontogenic tumor. In the recent classification of malignant epithelial odontogenic tumors by Eversole,[3] the tumor is recognized as an entity of the odontogenic carcinoma group. A summary of 12 previously reported cases, in addition to 4 cases from their own files, was published by Lu et al.[4] Details of the cases are summarized in a table within the report, but one case appears to have been reported twice. Despite obvious clinical similarities in the two reports, the post-treatment details differed significantly. Irrespective of this discrepancy, the present authors consider both cases to be the same case. Two recent cases[5,6] in the English language literature and seven other cases (six Chinese and one Japanese) in the non-English literature were not included in Lu et al's review. Information about 18 GCOC cases reported in English and accepted by the present authors form the basis of this chapter.

2. Clinical and radiologic profile

Clinical features of the GCOC include swelling with or without pain, osseous destruction with paresthesia being a frequent finding. Most typically, the radiographic features include a poorly demarcated radiolucency mixed with radiopaque material. The biologic behavior of the GCOC varies and probably reflects a spectrum of growth patterns from a slowly growing, locally invasive tumor to a highly aggressive, rapidly growing neoplasm.

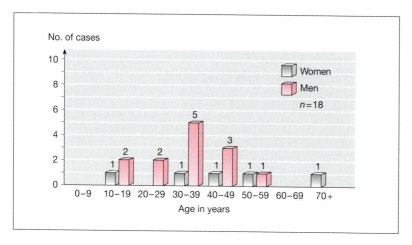

Fig 28-1 Age and gender distribution of 18 cases of GCOCs.

3. Epidemiological data

3.1 Prevalence, incidence, and relative frequency

Because of the extreme rarity of this tumor, few data are available as yet. Lu et al[4] mentioned that the GCOC appears to be more common in Asians than in other races, although the true prevalence remains unknown. In a demographic study of 759 cases of odontogenic tumors in a Chinese population, Lu and coworkers[7] found a relative frequency of 0.4% for the GCOC.

3.2 Age

Distribution of age at the time of diagnosis for the 18 reviewed cases (Fig 28-1) shows that 55.6% occur in the 4th and 5th decades. Ages ranged from 13 to 72 years with a mean age of 37.3 years (women, 43.8 years; men, 34.8 years).

3.3 Gender

The male:female ratio for the 18 cases was 2.6:1. (See Fig 28-1).

3.4 Location

The GCOC occurs more commonly in the maxilla than in the mandible with a ratio of 2:1.

4. Pathogenesis

The origin of the GCOC is not fully known. However, Lu et al[4] stated that the immunophenotype of the malignant cells supports an epithelial origin. Three patterns of development seem likely.[4] Most commonly, the tumor histologically presents de novo but with a benign COC and a malignant epithelial component present in the same lesion. Less commonly, the GCOC occurs after the recurrence of a benign COC. It is unclear whether these two patterns represent the same process but with temporally distinct development. A third pattern is the GCOC arising from another odontogenic tumor such as an SMA. In all cases, however, a typical benign COC can be identified either admixed or separate from the malignant cell and irrespective of the developmental pattern.

5. Pathology

5.1 Macroscopy

No macroscopic information for GCOCs is available.

5.2 Microscopy

5.2.1 Histologic definition

The CGCOC was not included in the WHO's classification,[8] but the present authors use the following definition:

A malignant neoplasm generally characterized by two types of epithelial cells. The malignant component of some tumors is found in nests, strands, and islands of varying size dominated by small, round, undifferentiated basaloid cells with hyperchromatic nuclei, frequent mitoses, and cytologic atypia. Masses of ghost cells, some of which may show dystrophic calcification, often intermingle with the small basaloid cells. Small deposits of dentinoid in close association with ghost cells may or may not be present. In some tumors, the epithelial component is formed predominantly by large cells with vesicular nuclei admixed with few cells showing squamous differentiation. Areas of necrosis with an acute and chronic inflammatory cell infiltrate are frequent findings.

5.2.2 Histopathologic findings

The preceding histologic definition is based on current (insufficient) knowledge. Too few cases have been reported to establish definitive histologic criteria. In addition to the malignant epithelial component, one may find a typical, simple unicystic type of COC. The cyst is lined with stratified epithelium that has a distinct basal cell layer of columnar cells overlaid by a loose, stellate reticulum–like epithelium of variable thickness.

Foci of ghost cells are scattered within the epithelial lining. Nests of tumor cells invade and destroy the surrounding bone, skeletal muscle, and connective tissue. The occurrence of tumor tissue necrosis may be marked. Folpe et al[9] stated that approximately 40% of their reported tumors were necrotic. The stroma consists of a mature, fibrous connective tissue which may occasionally show desmoplasia.[9]

5.2.3 Immunohistochemical findings

A number of authors have included immunohistochemical analysis in their reports. Due to the small number of reported GCOC cases with an immunohistochemical profile, the heterogeneity of the tumor cells, differences in methodologies, and antibody specificities, no definite profile can be determined as yet. Takata et al[10] assessed the proliferative activity of 25 cases of COC, including 4 cases of GCOCs, using the proliferative cell nuclear antigen (PCNA) labelling index (LI; the percentage of positive nuclei). The PCNA LI of the GCOC (65.2 ± 5.6) was significantly higher than that of the benign COC ($11.6 \pm 9.0; p = 0.002$). The authors concluded that PCNA LI is a possible parameter for differentiating GCOCs from benign COCs. Kim et al[6] used a series of immunohistochemical stains for apoptosis-related proteins such as bcl-2, bcl-X_L, and Bax in addition to a positive reaction in the TUNEL assay and concluded that ghost cells undergo abnormal terminal differentiation as an apoptotic process.

5.2.4 Ultrastructural findings

Folpe et al[9] studied the ultrastructure of the GCOC and found that the tumor cells were loosely cohesive. Aggregates of intermediate filament material in a perinuclear distribution imparted the eosinophilia seen in the cytoplasm at the light microscopic level.

6. Notes on treatment and recurrence rate

Alcalde et al[11] and Kamijo et al[5] recommended initial radical surgery combined with radiation therapy. It is still unclear whether chemotherapeutic agents are effective. Long-term follow-up is mandatory.

The biologic behavior of the GCOC appears to be unpredictable. Some cases have been associated with long-term survival following definitive surgery,[11-13] whereas others have had poor clinical outcomes with locally recurrent disease or metastases.[2,8,12,13-15] Lu et al[4] found that the overall 5-year survival rate of 15 previously reported cases was 73%, although recurrence was common after initial surgery. Several more cases have to be published to estimate a possible recurrence rate.

References

1. Pindborg JJ, Kramer IRH. Histological Typing of Odontogenic Tumours, Jaw Cysts and Allied Lesions. Berlin: Springer-Verlag, 1971.

2. Ikemura K, Horie A, Tashiro H, Nandate M. Simultaneous occurrence of a calcifying odontogenic cyst and its malignant transformation. Cancer 1985;56:2861–2864.

3. Eversole LR. Malignant epithelial odontogenic tumors. Semin Diagn Pathol 1999;16:317–324.

4. Lu Y, Mock D, Takata T, Jordan RCK. Odontogenic ghost cell carcinoma: Report of four new cases and review of the literature. J Oral Pathol Med 1999;28:323–329.

5. Kamijo R, Miyaoka K, Tachikawa T, Nagumo M. Odontogenic ghost cell carcinoma: Report of a case. J Oral Maxillofac Surg 1999;57:1266–1270.

6. Kim J, Lee EH, Yook JI, et al. Odontogenic ghost cell carcinoma: A case report with reference to the relation between apoptosis and ghost cells. Oral Surg Oral Med Oral Pathol Oral Radiol Endod 2000;90:630–635.

7. Lu Y, Xuan M, Takata T, et al. Odontogenic tumors. A demographic study of 759 cases in a Chinese population. Oral Surg Oral Med Oral Pathol Oral Radiol Endod 1998;86:707–714.

8. Kramer IRH, Pindborg JJ, Shear M. Histological Typing of Odontogenic Tumours. 2nd ed. Berlin: Springer-Verlag, 1992.

9. Folpe AL, Tsue T, Rogerson L, et al. Odontogenic ghost cell carcinoma: A case report with immunohistochemical and ultrastructural characterization. J Oral Pathol Med 1998;27:185–189.

10. Takata T, Lu Y, Ogawa I, et al. Proliferative activity of calcifying odontogenic cysts as evaluated by proliferating cell nuclear antigen labeling index. Pathol Int 1998;48:877–881.

11. Alcalde RE, Sasaki A, Misaki M, Matsumura T. Odontogenic ghost cell carcinoma: Report of a case and review of the literature. J Oral Maxillofac Surg 1996;54:108–111.

12. Ellis GL, Shmookler BM. Aggressive (malignant?) epithelial odontogenic ghost cell tumor. Oral Surg Oral Med Oral Pathol 1986;61:471–478.

13. Grodjesk JE, Dolinsky HB, Schneider LC, et al. Odontogenic ghost cell carcinoma. Oral Surg Oral Med Oral Pathol 1987;63:576–581.

14. Scott J, Wood GD. Aggressive calcifying odontogenic cyst—a possible variant of ameloblastoma. Br J Oral Maxillofac Surg 1989;27:53–59.

15. Siar CH, Ng KH. Aggressive (malignant?) epithelial odontogenic ghost cell tumour of maxilla. J Laryngol Otol 1994;108:269–271.

Section Six

Malignant Ectomesenchymal Odontogenic Neoplasms (Odontogenic Sarcomas)

Introduction to Odontogenic Sarcomas

Odontogenic sarcomas are rare malignancies of the jaws, including the ameloblastic fibrosarcoma (AFS), the ameloblastic dentinosarcoma (AFDS), the ameloblastic odontosarcoma (AOS), and the odontogenic carcinosarcoma (OCS). The AFS, AFDS, and AOS are considered to represent the malignant counterparts of the ameloblastic fibroma, the ameloblastic fibrodentinoma, and the ameloblastic fibro-odontoma, respectively. In AFS, AFDS, and AOS, only the ectomesenchymal component has undergone malignant transformation, while in OCS both the ectomesenchymal and the epithelial components reveal malignant changes. Generally, the prognosis for odontogenic sarcomas is poor.

Chapter 29

Ameloblastic Fibrosarcoma

1. Terminology

The ameloblastic fibrosarcoma (AFS) was classified by the World Health Organization (WHO) in 1992[1] as an odontogenic sarcoma and is also known as the ameloblastic sarcoma. Other odontogenic sarcomas are the ameloblastic fibrodentinosarcoma (AFDS; see chapter 30), the ameloblastic odontosarcoma (AOS; see chapter 30), and the odontogenic carcinosarcoma (see chapter 31). The distinction between odontogenic sarcomas with (AFDS, AOS) and without (AFS) formation of dental hard structures, as proposed by the WHO classification, is correct from the point of view of histopathologic diagnosis. However, a number of investigators have questioned this concept because the biologic profile and prognosis of the AFS, AFDS, and AOS appear to be identical. Therefore, the term *ameloblastic sarcoma* has been proposed.[2]

The ameloblastic fibrosarcoma is a rare malignant neoplasm composed of benign odontogenic, ameloblastomatous epithelium and malignant ectomesenchyme which resembles a fibrosarcoma. The ameloblastic fibrosarcoma is generally considered to be the malignant form of the ameloblastic fibroma (AF; see chapter 12) in which the ectomesenchymal cells have retained their embryonic appearance and develop malignant characteristics.

The first report of an AFS was published by Heath[3] in 1887 in which he described a "spindle-celled sarcoma" of the mandible containing scattered masses and cylinders of epithelial cells that resembled epithelial elements of the enamel organ. Pindborg[4] published the first thorough review of the literature prior to 1960; a total of nine cases including his own were included. Since that time several reviews have been published[2,5-7] and more cases have been added. The most comprehensive review is that of Muller et al[7] who analyzed the data of 51 cases of AFS, including cases of AFDS and AOS. Their review encompassed published cases through 1993. Since then at least 11 new cases have been published: Dallera et al[8] reported 5 cases of AFSs from Italy, and single case reports were published by Park et al,[9] De Oliveira Nogueira et al,[10] Tajima et al,[11] Sano et al,[12] De Nittis et al,[13] Hayashi et al,[14] and Bregni et al.[15]

2. Clinical and radiologic profile

Clinical signs and symptoms were not described in great detail in a number of case reports. Leider et al[17] recorded signs and symptoms of their six patients; pain and swelling were the most constant findings. Ul-

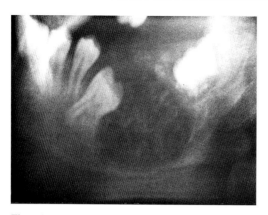

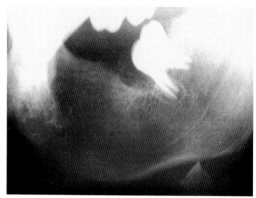

Fig 29-1 Lateral oblique radiograph of the left mandible of a 13-year-old boy showing an ameloblastic fibroma. The first mandibular molar is impacted, and the second molar is missing. The AF was enucleated.

Fig 29-2 Patient shown in Fig 29-1 at age 16 years. The patient presented with a large intraoral soft tissue mass in the left mandible. Radiographically, most of the previous defect has been replaced by bone and the third molar has developed. Alveolar bone destruction is evident mesially to the crown of the third molar. The histologic diagnosis was AFS.

ceration and bleeding, as well as paresthesia of the lower lip, were also reported. These findings were in agreement with those of Altini et al,[2] who evaluated signs and symptoms of cases of ameloblastic sarcomas (AFSs, AFDSs, and AOSs). Swelling was observed in all cases, and pain was a frequent complaint. Mobility of the teeth, a frequent finding in malignant jaw neoplasms, was seen in some cases.

Since 44% of AFS cases arise in previously benign ameloblastic fibromas, the history of patients with an AFS must be taken with great care in order to classify the neoplasm as de novo or as transformation from AF to AFS. In this context, the recurrence rate of AFs has been regarded as important; it has been reported to be as high as 18.3%.[18] Frequent recurrences and multiple surgical interventions have been considered possible supporting factors of malignant transformation.

Dallera et al[8] reported measurements of the tumors in their five AFS patients. The smallest was 4 x 4 x 3 cm and the largest was 7 x 6 x 4 cm.

Involvement of the cervical or submandibular lymph nodes in cases of AFS seems to be uncommon. Among 49 AFS cases, only 1 case with histologic documentation of metastasis involving the lung, liver, and mediastinal lymph nodes was reported.[7]

Radiographically, radiolucencies with irregular and indistinct margins are characteristic (Figs 29-1 and 29-2). Large radiolucencies with a multilocular appearance and gross expansion and thinning of the cortical bone may be seen. In cases where radiopacities are observed within radiolucent areas, a diagnosis of ameloblastic fibrodentinosarcoma or ameloblastic fibroodontosarcoma is likely. Park et al[9] examined their patient using computed tomography (CT) scans. These showed a well-defined heterogeneous mass of soft tissue density and a thin enhancing capsule in the submandibular area. Radionucleotide bone scans showed increased 99m Tc and 67 Ga uptake in the affected region. Both CT scans and magnetic resonance imagery (MRI) have become important tools in the diagnosis of odontogenic tumors such as AFSs.

3. Epidemiological data

3.1 Prevalence, incidence, and relative frequency

Although 62 cases of AFS (excluding AFDSs and AOSs) have been published according to Bregni et al,[15] this neoplasm must still be considered exceedingly rare, particularly since these cases have been published roughly over the last 100 years. No figures on incidence, prevalence, and relative frequency are presently available.

3.2 Age

The mean age at the time of diagnosis for 49 cases[7-16] of AFS (excluding AFDSs and AOSs) was 24.9 years with a range of 3 to 78 years (Fig 29-3). In contrast, the reported mean age of patients with ameloblastic fibromas ranged from 15 to 22 years.[7]

3.3 Gender

The male:female ratio of 49 cases[7-16] of AFS was 2:1 (see Fig 29-3).

3.4 Location

Based on 49 cases,[7-16] the mandible is the most common location for the AFS, with the mandible:maxilla ratio being 2.3:1. The posterior regions of both jaws were more frequently affected (Fig 29-4).

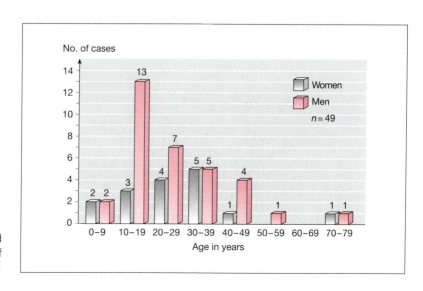

Fig 29-3 Age and gender distribution of 49 cases of AFS.[7-16]

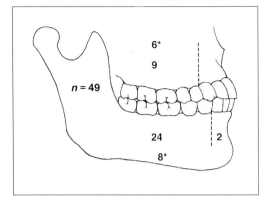

Fig 29-4 Topographic distribution of 49 cases of AFSs.[7-16] Asterisk indicates AFS without specific location in maxilla or mandible.

4. Pathogenesis

The pathogenesis of the ameloblastic fibrosarcoma has not been fully established. Out of 36 cases of AFS, 13 had a previous diagnosis of AF according to data compiled by Muller et al.[7] Thus, in a number of cases, gradual transformation of an AF to an AFS has been documented over time. The difference in the mean age at the time of diagnosis for AF (15 to 22 years[7]) and AFS cases (24.9 years) supports a stepwise progression of a benign to a malignant neoplasm as opposed to a de novo malignancy. Several investigators have tried to correlate AFS development with the stages of developing teeth histologically. In one case, Yamamoto et al[5] observed two characteristic features at the epithelium-ectomesenchyme interface: epithelium that was surrounded by both a cellular stroma and a cell-free zone, and a few aperiodic fibrils arranged near the basal lamina. The authors interpreted these findings as corresponding to the early bell stage of odontogenesis. Chomette et al[19] have sug-

gested that the epithelial component, being unable to assume its functions of organization and induction, may initiate the malignant transformation of its odontogenic ectomesenchyme.

5. Pathology

5.1 Macroscopy

The macroscopic findings of resected specimens were described by Eda et al[20] and Dallera et al[8] in detail. The specimens were tender but solid and whitish at the cut surfaces. The buccal and lingual cortices of the mandible were extremely thin.[20] Dallera et al[8] described the specimens as tough and rubbery; some calcified spicules of bone were detected. Cortical plates were focally perforated, thinned, or destroyed. In other cases,[5] the cut surface of the tumor was soft and pale with a few hemorrhagic areas; in some parts, a capsule was detected.

5.2 Microscopy

5.2.1 Histologic definition

Both the 1992 WHO classification[1] and the present authors define the AFS as follows: "A neoplasm with a similar structure to ameloblastic fibroma, but in which the ectomesenchymal component shows the features of a sarcoma."

5.2.2 Histopathologic findings

The histopathology of the AFS is characterized by a consistent appearance in which a malignant ectomesenchymal component is mixed with a benign epithelial odontogenic component. The malignant ectomesenchy-

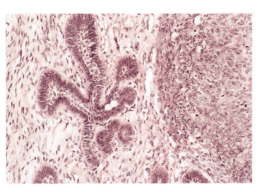

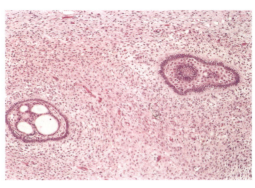

Fig 29-5 Ameloblastic fibrosarcoma exhibiting strands of ameloblastic epithelium in a malignant ectomesenchymal tissue of variable cellularity and polymorphism (hematoxylin-eosin [H&E], x100).

Fig 29-6 Islands of ameloblastic epithelium, one of which shows microcystic degeneration. The sarcomatous ectomesenchymal component is hypercellular (H&E, x60).

mal component consistently takes up more than 70% of the tumor area compared to 30% by the odontogenic epithelium.[8] The benign epithelial component shows budding and slender cords, usually only two layers thick, composed of small polygonal epithelial cells. In addition, epithelial islands and nests with the same histopathologic appearance as ameloblastic fibromas are evident. Columnar or cuboidal epithelial tumor cells resembling preameloblasts are arranged at the periphery in a palisading pattern. The nuclei are hyperchromatic and are polarized away from the basement membrane; the cytoplasm is clear and vacuolated (Figs 29-5 and 29-6). Polyhedral cells resembling stellate reticulum–like epithelial cells are seen in the center of the epithelial islands. No mitoses or malignant cytologic features are detected in the epithelial component. The ectomesenchymal component of the neoplasms shows a marked increase in cellularity. The fibroblast-like cells are pleomorphic, rounded, or fusiform and display increased, sometimes atypical, mitotic activity. Cytologically, these cells show hyperchromatic nuclei and scant cytoplasm. Cells with marked polymorphism, as

seen in pleomorphic malignant fibrous histiocytoma, have occasionally been described in AFS cases.[21]

Collagen is usually present only in small amounts. In some cases, a homogeneous, eosinophilic material is found in the ectomesenchymal component surrounding the epithelial islands. Ameloblastic fibrosarcomas typically display the greatest density of ectomesenchymal malignant tumor cells around the epithelial islands. In some cases,[8] areas of osteoid matrix have been identified in a lacelike pattern between the malignant ectomesenchymal cells; the authors interpreted this as evidence of an osteogenic sarcoma–like appearance. Both benign and malignant giant cells may occasionally be found. The vascular component is usually inconspicuous. The malignant component may reveal different grades of malignancy from low to high.

In some cases of AFS,[11,13] cords of odontogenic epithelium have been observed resembling those seen in odontogenic fibromas rather than ameloblastic fibromas. These cases of odontogenic fibroma–like sarcomas were clinically aggressive or caused death.[21] Slater[21] considered these cases to be possible nonodontogenic sarcomas arising adjacent to "normal" gingival odontogenic epithelium.

Of further interest is that the epithelial component of the AFS eventually becomes less prominent and may disappear altogether after local recurrences. Park et al[9] reported a case of highly malignant AFS which revealed that sheets of more anaplastic and poorly differentiated cells were not associated with the benign odontogenic epithelium, whereas less anaplastic mesenchymal tissue was closely associated with it. The authors suggested that the anaplasia of mesenchymal tissue correlates with the degeneration of benign odontogenic epithelium and that the loss of benign odontogenic epithelium results from an overgrowth of the malignant mesenchymal portion of the lesion.

5.2.3 Histochemical/immunohistochemical findings

Leider et al[17] studied their cases by histochemical methods using Wilder reticulum stain, Masson trichrome stain, alcian blue stain for mucopolysaccharides, and Mowry colloidal iron technique for acid mucopolysaccharides with and without hyaluronidase digestion. The findings were compared to cases of AFS and nonodontogenic fibrosarcomas. Staining characteristics of the mesenchymal component did not reveal any difference between the different neoplasms. Chomette et al[19] found that, compared to classic fibrosarcomas, a high level of alkaline phosphatase and adenosinetriphosphatase (ATPase) activities was present in cases of AFS.

Yamamoto et al[5] found that keratin could be demonstrated in the columnar and polyhedral cells of the epithelial component. The intensity of the staining reaction was not uniform; the polyhedral cells were more intensely stained. The basal part of some columnar cells revealed positive staining for tissue polypeptide antigen. The spindle-shaped fibroblastic cells were positive for vimentin. Sano et al[12] assessed the growth potential of ameloblastic fibrosarcomas in relation to ameloblastic fibromas (AFs) and related lesions by MIB-1 immunohistochemistry. Positive reactions for MIB-1 were observed in the nuclei of tumor cells in both the epithelial and ectomesenchymal components. Labeling indices were considered higher in the ectomesenchymal components in the AFS and in AFS with later recurrence. The labeling indices of ectomesenchymal components were significantly different between the nonrecurrent AF and the ameloblastic fibro-odontoma and AFS. The authors concluded that evaluation of the growth potential in AFS and related lesions could help in understanding tumor aggressiveness and in selecting appropriate surgical procedures.

Muller et al[7] performed a DNA ploidy analysis of their patients with AFS. Measurement of DNA ploidy by flow cytometry or image analysis has been considered useful in distinguishing benign from malignant neoplasms and providing an objective means of histologic grading. In their study, four of five cases were diploid, as were three cases of AFS which were used as controls. Although there is a relationship between increased histologic grade and DNA aneuploidy for many histologic types of sarcomas, the authors were unable to demonstrate this association with their AFS cases.

5.2.4 Ultrastructural findings

The ultrastructure of ameloblastic fibrosarcomas has been studied by several research groups.[5,9,20,22] Yamamoto et al[5] observed two cell types—columnar and polyhedral—in the epithelial component. The columnar cells had slightly enlarged oval nuclei located apically within the cells. The cytoplasm showed small processes and infolding toward the basal lamina; the number of mitochondria was moderately increased. The Golgi apparatus appeared less well developed. Rough and smooth endoplasmic reticulum were seen; the number of glycogen granules was moderately increased. Tonofilaments were well preserved, revealing typical arrangements in bundles. Desmosomes were also detected. The polyhedral cells displayed large amounts of tonofilaments and glycogen granules. The mesenchymal spindle-shaped, fibroblast-like cells showed irregular nuclei with one or two nucleoli and a variable amount of heterochromatin. Some lipid granules and filaments with focal condensation were also observed. The authors interpreted their ultrastructural findings as features of sarcomas. The ultrastructural study by Chomette et al[19] demonstrated clear cells with numerous microfilaments, secretory cells, fibroblasts, and myofibroblasts. In addition to these pleomorphic cells, many peculiar granular cells with numerous lysosomal bodies were also found.

6. Notes on treatment and recurrence rate

The information available concerning treatment, course, and prognosis of the AFS is limited due to the paucity of cases reported. When considering treatment modalities, one must keep in mind that an AFS may develop from a preexisting AF or AFO, or it may arise de novo. Since 36% of reviewed cases arose in previously benign ameloblastic fibromas,[7] some authors have suggested that ameloblastic fibromas be treated more radically to prevent recurrences and possible transformation to AFSs. Muller et al[7] supported this view based on the data they accumulated on ameloblastic fibrosarcomas: "Rather than

enucleation or curettage of AF, wide local excision ensuring complete removal may be warranted in view of the high recurrence rate. Regardless of therapy, a patient who has undergone therapy for an AF must be followed-up by regular clinical and radiographic exams for at least 10 years."

The vast majority of authors recommend radical extensive surgery for ameloblastic fibrosarcomas, usually necessitating partial or total mandibulectomy or maxillectomy. In some recently published cases, postsurgical radiotherapy[10] or adjuvant chemotherapy with cyclophosphamide, vincristine, and doxorubicin[9] were administered. In the latter case, chemotherapy and subsequent radiotherapy were ineffective.

Metastasis seems to be rare in AFSs; of 49 AFS cases,[7] there was only 1 case with histologic documentation of metastasis to the mediastinal lymph nodes, lung, and liver. Muller et al[7] suggested that routine neck dissection for AFS would therefore not be indicated.

Recurrences with adequately documented follow-up occurred in 20 of 49 adequately treated patients.[7] Two- and 5-year survival rates are not available, but 20.4% of patients with AFS died within 2 to 19 years.[7]

The prognosis for the AFS seems better than that for other fibrosarcomas of the orofacial region. Due to the fact that metastasis is rare in AFS cases and survival seems to be comparably good, some authors[16,23] have theorized that the AFS may be considered a low-grade fibrosarcoma. Prein et al[24] suggested that the AFS be considered "semimalignant"; they proposed calling the AFS a "proliferative ameloblastic fibroma."

References

1. Kramer IRH, Pindborg JJ, Shear M. Histologic Typing of Odontogenic Tumours. 2d ed. Berlin: Springer-Verlag, 1992.

2. Altini M, Thompson St, Lownie J, Berezowski BB. Ameloblastic sarcoma of the mandible. J Oral Maxillofac Surg 1985;43:789–794.

3. Heath C. Certain diseases of the jaws. Br Med J 1887;2:5–13.

4. Pindborg JJ. Ameloblastic sarcoma of the maxilla: Report of a case. Cancer 1960;13:917–920.

5. Yamamoto H, Caselitz J, Kozawa Y. Ameloblastic fibrosarcoma of the right mandible: Immunohistochemical and electron microscopical investigations on one case, and a review of the literature. J Oral Pathol 1987;16:450–455.

6. Wood RM, Markle T, Barker BF, Hiatt WR. Ameloblastic fibrosarcoma. Oral Surg Oral Med Oral Pathol 1988;66:74–77.

7. Muller S, Parker DC, Kapadia SB, et al. Ameloblastic fibrosarcoma of the jaw. A clinicopathologic and DNA analysis of five cases and review of the literature with discussion of its relationship to ameloblastic fibroma. Oral Surg Oral Med Oral Pathol Oral Radiol Endod 1995;79:469–477.

8. Dallera P, Bertoni F, Marchetti C, Bacchini P, Campobassi A. Ameloblastic fibrosarcoma of the jaw: Report of five cases. J Craniomaxillofac Surg 1994;22:349–354.

9. Park HR, Shin KB, So MY, et al. A highly malignant ameloblastic fibrosarcoma. Report of a case. Oral Surg Oral Med Oral Pathol Oral Radiol Endod 1995;79:478–481.

10. De Oliveira Nogueira T, Carvalho YR, Blumer Rosa LE, et al. Possible malignant transformation of an ameloblastic fibroma to ameloblastic fibrosarcoma: A case report. J Oral Maxillofac Surg 1997;55:180–182.

11. Tajima Y, Utsumi N, Suzuki S, Fujita K, Takahashi H. Ameloblastic fibrosarcoma arising de novo in the maxilla. Pathol Int 1997;47:564–568.

12. Sano K, Yoshida S, Nimoiyma H, et al. Assessment of growth potential by MIB-1 immunohistochemistry in ameloblastic fibroma and related lesions of the jaws compared with ameloblastic fibrosarcoma. J Oral Pathol Med 1998;27:59–63.

13. De Nittis A, Stambaugh M. Ameloblastic fibrosarcoma of the maxilla: Report of a case. J Oral Maxillofac Surg 1998;56:672–675.

14. Hayashi Y, Tohnai I, Ueda M, Nagasaka T. Sarcomatous overgrowth in recurrent ameloblastic fibrosarcoma. Oral Oncol 1999;35:346–348.

15. Bregni RC, Mosqueda TA, Garcia AM. Ameloblastic fibrosarcoma of the mandible: Report of two cases and review of the literature. J Oral Pathol Med 2001;30:316–320.

16. Motegi K, Banba S, Totuska M, Michi K, Yamazato S. Ameloblastic sarcoma of the maxilla: Report of a case. Nippon Koku Geka Gakkai Zasshi 1975; 21:176–179.

17. Leider AS, Nelson JF, Trodahl JN. Ameloblastic fibrosarcoma of the jaws. Oral Surg Oral Med Oral Pathol 1972;33:559–569.

18. Zallen R, Preskar M, McClary S. Ameloblastic fibroma. J Oral Maxillofac Surg 1982;40:513–517.

19. Chomette G, Auriol M, Guilbert F, et al. Fibrosarcoma améloblastique. Étude clinique et anatomopathologique de trois observations données histo-enzymologiques et ultrastructurales. Arch Anat Cytol Pathol 1982;30:172–178.

20. Eda S, Saito T, Morimura G, et al. A case of ameloblastic fibrosarcoma with an electron-microscopic observation. Bull Tokyo Dent Coll 1976; 17:11–25.

21. Slater LJ. Odontogenic sarcoma and carcinoma. Semin Diagn Pathol 1999;16:325–332.

22. Takeda Y, Kaneko R, Suzuki A. Ameloblastic fibrosarcomas in the maxilla, malignant transformation of ameloblastic fibroma. Virchows Arch A Pathol Anat Histopathol 1984;404:253–263.

23. Reichart PA, Zobl H. Transformation of ameloblastic fibroma to fibrosarcoma. Int J Oral Surg 1978;7:503–507.

24. Prein J, Remagen W, Spiessl B, Schafroth U. Ameloblastic fibroma and its sarcomatous transformation. Pathol Res Pract 1979;166:123–130.

Chapter 30

Ameloblastic Fibrodentinosarcoma and Fibro-odontosarcoma

1. Terminology

Ameloblastic fibrodentinosarcomas (AFDSs) and ameloblastic fibro-odontosarcomas (AOSs) are exceedingly rare malignant odontogenic sarcomas, which are also called ameloblastic sarcomas. The World Health Organization (WHO) classification of 1992[1] differentiated between odontogenic sarcomas without dental hard tissues (ameloblastic fibrosarcomas) and those revealing evidence of dentinoid (ameloblastic fibrodentinosarcomas) or dentinoid plus enameloid (ameloblastic odontosarcomas). The presence or absence of dentinoid and enameloid, however, seems to be of no prognostic significance.[1]

Slater[2] recently reviewed the morphologic criteria of both AFDSs and AOSs. Altini and Smith[3] described the first case of ameloblastic dentinosarcoma in 1976. In 1985, Altini et al[4] reported another case of ameloblastic dentinosarcoma and reviewed the literature on ameloblastic sarcomas. They found 28 cases of AFS, one case of AFDS, and 7 cases of AOS in the literature.

To determine the exact number of reported cases of AFDSs and AOSs is difficult because some authors feel that subclassification is not indicated. Corominas-Villafañe et al[5] described a case of AOS; however, no enameloid was described histologically, which according to Altini and Smith[3] would

classify this lesion as AFDS. Also, cases have been described as AOSs which only revealed focal formation of a predentin-like hyaline substance but no calcified dentinoid material.[6] Since Altini et al[4] did not believe these periepithelial hyaline deposits were forming a matrix material for dental hard tissues, such lesions should be classified as ameloblastic fibrosarcomas and not as AOSs.

Phillips et al[7] reported a case of AOS in 1988, and Takeda et al[8] described a case in 1990 with adequate demonstration of the histopathologic features of ameloblastic fibrosarcoma, dentinal matrix, and dysplastic dentine, as well as a small amount of abortive enamel matrix. At the time of the latter report, fewer than 10 cases of AOS had been reported since Thoma first described a case in 1954.[9] In 2001, Bregni et al[10] reported another case of AFDS.

2. Clinical and radiologic profile

In their review of ameloblastic sarcomas, Altini et al[4] summarized the clinical findings, including those for cases of AFDSs and AOSs. Swelling was reported in all cases of ameloblastic sarcomas. Pain was frequently associated with the lesions. Oral mucosal ulceration and/or bleeding was usually related to occlusal trauma. Mobility of the teeth and/or tissue proliferation through extraction sockets were noted in some cases. The growth rate was usually moderate, although rapid growth was also reported. Clinically, regional lymph nodes did not show signs of metastatic involvement.

Radiographically, the AFDS and AOS have to be differentiated from the ameloblastic fibrosarcoma (AFS) by the presence of radiopaque foci in an otherwise radiolucent lesion. In the two cases of AFDSs described to date the mandibular lesion was irregular but relatively well circumscribed in one case.[3] The other case revealed a large multilocular radiolucency containing an unerupted molar and a radiopaque mass at the lower border of the mandible.[4] Ameloblastic odontosarcomas have a similar radiographic appearance with irregular or well-defined margins and focal radiopacities within a radiolucent area. Computed tomography (CT) and magnetic resonance imagery (MRI) help to define the lesions in more detail.

3. Epidemiological data

3.1 Prevalence, incidence, and relative frequency

Both the AFDS (two accepted cases) and the AOS are exceedingly rare malignant odontogenic tumors. Therefore, no figures on prevalence, incidence, or relative frequency are available.

3.2 Age

The AFDS patients were two men, ages 27 and 25 years.[3,4] The case reported by Bregni et al[10] was a 32-year-old man. The mean

age at the time of diagnosis of patients with AOSs reported by Altini et al[4] (six cases, age unknown for one) was 21 years. The patient described by Takeda et al[8] was a 23-year-old man, and that reported by Phillips et al[7] was a 29-year-old man.

3.3 Gender

Both patients with AFDSs were men.[3,4] Of the six AOS cases reported by Altini et al,[4] two were men and four were women.

3.4 Location

In both AFDS cases, the large lesions were located in the mandible.[3,4] In the six AOS cases, the lesions were all located in the mandible; of these, five were in the posterior mandible.[4]

4. Pathogenesis

The etiology/pathogenesis of the AFDS and AOS is unknown. As in ameloblastic fibrosarcoma, however, the lesions may theoretically occur as a synchronous or metachronous process at the site of an ameloblastic fibroma or ameloblastic fibro-odontoma. In some cases, the malignant process develops from a benign lesion (ameloblastic fibro-odontoma) which recurs and becomes malignant.[11,12]

Slater[2] discussed the term *ameloblastic odontosarcoma* and considered the notion of a "malignant tooth," as suggested by the word *odontosarcoma,* disturbing. The AOS term resulted from the observation that an odontogenic sarcoma can arise from an antecedent ameloblastic fibro-odontoma, and it follows that such a neoplasm would be called ameloblastic fibro-odontosarcoma. Grossly identifiable tooth structures, however, usually are not formed. Eda et al[13] described a small complex odontoma associated with an ameloblastic fibrosarcoma, although the evidence of this combination is not clear from their report.

5. Pathology

5.1 Macroscopy

No detailed descriptions of the macroscopic aspects of AFDSs or AOSs have been reported. The resection specimens are usually large, resulting from hemimandibulectomies.

5.2 Microscopy

5.2.1 Histologic definition

Both the 1992 WHO classification[1] and the present authors use the following definition for AFDSs and AOSs: Neoplasms similar to ameloblastic fibrosarcomas in which limited amounts of dysplastic dentin (dentinoid) have formed and, in ameloblastic fibro-odontosarcoma, enamel as well.

5.2.2 Histopathologic findings

Histologically, the AFDS consists of an epithelial and an ectomesenchymal component, both including dentinoid, some of which may be dysplastic (Fig 30-1). The epithelial component is composed of follicles and strands of odontogenic epithelium as observed in ameloblastic fibromas. Intraepithelial and stromal microcysts may form.

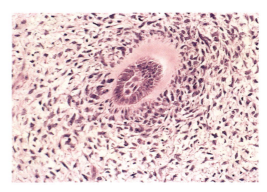

Fig 30-1 Ameloblastic fibrodentinosarcoma exhibiting an epithelial component with adjacent initial dentinoid formation. The surrounding malignant ectomesenchyme is characterized by increased cellularity, hyperchromatism, and some polymorphism (hematoxylin-eosin [H&E], x125). (Courtesy of Professor M. Altini, Johannesburg, RSA.)

Some epithelial islands may show ghost cells representative of a form of intracellular keratinization. In some areas, the odontogenic epithelium may induce the deposition of dentinoid (Fig 30-2). Deposits of dentinoid may be found adjacent to ameloblastomatous islands. These deposits rarely show dentinal tubules. The malignant ectomesenchymal component is characterized by increased cellularity, pleomorphism, hyperchromatism, and increased abnormal mitotic activity, as in ameloblastic fibrosarcomas. In both cases of AFDSs studied,[3,4] areas of apparently benign ectomesenchymal tissue were also present.

The histologic features of the AOS are identical to those of the AFDS except that enameloid is found in the former in addition to dentinoid. The histologic presence of prismatic or dysplastic enamel has been considered sufficient to justify the prefix *odonto*, although no grossly discernible tooth formation takes place in the AOS. As described in the literature,[3] extensive sampling may be

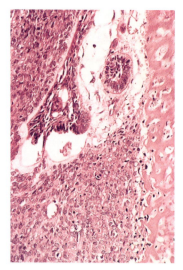

Fig 30-2 Ameloblastic fibrodentinosarcoma producing an area of dysplastic dentinoid closely associated with the sarcomatous ectomesenchyme (H&E, x125). (Courtesy of Professor M. Altini, Johannesburg, RSA.)

necessary to identify deposits of dentinoid or enameloid. As in the AFDS, ghost cell keratinization may be present. The benign odontogenic epithelium in the AOS may reveal mitotic activity or cytologic atypia.

5.2.3 Histochemical/immunohistochemical

Due to the small number of reported cases of AFDSs and AOSs, no studies on histochemistry or immunohistochemistry have been published.

5.2.4 Ultrastructural findings

No studies on the ultrastructure of the AFDS or AOS have been reported.

6. Notes on treatment and recurrence rate

The treatment of choice for both AFDSs and AOSs is radical surgery. In the two cases of AFDSs,[3,4] there were no recurrences. Recurrences have been noted (three, in some cases multiple, recurrences) in patients with AOSs and metastasis has been observed. Survival time has only been recorded in a few instances and was 3 years in one case.[13] The total number of AFDSs and AOSs at present is much too small to define the biologic behavior patterns of these neoplasms.

References

1. Kramer IRH, Pindborg JJ, Shear M. Histologic Typing of Odontogenic Tumours. 2d ed. Berlin: Springer-Verlag, 1992.

2. Slater LJ. Odontogenic sarcoma and carcinosarcoma. Semin Diagn Pathol 1999;16:325–332.

3. Altini M, Smith I. Ameloblastic dentinosarcoma—a case report. Int J Oral Surg 1976;5:142–147.

4. Altini M, Thompson SH, Lownie J, Berezowski BB. Ameloblastic sarcoma of the mandible. J Oral Maxillofac Surg 1985;43:789–794.

5. Corominas-Villafañe O, Cuesta-Carnero R, Corominas O, Gendelman H. Ameloblastic odontosarcoma: Report of a case. Acta Stomatol Belg 1993;90:149–156.

6. Herzog U, Putzke HP, Bienengräber V, Radke C. Das ameloblastische Fibroodontom—ein odontogener Mischtumor mit Übergang in ein odontogenes Sarkom. Dtsch Z Mund Kiefer Gesichtschir 1991;15:90–93.

7. Phillips VM, Grotepass FW, Hendricks R. Ameloblastic odontosarcoma with epithelial atypia: A case report. Br J Oral Maxillofac Surg 1988; 26:45–51.

8. Takeda Y, Kuroda M, Suzuki A. Ameloblastic odontosarcoma (ameloblastic fibro-odontosarcoma) in the mandible. Acta Pathol Jpn 1990; 40:832–837.

9. Thoma KH. Oral Pathology. 4th ed. St. Louis: CV Mosby, 1954:1234–1235.

10. Bregni RC, Taylor AM, García AM. Ameloblastic fibrosarcoma of the mandible: Report of two cases and review of the literature. J Oral Pathol Med 2001;30:316–320.

11. Müller S, Parker DC, Kapadia SB, et al. Ameloblastic fibro-sarcoma of the jaws. A clinicopathologic and DNA analysis of five cases and review of the literature with discussion of its relationship to ameloblastic fibroma. Oral Surg Oral Med Oral Pathol Oral Radiol Endod 1995;79:469–477.

12. Howell RM, Burkes EJJ. Malignant transformation of ameloblastic fibro-odontoma to ameloblastic fibrosarcoma. Oral Surg Oral Med Oral Pathol 1977;43:391–401.

13. Eda S, Saito T, Morimura G, et al. A case of ameloblastic fibrosarcoma, with an electron-microscopic observation. Bull Tokyo Dent Coll 1976;17:11–25.

Chapter 31

Odontogenic Carcinosarcoma

The 1992 World Health Organization (WHO) classification[1] of odontogenic tumors defined the odontogenic carcinosarcoma (OCS) as "a very rare neoplasm, similar in pattern to ameloblastic fibrosarcoma, but in which both the epithelial and the ectomesenchymal components show cytological features of malignancy." No further comments accompanied this definition and no examples of the histopathology of the OCS were given.

In 1999, Slater[2] stated that "such a tumour has not been reported as yet, to the best of my knowledge." A literature search in 2001 did not reveal any case reports or mentions of this neoplasm.

In his review, however, Slater[2] presented a case of OCS from his own files:

A 55-year-old man living in Saudi Arabia had an 8.0 x 6.2 x 5.0 cm tumour of the right mandibular body and ramus excised by hemimandibulectomy. Histology revealed an ameloblastic fibroma-like pattern with strands and cords of odontogenic epithelium separated by hypercellular fibrous connective tissue. The ameloblastomatous component displayed peripheral large cells with crowded large hyperchromatic nuclei; mitotic figures were observed among these large basaloid cells as well as among plump cells in the central stellate reticulum area. The sarcomatous component showed closely packed mitotically active polygonal cells

with hyperchromatism and moderate nuclear polymorphism. Slater[2] considered the mitotic rate of the epithelial component to be similar to that of the malignant ectomesenchymal tissue component (Figs 31-1 and 31-2).

Slater[2] further pointed out that a carcinosarcoma lacking the ameloblastic fibroma–like pattern could still be recognized as odontogenic if the epithelial component resembled that of an ameloblastoma. He considered a tumor of this type to be a sarcomatoid carcinoma arising in an amelo-

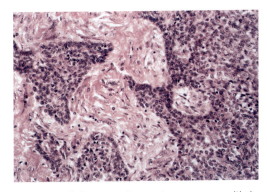

Fig 31-1 Odontogenic carcinosarcoma with irregular epithelial sheets and islands characterized by cellular atypia and increased mitotic activity. In this field, the ectomesenchymal component is predominantly fibrous and poor in cells with malignant features (hematoxylin-eosin [H&E], x75). (Courtesy of Professor J.J. Sciubba, Baltimore, MD.)

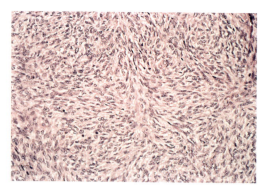

Fig 31-2 Area of an OCS exhibiting only the ectomesenchymal component where spindle-shaped fibroblasts arranged in whirled configurations show distinct sarcomatoid features (H&E, x75). (Courtesy of Professor J.J. Sciubba, Baltimore, MD.)

blastoma (a variant of ameloblastic sarcoma) and not an ameloblastic carcinosarcoma. Sarcomatoid carcinomas or carcinosarcomas have been reported as malignant mixed tumors (malignant ameloblastomas and fibrosarcomas) and as odontogenic carcinomas with sarcomatous proliferation.[3,4]

It seems evident that a consensus as to the definition of this obviously extremely rare tumor must be arrived at and cases of OCS must be published before conclusions about their etiology and biologic behavior can be made.

Comment

At the Consensus Conference held in Lyon (IARC/WHO) in July 2003 in conjunction with the preparation of chapter 6 (odontogenic tumors) for the forthcoming WHO volume *Tumours of the Head and Neck*, it was unanimously decided *not* to include the odontogenic carcinosarcoma in the new WHO classification due to the present lack of substantiated evidence.

References

1. Kramer IRH, Pindborg JJ, Shear M. Histologic Typing of Odontogenic Tumours. 2d ed. Berlin; Springer-Verlag, 1992.

2. Slater LJ. Odontogenic sarcoma and carcinosarcoma. Semin Diagn Pathol 1999;16:325–332.

3. Tanaka T, Ohkubo T, Fujitsuka H, et al. Malignant mixed tumor (malignant ameloblastoma and fibrosarcoma) of the maxilla. Arch Pathol Lab Med 1991;115:84–87.

4. Yoshida T, Shingaki S, Nakajima T, et al. Odontogenic carcinoma with sarcomatous proliferation. A case report. J Craniomaxillofac Surg 1989;17: 139–142.

Neoplasms and Other Lesions Occurring in the Maxillofacial Skeleton

Introduction to Neoplastic and Non-neoplastic Osseous Lesions

The term *fibro-osseous lesions* refers to several lesions representing a diverse process in which the normal bone architecture is replaced by fibroblasts and collagen fibers containing variable amounts of mineralized material. The term is not a specific diagnosis, indicating only a broad group of several entities. Although there is no completely satisfactory classification, it is generally accepted that benign fibro-osseous lesions in the oral and maxillofacial regions can be divided into three categories: the *benign fibro-osseous neoplasms,* the non-neoplastic *fibrous dysplasias*, and *reactive (dysplastic) lesions.*[1–3]

Cementum is a mineralized dental hard tissue covering the root surface of teeth. It is avascular and may present a structural similarity to woven bone. Cementoblasts are considered to be derived from ectomesenchyme

of the dental follicle, which also gives rise to the periodontal ligament. Cementoblasts synthesize an organic matrix—cementoid—which is deposited on the dentin during odontogenesis. Calcified cementum is mostly avascular. The apical third of the root may incorporate cementoblasts. In the normal periodontal ligament, it is common to find round, strongly basophilic, calcified masses known as cementicles, which are produced in that location. Lesions derived from cementoblasts may be either neoplastic or dysplastic.

One of these groups is the cemento-osseous lesions. These are non-neoplastic lesions of the jaws and include a variety of lesions characterized histopathologically by the presence of cementum-like tissues. The World Health Organization (WHO) classification of 1971[4] used the unifying concept of cementomas to group together lesions containing cementum-like tissue, thus forming a complex group of lesions with ill-defined characteristics. Therefore, in this classification both neoplastic (benign cementoblastomas, cemento-ossifying fibromas) and non-neoplastic lesions (periapical cemental dysplasias, gigantiform cementomas) formed one group.

The WHO classification of 1992[1] clearly separated neoplastic from non-neoplastic lesions containing cementum-like tissue. Several lesions were considered to belong to this category and were grouped together under the term *cemento-osseous dysplasias*. To this group belong lesions such as periapical cemental dysplasias (periapical fibrous dysplasias), florid cemento-osseous dysplasias (gigantiform cementomas and familial multiple cementomas) and other cemento-osseous dysplasias. These entities were considered as "lesions which share some of the features of periapical cemental dysplasias and/or florid cemento-osseous dysplasia, but do not have their characteristic clinicopathological patterns of presentation."[2]

In recent years, suggestions have been made to change the nomenclature of some of these lesions. The term *focal cemento-osseous dysplasia,* for example, has been coined to replace the term *periapical cemental dysplasia*. Some researchers consider focal cemento-osseous dysplasia and florid cemento-osseous dysplasia the same lesion. Details on recent advances relating to cemento-osseous dysplasias are described in chapters 34 and 35.

Comment

During the July 2003 Consensus Conference, held in conjunction with the preparation of the new WHO volume *Tumours of the Head and Neck*, a number of changes in terminology were introduced. Osseous neoplasms and non-neoplastic lesions were categorized under the section "Neoplasms and Other Lesions Occurring in the Maxillofacial Skeleton." The section on osseous neoplasms includes ossifying fibroma (formerly cemento-ossifing fibroma). The section on non-neoplastic lesions comprises fibrous dysplasia, osseous dysplasias, central giant cell lesion/granuloma, cherubism, aneurysmal bone cyst, and simple bone cyst.

Osseous dysplasias were defined as idiopathic processes located in the periapical region of the tooth-bearing jaw areas. These conditions include different clinical variants. When occurring in the anterior mandible and involving only a few teeth, the lesion is termed *periapical osseous dysplasia*. A similar lesion occurring in the posterior jaw is termed *focal osseous dysplasia* (formerly focal cemento-osseous dysplasia). Two additional types of osseous dysplasia are more extensive and occur bilaterally in the mandible. One is known as *florid osseous dysplasia* and mainly occurs in middle-aged black females. The second variant is called *familial gigantiform cementoma*. Regrettably, because the final production of this book coincided with the Consensus Conference, rewriting some of the following chapters was not possible.

References

1. Kramer IRH, Pindborg JJ, Shear M. Histological Typing of Odontogenic Tumours. 2d ed. Berlin: Springer-Verlag, 1992.

2. Su L, Weathers DR, Waldron CA. Distinguishing features of focal cemento-osseous dysplasias and cemento-ossifying fibromas. I. A pathologic spectrum of 316 cases. Oral Surg Oral Med Oral Pathol Oral Radiol Endod 1997;84:301–309.

3. Su L, Weathers DR, Waldron CA. Distinguishing features of focal cemento-osseous dysplasia and cemento-ossifying fibromas. II. A clinical and radiologic spectrum of 316 cases. Oral Surg Oral Med Oral Pathol Oral Radiol Endod 1997;84: 540–549.

4. Pindborg JJ, Kramer IRH. Histological Typing of Odontogenic Tumours, Jaw Cysts and Allied Lesions. Berlin: Springer-Verlag, 1971.

Chapter 32

Ossifying Fibroma

1. Terminology

Lack of standardized terminology and classifications of central or intraosseous cemento-osseous lesions of the jaws have long posed a dilemma for pathologists and clinicians. Montgomery[1] appears to have been the first to designate jaw lesions of this type as ossifying fibromas. To some observers, all of these lesions were actually examples of monostotic manifestations of fibrous dysplasias. Jaffe[2] originally believed this to be the case, although 5 years later[3] he considered the ossifying fibroma—which he called fibrocementoma—as a separate entity from fibrous dysplasia.

Various terms have been applied to these benign fibro-osseous neoplasms over the years. When bone predominates in a particular lesion, it is called an *ossifying fibroma*; the term *cementifying fibroma* is used when curved/linear trabeculae or spheroidal (psammoma-like) calcifications are encountered. When tumors contain both bone and cementum-like material, with or without psammoma-like bodies, and are well circumscribed radiographically, a diagnosis of *cemento-ossifying fibroma* (COF) is made.[4] Previously, many investigators classified cementifying fibromas separately from ossifying fibromas because the former were considered to be of odontogenic origin and the latter to be osteogenic. It is now agreed that both types fall under the same classification

as osteogenic neoplasms. On the basis of an analysis of 64 cases classified as ossifying and/or cementifying fibroma, Eversole et al[5] decided that a distinction between these two variants would be academic, as no behavioral differences exist. The authors suggested consequently that the nomenclature could be simplified by referring to all lesions in this group as ossifying fibromas. It should be stressed that differentiating between the COF and fibrous dysplasia based on clinical/radiologic and histopathologic features may be difficult. The erroneous view that both lesions are part of the same spectrum still persists.[6]

The term *juvenile aggressive (or active ossifying) fibroma* (JOF) is used for an actively growing lesion that mainly affects individuals younger than 15 years of age.[4] This lesion behaves in an aggressive fashion, reaching massive proportions with extensive cortical expansion. Slootweg and coworkers,[7] in an analysis of 33 cases of JOFs, were able to separate the lesions into two distinct groups which they designated as *juvenile ossifying fibroma—WHO type* (JOF-WHO) and *juvenile ossifying fibroma with psammoma-like ossicles or cementicles* (JOF-PO). Further information about these lesions appears later in this chapter.

It should be stressed that the extraosseous or peripheral lesion known as *peripheral ossifying fibroma* (synonyms include soft fibroma, peripheral fibroma with calcification, peripheral odontogenic fibroma, and calcifying fibroblastic granuloma) is reactive in nature and is *not* the extraosseous counterpart of the COF.[8]

2. Clinical and radiologic profile

In an analysis of 75 cases of COFs in an American population, Su et al[9] identified a slow-growing, buccolingual jaw expansion or mild tenderness in 51% of patients; the remaining 49% were asymptomatic. However, the clinical presentation is variable.[10] Small lesions are often discovered incidentally. Bilateral and multiple COFs have been reported.[11-13] If untreated, lesions may become large and cause considerable cosmetic and functional problems.

Radiographically, Eversole et al[5] found that the 64 COF cases they examined were all well-defined unilocular, round, or oval structures (Fig 32-1). Larger tumors may have a multilocular radiographic appearance. MacDonald-Jankowski[10] described

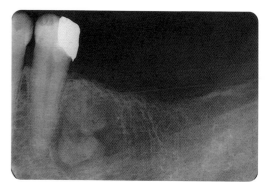

Fig 32-1 Radiograph showing a well-defined, unilocular COF in the edentulous left mandibular area of a 45-year-old man. Small radiodensities (*arrow*) are seen in the lower part of the radiolucency.

Fig 32-2 Mixed radiolucency and opacity in the edentulous area distal to the mandibular left second premolar.

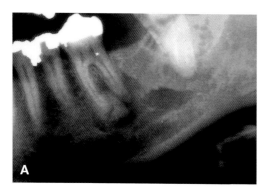

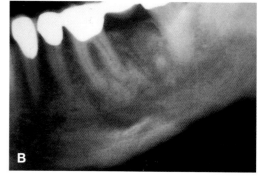

Fig 32-3 Radiographic stages of a COF. A: Mixed radiolucency/radiopacity in the periapical mandibular right molar region. B: The same tumor after 7 years. The radiopacities have increased significantly with age.

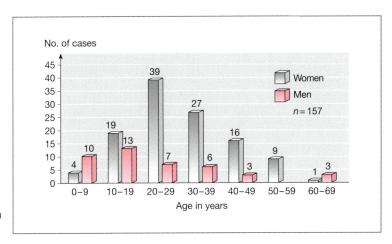

Fig 32-4 Age distribution of 157 cases of COFs.

three stages in the radiographic appearance of the COF. The initial appearance is radiolucent, which then becomes progressively radiopaque as the stroma mineralizes (Figs 32-2 and 32-3). Eventually, the individual radiopacities coalesce to the extent that the mature lesion may appear sclerotic. The author also presented a summary of the radiologic features in 177 reported cases of COFs from the literature and his own files,[9,10,14,15] demonstrating that 42% were radiolucent, 24% were radiopaque, and 34% had a mixed appearance. The presence of a well-defined margin was held by Sciubba and Younai[15] to be a consistent and reliable radiologic marker for COF.

Su et al[9] reported that the average lesion diameter was 3.8 cm, with a range of 0.2 to 15 cm in 54 cases of COFs. A majority (93%) of COFs failed to demonstrate an association with the tooth apex but often caused divergence of the involved roots. Root resorption was not a common finding. This raises doubt as to whether the COF originates in the periodontal ligament. Su et al also noticed three different patterns of radiographic borders: a defined lesion without a sclerotic border (40%), a well-defined lesion with a sclerotic border (45%), and a lesion with an ill-defined border (15%). None of the 64 cases of COFs examined by Eversole et al[5] were associated with the crowns of impacted teeth and 35% of the tumors were detected in edentulous areas.

3. Epidemiological data

3.1 Prevalence, incidence, and relative frequency

No data on these aspects of COFs are available.

3.2 Age

Based on pooled, comparable data retrieved from three reports on COFs (n = 157),[5,9,15] 79.6% of tumors were diagnosed before 40 years of age, and 58.6% before 30 years of age (Fig 32-4). There is a distinct peak in the 3rd decade for women, with cases in men occurring slightly earlier. The mean ages for patients in the cited studies[5,9,15] were 36, 32, and 30 years, respectively. A mean age of 39 was found in a study of 20 Hong Kong Chinese patients (all women).[10]

275

3.3 Gender

In the same three studies,[5,9,15] occurrence was far more common in female patients, with the male:female ratio varying from 1:3.2 to 1:4.3. Several authors[5,9,16] have indicated that there appears to be no ethnic predilection for COFs.

3.4 Location

In a summary of data from 11 studies on COFs,[10] it was found that between 70% and 90% of all tumors were located in the mandible. In one study from Nigeria,[17] the tumor was found to be slightly more common in the maxilla with a maxilla:mandible ratio of 10:9. However, the criteria for diagnosing COFs more than 30 years ago when the study was done may not meet today's criteria. Su et al[9] reported that 52 (70%) of their 75 cases of COFs were located in the mandible, with 43% located in the posterior region—including the ramus area, followed by 22% in the posterior maxilla (Fig 32-5). The same authors also found that COFs did not display a significant association with tooth apex or in edentulous areas (7% and 8%, respectively, in these locations), whereas the focal cemento-osseous dysplasia (also known as periapical cemental dysplasia[4]) arose either in close proximity to the apex of the teeth or in a site of previous extraction (70% and 21%, respectively, in these locations).

4. Pathogenesis

The pathologic nature of COFs is not clearly understood. The close proximity to the periodontal ligament has led to a presumption that COFs originate in the periodontal ligament with the potential for both osseous and cemental differentiation. There is, however, no scientific evidence to support this hypothesis.[9] As already mentioned, only 7% of COFs demonstrated a relationship to periapical sites[9]; furthermore, lesions that are histopathologically identical to COFs have also been found in other bones of the body.[18] Studies aimed at elucidating the pathogenesis of the COF are strongly needed.

5. Pathology

5.1 Macroscopy

The cut surface of the tumor is whitish yellow, and the consistency of the lesion varies with the amount of calcified material. The generally sharp delineation of the COF is also apparent in surgery when it tends to be enucleated as either large intact specimens or large surgically dissected fragments. Su et al[19] reported that 88% of COFs in their study exhibited a single or large enucleated fragment, whereas 12% had multiple curetted fragments that were not a result of incisional

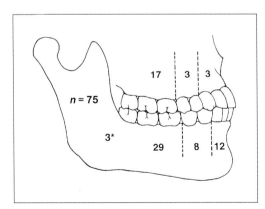

Fig 32-5 Topographic distribution of 75 COFs. Asterisk indicates cases localized in the ascending ramus.

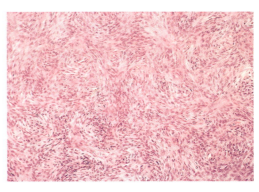

Fig 32-6 Cellularity and mitotic activity within a COF (hematoxylin-eosin [H&E], x80).

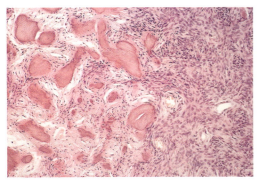

Fig 32-7 COF with hypercellular stroma (*right*) and a combination of bone trabeculae and cementum-like spherical structures (*left*). (H&E, x80).

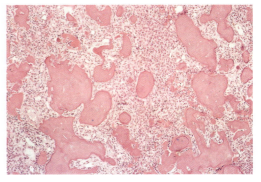

Fig 32-8 Irregular cementum-like structures, some of which exhibit fringelike osteoid rims. The fibrous stroma in this COF is of variable cellularity (H&E, x80).

biopsy procedure. A fibrous capsule was identified in 44% of the lesions.

5.2 Microscopy

5.2.1 Histologic definitions

According to the 1992 World Health Organization (WHO) classification,[4] a COF is a "demarcated or rarely encapsulated neoplasm consisting of fibrous tissue containing varying amounts of mineralized material resembling bone an/or cementum."

The definition used by the present authors is as follows:

A benign osteogenic, well-demarcated neoplasm composed of calcified material and a fibroblastic stroma, which may be very cellular (Fig 32-6). The calcified component is usually a combination of bone trabeculae and strongly basophilic cementum-like structures with variable osteoblastic rimming (Figs 32-7 and 32-8). Osteoclast-like giant cells and occasional aneurysmal bone cavity components characterized by sinusoid blood spaces may be present.

5.2.2 Histopathologic findings

In their 75 cases of COFs, Su et al[19] found three histologic subtypes. The first and most common subtype has an equal amount of calcified material and fibroblastic stroma. The calcified structures consist of both separate and retiform bony trabeculae with a prominent osteoblastic rim and occasional osteoclasts. Rounded or lobulated cementum-like bodies may be scattered throughout the lesion and may constitute a major component, such as in a cementifying fibroma. The connective tissue consists of sheets of spindle-shaped, fibroblastic, or stellate cells with focal areas of storiform pattern (a typical radiograph would show a well-defined mixed radiolucency and radiopacity).

The second and least common subtype of COF is characterized by predominantly storiform cellularity in the stroma containing scant separate osteoid or bony trabeculae, often without osteoblastic rimming. Some cells in the storiform pattern exhibit stellate or rounded nuclei which may resemble potential osteoblasts, and dense collagen fibers are sometimes intermingled with the storiform pattern (a corresponding radiograph is mainly radiolucent).

The third subtype of COF represents a combination of the first two, which are each seen in different areas of large lesions. It is important to stress that the COF is a sharply demarcated lesion. The hard tissues of the tumor *do not* fuse with the surrounding bone, except occasionally in limited areas.[4] This is a significant feature in distinguishing a COF from a fibrous dysplasia, in which it is common to find that the metaplastic bone of the lesion fuses directly to the bordering cortical bone.

Eversole et al[5] assessed the histologic features of a series of 64 cases of COFs using both light and polarization microscopy. The use of polarized light enabled the authors to study and differentiate between four different fiber patterns in the hard tissue elements, including woven bone trabeculae, lamellar bone trabeculae, ovoid-curvoid deposits, and anastomosing curved/linear trabeculae.

6. Notes on treatment and recurrence rate

Surgical curettage or enucleation are the initial treatment of choice for most small COFs. In the absence of a reliable diagnostic or prognostic predictor to indicate the potential of COF for aggressive behavior or the likelihood of recurrence, periodic clinical and radiographic follow-up should be pursued. For larger tumors or a sudden growth spurt connoting aggressive behavior, en bloc resection should be considered as secondary definitive therapy. If the tumor is only partially removed, continued growth does not necessarily follow. Nevertheless, Eversole et al[5] reported a 28% overall recurrence rate following curettage in 22 patients with a mean follow-up period of 38 months.

7. Juvenile ossifying fibroma

The juvenile ossifying fibroma is a well-defined clinical and histologic entity that has recently been separated from other central fibro-osseous lesions, including the COF.[7] It is described in the WHO classification[4] as "an actively growing lesion consisting of a cell-rich fibrous stroma, containing bands of cellular osteoid without osteoblastic rimming together with trabeculae of more typical woven bone. Small foci of giant cells may also be present, and in some parts there may be

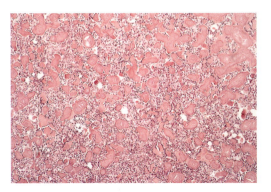

Fig 32-9 Juvenile COF with psammoma-like ossicles or "cementicles" exhibiting osteoid rimming in a 26-year-old woman (H&E, x80).

abundant osteoclasts related to the woven bone. Usually no fibrous capsule can be demonstrated, but like the ossifying fibroma (and unlike fibrous dysplasia), the JOF is well demarcated from the surrounding bone."

As mentioned earlier, Slootweg et al[7] distinguish between two distinct groups of JOFs, the JOF-WHO and the JOF with psammoma-like ossicles, the latter being histologically similar to those described in the maxillary sinuses.[20-22] The authors found that JOF-WHO lesions occurred in a young age group (mean, 11.8 years), whereas JOF-PO lesions occurred in about a decade later (mean, 22.6 years) and showed a more cellular stroma (Fig 32-9). Williams et al[23] recently studied a total 8 cases of JOF (mean age of 10 years with a range of 5 to 15 years). Histologically, they found the typical features described in the WHO classification[4] with a few modifications: there were cases of osteoblastic rimming of osteoid trabeculae; the stroma showed pseudocysts associated with giant cells; and no cementicles were seen.

Slootweg et al[7] observed that COFs contained cementicles identical to the ossicles in JOF-POs, which led the authors to suggest that the JOF-PO should be classified within the spectrum of cemento-ossifying fibroma separate from the JOF-WHO. Williams et al[23] confirmed these findings. It should be mentioned that the JOF-PO in the German language literature has for some years been known as "psammöses Desmoosteoblastom" (psammotoid ossifying fibroma)[24] and is considered a semimalignant bone tumor of the maxillofacial skeleton.

References

1. Montgomery AH. Ossifying fibromas of the jaw. Arch Surg 1927;15:30–44.

2. Jaffe HL. Giant cell reparative granuloma, traumatic bone cyst and fibrous (fibro-osseous) dysplasia. Oral Surg Oral Med Oral Pathol 1953;6:159–175.

3. Jaffe HL. Tumors and Tumorous Conditions of the Bones and Joints. London: Henry Kimpton, 1958.

4. Kramer IRH, Pindborg JJ, Shear M. Histological Typing of Odontogenic Tumours. 2d ed. Berlin: Springer-Verlag, 1992.

5. Eversole LR, Leider AS, Nelson K. Ossifying fibroma: A clinicopathologic study of sixty-four cases. Oral Surg Oral Med Oral Pathol 1985;60:505–511.

6. Voytek TM, Ro JY, Edeiken J, Ayala AG. Fibrous dysplasia and cemento-ossifying fibroma. A histological spectrum. Am J Surg Pathol 1995;19:775–778.

7. Slootweg PJ, Panders AK, Koopmans R, Nikkels PG. Juvenile ossifying fibroma. An analysis of 33 cases with emphasis on histopathological aspects. J Oral Pathol Med 1994;23:385–388.

8. Buchner A, Hansen LS. The histomorphologic spectrum of peripheral ossifying fibroma. Oral Surg Oral Med Oral Pathol 1987;63:452–461.

9. Su L, Weathers DR, Waldron CA. Distinguishing features of focal cemento-osseous dysplasia and cemento-ossifying fibromas. II. A clinical and radiologic spectrum of 316 cases. Oral Surg Oral Med Oral Pathol Oral Radiol Endod 1997;84:540–549.

10. MacDonald-Jankowski DS. Cemento-ossifying fibromas in the jaws of Hong Kong Chinese. Dentomaxillofac Radiol 1998;27:298–304.

11. Wei-Yung Y, Pederson GT, Bartley MH. Multiple familial ossifying fibromas: Relationship to other osseous lesions of the jaws. Oral Surg Oral Med Oral Pathol 1989;68:754–758.

12. Hauser MS Freije S, Payne RW, Timen S. Bilateral ossifying fibroma of the maxillary sinus. Oral Surg Oral Med Oral Pathol 1989;68:759–763.

13. Sakoma T, Kawasaki T, Watanabe K. Concurrent cementifying and ossifying fibromas of the mandible. Report of a case. J Oral Maxillofac Surg 1998;56:778–782.

14. Eversole LR, Merrell PW, Strub D. Radiographic characteristics of central ossifying fibroma. Oral Surg Oral Med Oral Pathol 1985;59:522–527.

15. Sciubba JJ, Younai F. Ossifying fibroma of mandible and maxilla: Review of 18 cases. J Oral Pathol Med 1989;18:315–328.

16. Summerlin D-J, Tomich CE. Focal cemento-osseus dysplasia: A clinicopathologic study of 221 cases. Oral Surg Oral Med Oral Pathol 1994;78:611–620.

17. Anand SV, Dabey WW, Cohen B. Tumours of the jaws in West Africa: A review of 256 patients. Br J Surg 1967;54:901–917.

18. Slootweg PJ. Maxillofacial fibro-osseous lesions: Classification and differential diagnosis. Semin Diagn Pathol 1996;13:104–112.

19. Su L, Weathers DR, Waldron CA. Distinguishing features of focal cemento-osseous dysplasias and cemento-ossifying fibromas. I. A pathologic spectrum of 316 cases. Oral Surg Oral Med Oral Pathol 1997;84:301–309.

20. Fu YS, Perzin KH. Non-epithelial tumours of the nasal cavity, paranasal sinuses and nasopharynx: A clinicopatholigic study. II. Osseous and fibro-osseous lesions including osteoma, fibrous dysplasia, ossifying fibroma, osteoblastoma, giant cell tumour and osteosarcoma. Cancer 1974;33:1289–1305.

21. Hyams VJ, Batsakis JG, Michaels L. Tumours of the upper respiratory tract and ears. Atlas of Tumours Pathology, 2d ser., fascicle 25. Washington, DC: Armed Forces Institute of Pathology, 1988:181.

22. Johnson LC, Yousefi M, Vinh TN, et al. Juvenile active ossifying fibroma its nature dynamics and origin. Acta Otolaryngol Suppl 1991;488:1–40.

23. Williams HK, Maugham C, Speight PM. Juvenile ossifying fibroma. An analysis of eight cases and a comparison with other fibro-osseous lesions. J Oral Pathol Med 2000;29:13–18.

24. Adler C-P, Neuburger M, Herget GW. Psammöses Desmoosteoblastom des rechten Oberkiefers. Fallbericht und Differenzialdiagnose einer seltenen Tumorentität. Mund Kiefer Gesichtschir 2001;5:150–154.

Chapter 33

Fibrous Dysplasia

1. Terminology

Fibrous dysplasia (FD) is a benign non-neoplastic developmental bone disease of fibro-osseous origin that may involve one or more bones of the cranial or extracranial skeleton. It is considered an uncommon developmental anomaly and may be divided into three variants: *monostotic, polyostotic,* and *craniofacial.*[1] Some authorities have suggested five main clinical subgroups of FD: a monostotic form (I), a polyostotic form (II), a polyostotic form accompanied by pigmented skin lesions (Jaffe type; III), a polyostotic form accompanied by pigmented skin lesions and endocrine dysfunction presenting as precocious puberty in women (Albright syndrome; IV), and a craniofacial form confined to the bones of the craniofacial complex (V).[2]

In 1891, von Recklinghausen reported on three groups of bone diseases, one of which most likely contained cases of what is currently called polyostotic fibrous dysplasia (PFD).[1] Subsequent to von Recklinghausen's description, a number of cases were described under the term *ostitis fibrosa generalisata.* In 1937, Albright and coworkers, as well as McCune and Burch, recorded cases of FD with multiple disseminated lesions of bone, skin pigmentation, and precocious puberty in female patients.[1]

In 1938, Lichtenstein described eight cases of osteofibrotic bone lesions without extraskeletal manifestations and called the process polyostotic fibrous dysplasia.[3] In 1942, Lichtenstein and Jaffe[4] recognized FD as a disease entity and noted that a monostotic form of FD may occur.

Pritchard[5] reviewed 256 cases of FD published between 1929 and 1949 and noted an equal gender distribution. In 1972, Eversole et al[1] reviewed 228 cases of monostotic FD, 41 cases of polyostotic FD, and 40 cases of craniofacial FD. Numerous reports on smaller and larger series of FD, including cases from different geographic areas and ethnic groups, have been reported over the last several decades. Dahlgren et al[6] described 20 Swedish patients with FD. Waldron and Giansanti[7] reported on 22 cases of FD.

Daramola et al[8] described clinicoradiologic features of 47 Nigerian patients with FD.[8] In 1992, Awange[9] reviewed 333 cases of FD in Africa. Other reports have been made from researchers in Switzerland ($n = 6$),[10] South Korea ($n = 31$),[11] and Holland ($n = 12$).[12] MacDonald-Jankowski[13] described 7 cases of FDs from Hong Kong and derived a systematic review of 104 individual cases from nine reports.

The literature on fibrous dysplasia and its subtypes is extensive; a 2001 online literature search using the term *fibrous dysplasia* yielded 2,423 results. Of particular significance is that considerable progress has been made in clarifying the etiology of fibrous dysplasia and Albright syndrome (also known as McCune-Albright syndrome).[14]

2. Clinical and radiologic profile

Clinically, monostotic FD (MFD) may exhibit a slow-growing, usually painless swelling of the affected bone which causes deformity. The growth often slows or ceases after the onset of puberty and as such is considered self-limiting.

Involvement of the maxilla is more common than involvement of the mandible. Maxillary cases often involve a group of contiguous bones separated by sutures—such as the maxilla and the zygomatic, sphenoid, and occipital bones—and in this sense are not strictly monostotic. The designation *cranio-facial FD* has been suggested for such cases. In certain conditions such as pregnancy, FD may be reactivated. Fibrous dysplasia is nonencapsulated and essentially benign both in its clinical and biologic course and in its histologic components.

MacDonald-Jankowski[13] systematically evaluated nine series of FD (including monostotic, polyostotic, and craniofacial variants) of the jaws, totaling 104 cases from various populations. He recorded swelling in 95% and pain in 15% of the cases in which adequate information was available.

Generally, minor occurrences do not produce any patient complaints and are sometimes detected accidentally on radiographs. When swelling occurs, it involves the corpus of the mandible more often than the ramus or temporomandibular joint. In the maxilla, the alveolar process is involved to varying extents (Fig 33-1). Foci are often localized around the canine fossae and may involve the zygomatic bones, where they usually produce marked facial asymmetry. Frequently,

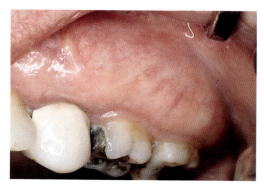

Fig 33-1 Clinical photograph showing the left maxillary alveolar process of a 66-year-old woman. The alveolar process is bulky and bony hard; the overlying oral mucosa is normal.

maxillary growth may extend diffusely in the bony walls of the maxillary sinuses, causing constriction. Swellings are immobile and are not tender to palpation. The oral mucosa overlying FD is unremarkable. Teeth may be displaced, producing some degree of malocclusion. Pathologic fractures of the jaw affected by FD are rare.[13]

The extent of skeletal involvement in cases of polyostotic FD ranges 5% to 60%.[2] A number of endocrine disturbances, including accelerated skeletal growth, hyperthyroidism, hyperparathyroidism, Cushing syndrome, diabetes mellitus, gynecomastia, café au lait skin pigmentation, and female sexual precocity, have been associated with PFD. The term *Albright syndrome* has been applied to patients who exhibit skin pigmentation, precocious puberty, or other endocrine disturbances. The definition of Albright syndrome, however, varies somewhat from author to author.

The frequency of jaw involvement in PFD is difficult to determine but was found to be 40.5% in one study.[2] Thickening of the occipital bone and the base of the skull are considered the most common craniofacial manifestations.

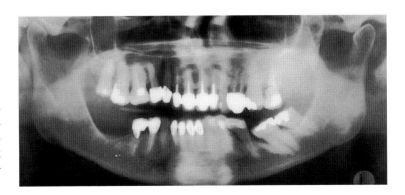

Fig 33-2 Panoramic radiograph showing diffuse radiopacity of the left maxillary complex and part of the left mandible.

Cases of fibrous dysplasia have been studied extensively by conventional radiography, computed tomography (CT), magnetic resonance imaging (MRI), and bone scintigraphy. Generally, the radiographic presentation of FD varies according to the degree of maturation of the individual lesion. In the early stages, predominantly destructive changes are visible in the form of thinning spongiosa with partly distinct and partly undefined delimitation from the surrounding bone. Even at the early stage, the border between cancellous and cortical bone is obliterated. At a later stage, the area becomes opaque. The most frequently used radiologic description of bone affected by FD is "ground glass," although it has also been called smoky, cloudy, whorled, or diffuse sclerotic[13] (Figs 33-2 and 33-3).

Radiologic features are especially important in differentiating between FD and fibro-osseous lesions, particularly cemento-ossifying fibromas (COFs). If the margin of the affected area is poorly defined, it is fibrous dysplasia; if the margin is well defined, it is a COF.[13] This distinction is considered important because FD is a self-limiting disease that may require surgical recontouring of the bone, whereas the COF (see chapter 32) is a benign neoplasm that must be treated by complete surgical removal. At the initial radiolucent stage, FD may be confused with a

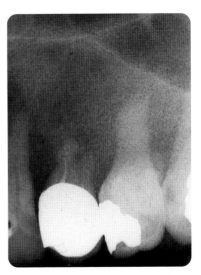

Fig 33-3 Fibrous dysplasia presenting with a characteristic ground-glass appearance of bone.

number of lesions, including central giant cell granulomas, traumatic bone cysts, and COFs. Paget disease, which affects older patients and frequently occurs bilaterally, is easily differentiated from FD; the latter is characterized by earlier onset and a normally unilateral distribution. The unilateral nature of fibrous dysplasia was recently demonstrated in a Chinese population.[13]

283

MacDonald-Jankowski[13] did extensive study on the radiologic features of 93 cases of FDs, and found 5% of the affected areas to be radiolucent and 95% to be of a ground-glass appearance. The shape of mandibular growths was ovoid in 91% of patients and multilocular in 9%. Expansion of the lower border of the mandible in a buccolingual direction was seen in 100% of patients, as was antral involvement in maxillary cases. Displaced teeth were seen in 41% of the evaluated cases.

Other radiographic findings that have been described in FD cases are loss of lamina dura and displacement of the inferior dental nerve canal. While some researchers considered an upward displacement of the canal to be unique for FD, others found a marked downward displacement of the inferior alveolar nerve canal.[13] Petrikowski et al[15] compared radiographic features of FD, osteogenic sarcomas, and osteomyelitis. Compared to osteogenic sarcomas and osteomyelitis, the authors found superior displacement of the mandibular canal and a fin-gerprint bone pattern pathognomonic for FD. Displacement of the maxillary sinus cortex, alteration of the lamina dura to the abnormal bone pattern, and narrowing of the periodontal ligament space were also distinguishing radiologic features.

While the typical plain film and CT changes (Figs 33-4 to 33-7) of fibrous dysplasia have been well described in the literature, findings with MRI and contrast-enhanced MRI have rarely been reported. Casselmann et al[16] studied MRI signal characteristics on T1- and T2-weighted images and a gadolinium-enhanced T1-weighted spin echo sequence in five patients with craniofacial FD. Low to intermediate signal intensity was usually seen in the largest part of the affected areas on both spin echo sequences. Smaller regions of hyperintensity on T1- and T2-weighted images and intermediate signal intensity throughout a growth on T1-weighted images were also seen. All areas were enhanced, but only two became hyper- or isointensive compared to fat. High levels of clinical and pathologic activity may cor-

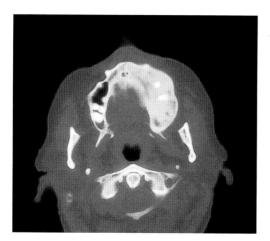

Fig 33-4 CT scan of an enlarged extended maxillary alveolar process.

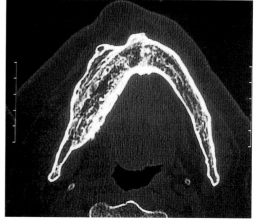

Fig 33-5 CT scan showing unilateral enlargement of the mandible.

relate with high signal intensity on spin echo performed normally and with enhancement. Varying signal intensity, including higher intensity on T2-weighted images, is explained by the complex histology and high levels of metabolic activity of FD.[16]

Bone scintigraphy of benign jaw lesions, including FDs, has been performed.[17] Abnormal scintigrams were found in all FD cases, as well as in patients in whom the disease was considered to be inactive. In addition, it has been shown that scintigraphy cannot be used to differentiate between FD and osteomyelitis.[17]

The radiographic appearance of jaw growths compared to those of other bones of the skeleton in both the monostotic and polyostotic variants of FD have been discussed by Gibson and Middlemiss.[18]

3. Epidemiological data

3.1 Prevalence, incidence, and relative frequency

Figures on prevalence and incidence for the monostotic and polyostotic variants of FD have not been published to date. Generally, MFD is considered to be uncommon and PFD is a relatively rare disease.[2] In their review of FD, Eversole et al[1] found MFD in 74%, PFD in 13%, and craniofacial FD in 13% of patients.

3.2 Age

Since the FDs throughout the patient's lifetime persist (if bone is not surgically remodelled), the onset of the disease is often difficult to establish. McDonald-Jankowski,[13] who studied nine series of FD which included all three variants, recorded 61 cases in which the age of the patient at the time of di-

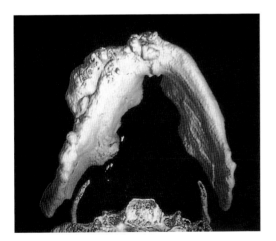

Fig 33-6 Three-dimensional reconstruction of the mandible as seen in Fig 33-5. Note the irregular surfaces of both the buccal and the lingual cortical plates.

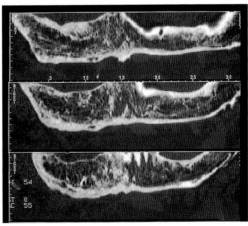

Fig 33-7 Denta CT scan showing the thickening of the lower border of the right mandible.

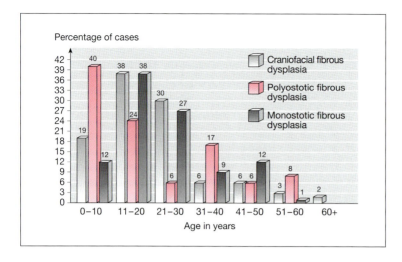

Fig 33-8 Age distribution of FD (monostotic, polyostotic, and craniofacial variants) according to Eversole et al.[1]

agnosis was stated; the mean age was 25 years. In other series, it was 27 years[1] and 28 years.[12] Eversole et al[1] reported on the mean age of the different variants of FD, the mean for MFD being 25.0 years, for PFD 23.6 years, and for craniofacial FD 21.0 years. Figure 33-8 shows the age distribution of the three FD variants according to Eversole et al.[1] To compile individual data and provide an updated age distribution for FD is beyond the scope of this book. It is noteworthy that age distribution in the Eversole et al study was recorded at the time of admission rather than at the onset of signs and symptoms. The mean age and age range seem to be similar in different ethnic groups.

The age at onset of polyostotic FD may vary widely, and reports range from vaginal bleeding in a 3-month-old girl (precocious puberty) to leg pain in a 68-year-old man.[2] The median age of onset of symptoms has been reported to be 8 years, with two thirds of patients reporting symptoms before the age of 10.

3.3 Gender

Monostotic FD of the jaws is seen with approximately equal frequency in men and women.[2] In the series reviewed by Eversole et al,[1] the male:female ratio was 1.6:1 for MFD, 1.2:1 for PFD, and 9.4:1 for craniofacial FD. McDonald-Jankowski[13] reported a male:female ratio of 1.3:1 with 41 cases in men and 51 cases in women.

3.4 Location

Generally, the maxilla is affected more often than the mandible. Of 92 cases that were evaluated by MacDonald-Jankowski,[13] 66% (61) were in the maxilla and 34% (31) were in the mandible, yielding a ratio of 1.97:1. In 47 Nigerian patients,[8] 62% of growths were located in the maxilla and 38% in the mandible, giving a ratio of 1.63:1. The unilateral nature of FD has been found in the majority of studies. In some reports[13] a predilection for the right side has been observed, but it has been argued that this may prove invalid as more cases are reported.

4. Pathogenesis

Fibrous dysplasia is a congenital, metabolic, nonfamilial disturbance of bone formation. It manifests as single or multiple bone growths that progressively enlarge. The etiology of FD was unknown until recently, and numerous factors have been discussed as probable causes of the disease. Activating mutations in the gene that encodes the alpha subunit of stimulatory G protein cause monostotic and polyostotic FD, pituitary adenoma, and Albright syndrome. The variants of FD are sporadically occurring disorders in which a mutation in the *GNAS=1* gene (guanine nucleotide-binding protein, alpha-stimulating activity polypeptide–1) occurs postzygotically in a somatic cell. All cells descended from the mutated cell can manifest as FD or Albright syndrome. Cells descended from nonmutated cells develop into normal bone tissue. Thus, the clinical pattern is variable in distribution and appearance.[14]

Essentially, FD growths are composed of non-encapsulated clonal proliferations of fibroblast-like osteoprogenitor cells with an activating mutation of *GNAS=1*, which demonstrate a constitutively high expression of the proto-oncogene *c-fos*. Cohen and Howell[14] reported that osteoprogenitor cells have an increased rate of proliferation and display markers of early osteoblastic differentiation but they undergo abnormal maturation and fail to express normal levels of late osteoblastic markers. The authors concluded: "These findings describe a lesion best categorized as a benign unencapsulated neoplasm." Several findings support the concept of FD as a neoplasm: FD growths may sometimes exhibit aggressive behavior; the same activating mutation causes pituitary adenoma, which is a neoplasm; and high levels of *c-fos* in FD may be comparable to *c-fos* expression in osteosarcomas. That osteosarcomas may develop in fibrous dysplasia has been well documented; osteosarcomas are known to develop in about 4% of patients with Albright syndrome and in about 0.5% of patients with FD.[14] Postirradiation osteosarcomas have also been observed in cases of FD. The combination of a *GNAS=1* mutation, increased *c-fos* expression, and radiation exposure in some cases suggests multistep carcinogenesis of osteosarcoma, which could account for the low frequency of tumors in cases of FD.[14]

5. Pathology

5.1 Macroscopy

The macroscopic features of FD are characterized by a gray-whitish tissue mainly involving the medullary portion of the jaws. Deformity of the affected bone is observed, and distinct thickening may be apparent. The consistency may range from soft to very hard. Even within different parts of the same growth, the consistency may vary considerably. The affected areas are clearly delimited from surrounding normal bone, but there is no encapsulation.

5.2 Microscopy

5.2.1 Histologic definition

Both the World Health Organization (WHO)[20] and the present authors classify FD as follows:

A benign, self-limiting, but nonencapsulated lesion occurring mainly in young subjects, usually in the maxilla, and showing replacement of the normal bone by a cellular fibrous tissue containing islands or trabeculae of metaplastic bone.

5.2.2 Histopathologic findings

The histopathologic features of FD vary with the duration of disease and stage of development. Fibrous dysplasia replaces normal bone with a cellular, fibrous tissue containing irregularly shaped bony trabeculae. The trabeculae consist of immature, nonlamellar (woven) bone without osteoid rims or osteoblasts (Fig 33-9). Early of FD growths are characterized by a fibroblastic tissue which is richly cellular, often revealing a whorled pattern with little bone. The trabecular arrangement has been compared to the appearance of Chinese characters and, therefore, is often referred to as "Chinese character trabeculae" (Fig 33-10). Affected bone usually fuses with the adjacent nonaffected bone, whether cortical or cancellous. As FD progresses, the amount of lamellar trabeculae increases. These trabeculae are slender and tend to run parallel to each other. They lie very close together in a moderately cellular fibrous stroma. The term *osseous keloid* has sometimes been used for this type of lesion. Monostotic FD of the jaws may exhibit varying amounts of spherical, amorphous calcifications and curved/linear, round, calcified trabeculae which tend to form conglomerate structures. These are considered by some researchers to be more representative of cementum than bone. Another feature that is generally not observed elsewhere in the skeleton of patients with FD but which may occur in the jaws is lamellar bone bordered by osteoblasts.

In cases where biopsy specimens do not contain surrounding tissue, the evaluation of the FD border cannot be made. In such cases, the observation that fibrous dysplasia shows a rather uniform appearance with a constant ratio of bone to fibrous tissue throughout the entire area may be helpful in diagnosis and classification.

Normally, there are no differences in the histologic appearance of MFD and PFD cases. However, there may be a higher incidence of lamellar bone in MFD.[21]

The differential diagnosis of fibro-osseous lesions, including fibrous dysplasia, has been discussed by a number of authorities for several decades.[1,2,7,12,21] Slootweg[21] described the differential diagnosis of maxillofacial fibro-osseous lesions and compared the histopathologic features of fibrous dysplasia, cemento-ossifying fibromas, and focal cemento-osseous dysplasia (focal and florid). Fibrous dysplasia, as has already

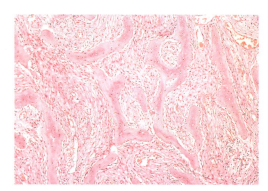

Fig 33-9 Irregularly shaped trabeculae of woven bone in a cellular, slightly vascular fibrous tissue stroma (hematoxylin-eosin [H&E], x80).

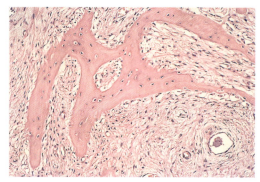

Fig 33-10 Higher magnification of a "Chinese character" trabecula (H&E, x120).

been discussed, is characterized by evenly distributed islands of woven bone that fuse with surrounding bone. The presence of lamellar bone and osteoblastic rimming does not exclude the diagnosis of FD as would be the case for lesions occurring outside the maxillofacial bones. Cemento-ossifying fibromas are encapsulated or well demarcated (see chapter 32). A broad range of mineralized material is found in cemento-ossifying fibromas; woven, as well as lamellar, bone may be found in addition to rounded cell-poor particles of cementum-like material. Juvenile and psammomatoid COFs are subtypes with cellular stroma showing mitotic activity. Cemento-ossifying fibromas may resemble well-differentiated osteosarcomas but it also may be more cellular and have a higher number of mitoses than osteosarcomas. Focal cemento-osseous dysplasia (see chapter 34) has histopathologic features similar to those of COFs but without demarcation.

5.2.3 Histochemical/immunohistochemical findings

Systematic histochemical or immunohistochemical studies of fibrous dysplasia have not been reported in the literature.

5.2.4 Ultrastructural studies

Ultrastructural studies of FD have not been reported in the literature. However, Donath[22] studied some fibro-osseous lesions of the jaws, including fibrous dysplasia, by electron microscopy. Ultrastructurally, FD tumor cells are of the osteoblast type and possess only short fragments of rough endoplasmic reticulum, a prominent Golgi apparatus, mitochondria, and free ribosomes. Collagen fibers attach to the bone surface at right angles. Newly formed osteocytes exhibit a few organelles but contain free ribosomes and little rough endoplasmic reticulum. Donath[22]

concluded that the diagnosis of FD is not a histologic or ultrastructural problem. On the other hand, he pointed out that the differentiation of fibro-osseous lesions using cytologic characteristics is not possible because fibroblasts, osteoblasts, and osteoclasts are identical in all these lesions.

6. Notes on treatment and recurrence rate

Clinical management of and therapy for FD of the facial skeleton and jaws may be a major problem, especially when associated with gross facial disfigurement. In most cases, however, FD tends to stabilize and essentially stops enlarging when skeletal maturation is reached. Small lesions, particularly those of the mandible, may be surgically resected. Due to the diffuse nature and large size of a number of lesions, particularly those of the maxillary complex, extensive surgical procedures may be necessary. The treatment of choice is principally surgical, depending on the size and consistency of the lesion. Surgical recontouring and surgical reduction of the dysplasia to an acceptable contour without complete removal is usually recommended.

Camilleri[23] suggested that surgery for craniofacial FD is indicated at any age if important functions are threatened; deformity becomes substantial; or complications such as obstruction and infection of paranasal sinuses, dental malocclusion, or severe epistaxis develop. During surgery on active-phase FD, excessive bleeding may occur.

Reliable data on the incidence of continued growth (no recurrence) after surgical reduction of FD of the jaws are difficult to determine,[24] but it has been estimated that between 25% and 50% of patients will experience some regrowth after a surgical recontouring procedure. Since regrowth after surgical reduction seems to be more common in younger individuals, surgery should be delayed as long as possible.[24]

Fractures and intraosseous infections have been described in patients with FD.[25] Infection is related to the sclerotic and avascular nature of mature FD and may result in the development of osteomyelitis.

In rare cases, malignant transformation of fibrous dysplasia may occur, resulting in osteosarcoma. Yabut et al[26] reviewed the literature of malignant transformation in patients with FD. While most of the diagnoses of 83 patients were made in childhood, malignancies developed during the 3rd to 4th decades of life. Approximately 0.4% of FD cases were estimated to undergo malignant transformation. Local irradiation is considered to be a main cause for malignant change; however, only 23 of 83 patients received irradiation, showing that this is not a prerequisite for malignancy. The prognosis for sarcomas is poor, with a mean survival time after diagnosis of 3.4 years.[26]

Patients with FD should be evaluated periodically, both clinically and radiographically, for growth and the late development of pain and swelling which may indicate possible malignant changes.

References

1. Eversole LR, Sabes WR, Rovin S. Fibrous dysplasia: A nosologic problem in the diagnosis of fibro-osseous lesions of the jaws. J Oral Pathol 1972;1:189–220.

2. Waldron C. Fibro-osseous lesions of the jaws. J Oral Maxillofac Surg 1985;43:249–262.

3. Lichtenstein L. Polyostotic fibrous dysplasia. Arch Surg 1938;36:874–898.

4. Lichtenstein L, Jaffe HL. Fibrous dysplasia of bone. Arch Pathol 1942;33:777–816.

5. Pritchard JE. Fibrous dysplasia of the bones. Am J Med Sci 1951;222:313–332.

6. Dahlgren SE, Lind PO, Lindbom A, Martensson G. Fibrous dysplasia of jaw bones. Acta Otolaryngol 1969;68:257–270.

7. Waldron CA, Giansanti JS. Benign fibro-osseous lesions of the jaws: A clinical-radiologic-histologic review of sixty-five cases. Oral Surg Oral Med Oral Pathol 1973;35:190–201.

8. Daramola JO, Ajagbe HA, Obisesan AA, Lagundoye SB, Oluwasanmi JO. Fibrous dysplasia of the jaws in Nigerians. Oral Surg Oral Med Oral Pathol 1976;42:290–300.

9. Awange DO. Fibrous dysplasia of the jaws: A review of literature. East Afr Med J 1992;69:205–209.

10. Obwegeser HL, Freihofer HPM, Horejs J. Variation of fibrous dysplasia in the jaws. J Maxillofac Surg 1973;1:161–171.

11. Yoon JH, Kim J, Lee CK, Choi J. Clinical and histopathological study of fibro-osseous lesions of the jaws. Yonsei Med J 1989;30:133–143.

12. Slootweg PJ, Müller H. Differential diagnosis of fibro-osseous jaw lesions. A histological investigation on 30 cases. J Craniomaxillofac Surg 1990;18:210–214.

13. MacDonald-Jankowski D. Fibrous dysplasia in the jaws of a Hong Kong population: Radiographic presentation and systematic review. Dentomaxillofac Radiol 1999;28:195–202.

14. Cohen MM, Howell RE. Etiology of fibrous dysplasia and McCune-Albright syndrome. Int J Oral Maxillofac Surg 1999;28:366–371.

15. Petrikowski CG, Pharoah MJ, Lee L, Grace MAG. Radiographic differentiation of osteogenic sarcoma, osteomyelitis, and fibrous dysplasia of the jaws. Oral Surg Oral Med Oral Pathol Oral Radiol Endod 1995;80:744–750.

16. Casselmann JW, De Jonge I, De Clercq C, Hont GD. MRI in craniofacial fibrous dysplasia. Neuroradiology 1993;35:234–237.

17. von Wowern N, Hjørting-Hansen E, Edeling C-J. Bone scintigraphy of benign jaw lesions. Int J Oral Surg 1978;7:528–533.

18. Gibson MJ, Middlemiss JH. Fibrous dysplasia of bone. Br J Radiol 1971;44:1–13.

19. Lathouwer C, Brocheriou C. Sarcoma arising in irradiated jawbones. Possible relationship with previous non-malignant bone lesions. Report of 6 cases and review of the literature. J Maxillofac Surg 1976;4:8–20.

20. Kramer IRH, Pindborg JJ, Shear M. Histological Typing of Odontogenic Tumours. 2d ed. Berlin: Springer-Verlag, 1992.

21. Slootweg P. Maxillofacial fibro-osseous lesions: Classification and differential diagnosis. Semin Diagn Pathol 1996;13:104–112.

22. Donath K. Ultrastrukturpathologie der "fibro-ossären Kieferläsionen." Dtsch Z Mund Kiefer Gesichtschir 1986;10:218–224.

23. Camilleri AE. Craniofacial fibrous dysplasia. J Laryngol Otol 1991;105:662.

24. Waldron CA. Fibro-osseous lesions of the jaws. J Oral Maxillofac Surg 1993;51:828–835.

25. Pierce AM, Sampson WJ, Wilson DF, Goss AN. Fifteen-year follow-up of a family with inherited craniofacial fibrous dysplasia. J Oral Maxillofac Surg 1996;54:780–788.

26. Yabut SM, Kenan S, Sissons HA, et al. Malignant transformation of fibrous dysplasia. Clin Orthop 1988;228;281.

Chapter 34

Focal Cemento-osseous Dysplasia

1. Terminology

The classification of fibro-osseous lesions of the jaws has long been an area of debate and confusion for both the pathologist and the clinician. Generally, classifications divide fibro-osseous lesions into *reactive* and *neoplastic* lesions. The focal cemento-osseous dysplasia (FocCOD), or periapical cemental dysplasia (PCD), is a non-neoplastic lesion that has been referred to in a number of different ways, including *periapical osteofibroma, periapical fibrous dysplasia, periapical fibro-osteoma, periapical fibro-osteocementoma, cementoma, fibrocementoma, sclerosing cementoma, cementoblastoma,* and *benign fibro-osseous lesions of periodontal ligament origin. Focal cemento-osseous dysplasia* is the term used in this chapter. The persistent changes in terminology reflect the problem of taxonomy and classification of this lesion and its relation to some of the other cemento-osseous dysplasias.

The classification of FocCOD is based on the gender and age of affected individuals together with location and radiographic and histologic features of the lesion. However, lesions are not necessarily typical and cannot always be satisfactorily assigned to a particular category. In the 1992 World Health Organization (WHO)[1] classification, FocCOD was classified as a separate entity under the name periapical cemental dysplasia. However, a number of authorities consider PCDs and florid cemento-osseous dysplasias (gigantiform cementomas) to be variants of the same lesion.[2] Neville et al[3] adopted the concept of benign fibro-osseous lesions of periodontal ligament origin – including FocCODs, cementomas, cementifying fibromas, ossifying fibromas, and gigantiform cementomas—encompassing lesions ranging from reactive to neoplastic. Summerlin and Tomich[4] and Su et al[5,6] published large series of cases of FocCODs and compared them to cemento-ossifiying fibromas. The authors considered FocCOD and PCD to be the same process affecting different locations.

Brophy[7] first described the periapical lesion currently known as the FocCOD in 1915. Two exhaustive studies of FocCODs were reported by Fontaine in 1955[8] and Zegarelli et al in 1964.[9] The latter series comprised 230 patients with 435 "cementomas." Neville et al[3] published a radiographic survey of 1,138 black women with benign fibro-osseous lesions of periodontal ligament origin, including FocCOD. Baden and Saroff[10] reviewed the FocCOD literature in 1987. Periapical cemental dysplasias with multiple lesions in Japanese patients were reported by Tanaka et al in 1987.[11] Ackermann and Altini[2] reappraised the cementomas in a clinicopathologic study of 127 cases and suggested a classification for cemental "tumors" that included cemento-ossifying fibromas

(COFs); cementoblastomas; cemento-osseous dysplasias with single, multiple, and florid subtypes. In their study, no cases of FocCODs were found. Slootweg[12] reviewed maxillofacial fibro-osseous lesions, their classifications, and differential diagnoses. He suggested dividing FocCODs into focal and florid variants.

Familial occurrence of FocCODs has been described.[13] They have also been observed in association with Crouzon syndrome and acanthosis nigricans.[14] In the last 20 years, several additional case reports of FocCODs have been published.[15–17]

2. Clinical and radiologic profile

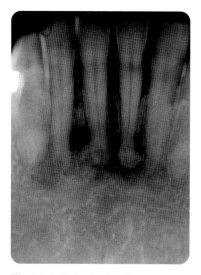

Fig 34-1 Periapical radiograph of mandibular incisors showing the characteristic features of a focal cemento-osseous dysplasia. The radiolucency involves the apices of the four central incisors. Radiopaque areas representing cementoid/osteoid material are seen at the tips of the roots.

Focal cemento-osseous dysplasia is usually asymptomatic and most often found accidentally on routine radiographs. Su et al,[5] however, stated that 38% of their patients with FocCODs had symptoms such as local jaw expansion and mild discomfort. Vitality tests of affected teeth are usually positive.

Radiographically, FocCODs present with three different appearances, according to their developmental stage. The initial osteolytic stage is characterized by radiolucency of the periapical areas of involved teeth, often in the anterior mandible. The radiographic appearance of FocCODs in this stage may easily be mistaken for periapical pathosis related to pulpal necrosis (eg, periapical granuloma or radicular cyst). Diagnostic problems may arise in cases of endodontically treated teeth and periapical radiolucencies that actually represent FocCODs.[18] The second intermediate stage is

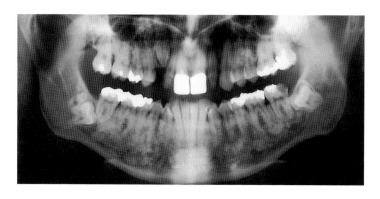

Fig 34-2 Panoramic radiograph of a patient with multiple FocCODs involving the molar roots.

characterized by radiopaque foci in an otherwise rarified translucent area. The final mature stage reveals a characteristic radiographic appearance: well-defined radiopacities surrounded by a radiolucent halo (Figs 34-1 and 34-2).

Among 120 cases of FocCODs for which radiographic information was available, Summerlin and Tomich[4] found 52 lesions with radiolucency with or without a sclerotic rim of bone. Mixed radiolucency/radiopacity was seen in 47 cases, and pure radiopaque lesions were found in 20 cases.

Radiographically, 53% of the FocCOD cases studied by Su et al[6] showed a well-defined border and 69% demonstrated an irregularly mixed radiopacity. FocCODs were closely associated with tooth apices (70.6% of cases) and previous extraction sites (21% of cases). The size of the FocCODs averaged 1.8 cm.

While diagnosis of FocCODs is usually based on radiographic findings and positive vitality tests, other diagnostic techniques have occasionally been applied. Taki et al[19] used scintigraphy in a case of multiple FocCODs in a Japanese woman. Intensive accumulation of Tc-99m and Ga-67 was observed in the areas of FocCODs. Chandler et al[20] used laser Doppler flowmetry to study blood flow in teeth affected by FocCODs and demonstrated that the pulps were vital and the periapical lesions were not of endodontic origin.

Differential radiographic diagnosis of FocCOD includes periapical pathosis (granuloma), radicular cyst, ameloblastoma, central giant cell lesion, odontogenic myxoma, and solitary bone cavity. The studies by Summerlin and Tomich[4] and Su et al[5,6] clearly showed that there are a number of parameters, including radiographic features that allow for differentiation between FocCODs and cemento-ossifying fibromas (COFs).

3. Epidemiological data

3.1 Prevalence, incidence, and relative frequency

Few studies have been conducted to determine the frequency of cementomas, and there are no reports of age-specific incidence rates. In radiographic surveys from 1934 and 1958,[2] prevalence rates of 0.24% and 0.29%, respectively, were reported for FocCODs.[2] The overall incidence of FocCODs has been estimated at 3 per 1,000 teeth occurring most often in the anterior mandible of black middle-aged women.[9] The radiographic study by Neville et al[3] documented 38 cases of benign fibro-osseous lesions of periodontal ligament origin in 491 black women (7.7%, age adjusted incidence rate). Of the 38 cases, 29 (5.5%, age adjusted incidence rate) presented with FocCODs.

The focal cemento-osseous dysplasia is considered an uncommon lesion, accounting for only 0.4% of the annual surgical excisions from 1982 to 1994 in one oral pathology laboratory.[6]

3.2 Age

One review of 350 cases indicated that FocCODs primarily affects middle-aged patients, with a mean of 42.5 years (range, 14 to 82 years).[10] The mean age at presentation was 37.8 years in the study by Summerlin and Tomich[4] and 38 years (range, 10 to 79 years) in the study by Su et al.[6] Figure 34-3 shows the age distribution of 420 cases pooled from these two studies. Both reports included white and black patients; gender distribution was not specified. Tanaka et al[11] reviewed the Japanese literature and found 26 cases of FocCODs with multiple lesions. The mean age at presentation was 45 years (range, 21 to 65 years). From the information available,

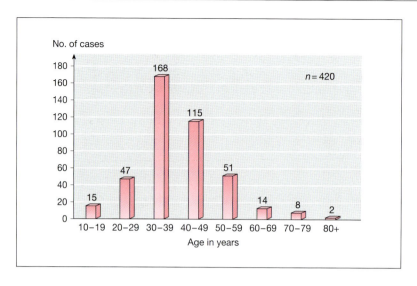

Fig 34-3 Age distribution of 420 Foc-COD cases.[4,6] No gender distribution was available.

the peak incidence of FocCODs is in the 4th and 5th decades.

3.3 Gender

Virtually all studies of FocCODs show a clear predilection for women. Of 339 cases of FocCOD reviewed by Baden and Saroff,[10] 309 (90.3%) were women. Of 221 FocCOD cases studied by Summerlin and Tomich,[4] 194 (88%) were found in women and only 24 (11%) in men. In three cases gender was not stated. Similar findings were obtained in the study by Su et al,[6] with 89% of lesions found in women and 11% in men. All 25 cases reviewed by Tanaka et al[12] were in women.

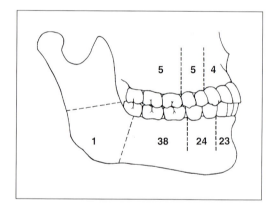

Fig 34-4 Topographic distribution of FocCODs. Numbers indicate percentages.

3.4 Location

The mandible is the most common location for FocCODs. In one study,[10] 595 of 873 Foc-CODs were located in the mandible (68.2%) compared to 278 lesions in the maxilla (31.9%). The mandible was also the site of preference in another study,[4] with 77% located in the posterior mandible (n = 171), 11% in the maxilla (n = 24), and 4% in the anterior mandible (n = 9). The site was not specified in 16 of these cases. Figure 34-4 shows the distribution of maxillary and mandibular FocCODs according to the findings by Su et al.[6] In Japanese patients, FocCODs occurred mainly in the premolar-molar area (66.2 %).[11]

3.5 Ethnic distribution

There seems to be a clear predilection for blacks compared to whites in most studies. For example, 69.1% of patients reviewed by Baden and Saroff[10] were black. The study by Su et al[6] involved 64% black patients (n = 139) and 36% white patients (n = 78). In contrast, 32% of patients were black (n = 70) in the study by Summerlin and Tomich[4] compared to 58% white patients (n =129). This finding is explained by the fact that generally only 7% of the surgical excisions in the particular hospital setting were in black persons.

The small series published by Tanaka et al[12] shows that FocCODs may also occur in Japanese populations.

4. Pathogenesis

The pathogenesis of FocCODs is largely unknown, but gender, age, ethnicity, and location seem to be of significance. Generally, FocCODs seem to occur predominantly in the mandible of black middle-aged women and are considered to be of periodontal ligament origin.

The development of FocCODs is characterized by three stages which have specific radiographic and morphologic appearances. Pathogenetically, the first stage is characterized by proliferation of a cellular fibrous connective tissue. During the second stage, bone and/or cementum is formed within the fibrous tissue, giving the lesion a characteristic radiolucent/radiopaque appearance. The final stage of maturation is characterized by continuous progressive formation of bone and/or cementum. A narrow rim of connective tissue usually surrounds the hard tissue masses.

Generally, the common circumstances in which excessive cementum may be formed are in response to chronic inflammation at the apex of a tooth, on nonerupted teeth, or on teeth subjected to excessive occlusal stress. This condition is known as hypercementosis. Whenever cementum is laid down away from its normal location—at the surface of roots—it may be difficult to distinguish from bone on histologic examination. Cementicles are another microscopic expression of aberrant formation of cementum.

Etiologic factors that may play a role in FocCOD development are unknown; however, chronic or slight trauma has been mentioned in the history of some patients with FocCODs.

5. Pathology

5.1 Macroscopy

The macroscopic aspect of FocCODs has been characterized as quite specific.[4,5] During surgery, the oral/maxillofacial surgeon will usually be able to remove only small, gritty hemorrhagic fragments of tissue that are curetted with some difficulty. Su et al[5] clearly showed that 92.5% of FocCOD specimens consisted of multiple small fragments of tissue, whereas 88% of COFs were large intact specimens.

5.2 Microscopy

5.2.1 Histologic definition

Both the 1992 WHO classification[1] and the present authors define the FocCOD as follows:

A non-neoplastic lesion affecting the periapical tissues of one or more teeth and with histologic features similar to those of the lesions of the cemento-ossifying fibroma group, but without a sharply defined margin.

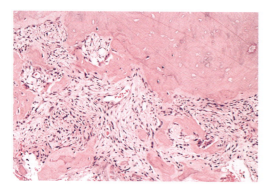

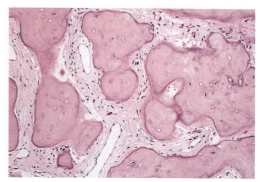

Fig 34-5 Photomicrograph of a FocCOD. The periphery of the lesion is characterized by dense fibrous tissue with small, newly formed islands of cemento-osseous tissue (hematoxylin-eosin [H&E], x60).

Fig 34-6 Intermediate-stage focal cemento-osseous dysplasia. Irregular islands and cementicle-like structures with basophilic reversal lines are embedded in a dense, collagenous tissue (H&E, x100).

5.2.2 Histopathologic findings

The histologic features of FocCODs are generally considered to be similar to those of cemento-ossifying fibromas; however, while COFs and fibrous dysplasias may occur anywhere in the maxillofacial skeleton, Foc-CODs are confined to the mandible and maxilla. As the name implies, FocCODs characteristically occur in the tooth-bearing areas of the jaws, and lesions are closely associated with the apices of teeth.

Since FocCODs go through three developmental stages, the ratio of fibrous tissue to mineralized material may vary; it has been demonstrated that FocCODs are initially fibroblastic but, over the course of several years, show increasing degrees of calcification. As with COFs, the mineralized material is an admixture of woven and lamellar bone in addition to cementum-like particles. Slootweg[12] considered a sharply defined margin the only distinguishing feature between COFs and FocCODs.

Studies of FocCODs and COFs[5] have shown that histopathologic distinction of

these lesions is possible in 94% of cases. Focal cemento-osseous dysplasias are characterized by thick, curved/linear bone trabeculae ("ginger root" pattern) or irregularly shaped cementum-like masses. The stroma of FocCODs displays cavernous channels associated with the trabeculae. Free hemorrhage in artifactual spaces is frequently caused by curettage. Similar findings were reported by Summerlin and Tomich.[4]

Histopathologically, specimens of Foc-CODs consist of dense fibrous tissue with varying amounts of hard tissue. Hard tissues consist of spherical and trabecular-shaped cementum-like structures with irregular, basophilic reversal lines. Smaller cementicle-like structures and trabecular woven bone may be observed at the periphery of the lesion (Figs 34-5 and 34-6).

The histologic features of the florid cemento-osseous dysplasia (gigantiform cementoma) are similar to those of the Foc-COD, except that the former tends to be more heavily mineralized with less fibroblastic tissue and more osseous/cementum-like material. Due to the similarity of features, some authorities have suggested grouping Foc-CODs and florid cemento-osseous dysplasias together, either as PCD with subtypes (focal and florid)[14] or as cemento-osseous dysplasia with subtypes (single, multiple, and florid).[2]

Summerlin and Tomich[4] stated that PCD and FocCOD are "closely related, if not identical conditions" and concluded that "periapical cemento-osseous dysplasia and focal cemento-osseous dysplasia are the same process." They also concluded that these "focal lesions may be the initial manifestation of the more generalized condition—the well-recognized condition called florid osseous (cemento-osseous) dysplasia." No histopathologic differences were observed between "conventional" PCD and FocCOD.[5]

5.2.3 Histochemical/immunohistochemical findings

Studies using histochemical and immunohistochemical methods have not been published to date.

5.2.4 Ultrastructural findings

Electron microscopic studies of FocCODs have not been published in the literature.

6. Notes on treatment and recurrence rate

Correct diagnosis of FocCODs is most important. Diagnosis is based on clinical and radiographic features. As soon as the diagnosis of FocCOD is clinically confirmed, the need for treatment—particularly endodontic treatment—is eliminated. Patients with Foc-CODs should be followed up regularly, and vitality tests of involved teeth should be performed. Occasional radiographs should

monitor the process of calcification and the possible development of a florid cemento-osseous dysplasia. Baden and Saroff[10] described complications that may arise in cases of FocCODs associated with chronic periodontitis. Since cementum and osteocementum are avascular and the fibrous component decreases in the later stage of Foc-COD development, the overall decrease in vascularization may result in tissue ischemia predisposing to necrosis, sequestrum formation, and osteomyelitis. Deep periodontal curettage in cases of periodontitis, open-flap surgery with recontouring of bone, and elimination of intrabony pockets all expose the hard tissue masses and may predispose the patient to necrosis and secondary infection.

References

1. Kramer IRH, Pindborg JJ, Shear M. Histologic Typing of Odontogenic Tumours. 2d ed. Berlin: Springer-Verlag, 1992.

2. Ackermann GL, Altini M. The cementomas—a clinicopathological reappraisal. J Dent Assoc S Afr 1992;47:187–194.

3. Neville BW, Albenesius RJ, Charleston SC. The prevalence of benign fibro-osseous lesions of periodontal ligament origin in black women: A radiographic survey. Oral Surg Oral Med Oral Pathol 1986;62:340–344.

4. Summerlin D-J, Tomich CE. Focal cemento-osseous dysplasia: A clinicopathologic study of 221 cases. Oral Surg Oral Med Oral Pathol 1994;8:611–620.

5. Su L, Weathers DW, Waldron CA. Distinguishing feature of focal cemento-osseous dysplasias and cemento-ossifying fibromas. I. A pathologic spectrum of 316 cases. Oral Surg Oral Med Oral Pathol Oral Radiol Endod 1997;84:301–309.

6. Su L, Weathers DR, Waldron CA. Distinguishing features of focal cemento-osseous dysplasia and cemento-ossifying fibromas. II. A clinical and radiological spectrum of 316 cases. Oral Surg Oral Med Oral Pathol Oral Radiol Endod 1997;84;540–549.

7. Brophy TW. A treatise on the diseases, injuries and malformations of the mouth and associated parts. Oral Surgery 1915:867–871, P. Blakinston and sons.

8. Fontaine J. Periapical fibro-osteoma or cementoma. J Can Dent Assoc 1955;21:10.

9. Zegarelli E, Kutscher AH, Napoli N, et al. The cementoma–a study of 230 patients with 435 cementomas. Oral Surg 1964;17:219.

10. Baden E, Saroff SA. Periapical cemental dysplasia and periodontal disease. A case report with review of the literature. J Periodontol 1987;58: 187–191.

11. Tanaka H, Yoshimoto A, Toyama Y, et al. Periapical cemental dysplasia with multiple lesions. Int J Oral Maxillofac Surg 1987;16: 757–763.

12. Slootweg PJ. Maxillofacial fibro-osseous lesions: Classification and differential diagnosis. Semin Diagn Pathol 1996;13:104–112.

13. Thakkar NS, Horner K, Sloan P. Familial occurrence of periapical cemental dysplasia. Case report. Virchows Archiv A Pathol Anat 1993;423: 233–236.

14. Suslak L, Glista B, Gertzman GB, et al. Crouzon syndrome with periapical cemental dysplasia and acanthosis nigracans: The pleiotropic effect of a single gene? Birth Defects 1985;21:127–134.

15. Ward RM. Periapical cemental dysplasia: A case report. Dent J 1989;89:53–54.

16. Smith S, Patel K, Hoskinson AE. Periapical cemental dysplasia: A case of misdiagnosis. Br J Dent 1998;185:122–123.

17. Long JE, Gordy FM, McGinnis JP, Krolls SO. Case presentation. Periapical cemental dysplasia. Miss Dent Assoc J 1999;55:28–29.

18. Wilcox LR, Walton RE. A case of mistaken identity: Periapical cemental dysplasia in an endodontically treated tooth. Endod Dent Traumatol 1989; 5:298–301.

19. Taki S, Tonami N, Taki J, et al. Intense accumulation of Tc-99m MDP and Ga-67 in multiple periapical cemental dysplasia. Ann Nucl Med 1995; 9:243–245.

20. Chandler NP, Love RM, Sundqvist G. Laser doppler flowmetry. An aid in differential diagnosis of apical radiolucencies. Oral Surg Oral Med Oral Pathol Oral Radiol Endod 1999;87:613–616.

Chapter 35

Florid Cemento-osseous Dysplasia

1. Terminology

The definition, classification, and terminology of cementomas, a group of odontogenic lesions derived from the cementum of teeth, have been subjects of debate for several decades. In the World Health Organization (WHO) classification of 1971,[1] cementomas were classified under four variants: *benign cementoblastomas, periapical cemental dysplasias, cementifying fibromas* and *gigantiform cementomas*. In the WHO classification of 1992,[2] neoplasms (cemento-ossifying fibromas) and non-neoplastic (dysplastic) bone lesions were separated. Among the non-neoplastic lesions, cemento-osseous dysplasias encompass periapical cemental dysplasia (PCD, or focal cemento-osseous dysplasia; see chapter 34), florid cemento-osseous dysplasia (FCOD), and other cemento-osseous dysplasias that share some features of both PCDs and FCODs.

In 1985, Waldron[3] suggested classifying fibro-osseous jaw lesions as five types: periapical cemental dysplasia, localized fibro-osseous cemental lesions, florid cemento-osseous dysplasia, ossifying and cementifying fibroma, and cementoblastoma. Most authorities have acknowledged that subclassification of cementomas is difficult and subjective, since clinical and morphologic features of "variants" often overlap and are therefore difficult to separate.[4] In fact, doubt

has been expressed whether the PCD is a distinct entity. In a study of 127 "cementomas," Ackermann and Altini[4] did not find a single case of PCD and therefore considered this lesion to be a variant of FCOD (gigantiform cementoma).

The confusion about how to define and classify cementomas is reflected by the plethora of terms that have been used to describe these lesions: *multiple cemento-ossifying fibromas, sclerosing osteitis, sclerosing osteomyelitis, chronic sclerosing osteomyelitis, multiple enostosis, multiple osteomas, periapical cementoblastoma, Paget disease of the mandible, sclerotic masses of the jaws, multiple periapical osteofibromatosis,[5] sclerotic cemental masses, monstrous cementoma, familial multiple cementomas,* and *periapical cemental dysplasia with multiple lesions.*[6] Some of these terms were certainly applied inappropriately. The pathobiology of Paget disease or chronic diffuse sclerosing osteomyelitis[6] have no relationship to FCOD.

The term *florid osseous dysplasia* was first suggested by Melrose et al[7] in 1976 to describe a condition of exuberant multiquadrant masses of cementum and/or bone in both jaws and, in some cases, simple bone cavity (SBC)–like lesions in affected quadrants. The word *florid* was introduced to describe the widespread, extensive manifestations of the disease. FCODs are not associated with any other extragnathic abnormalities, and there are no disturbances in the blood chemistry of affected patients.[8] The florid cemento-osseous dysplasia is essentially a benign non-neoplastic lesion.

The first case of "gigantiform cementoma" was probably reported by Agazzi and Belloni in 1953.[9] Since then one large series of 107 cases,[4] a small series of 7 Japanese patients with FCODs[10] and several case reports[5,11,12] have been published. The latter included one case of FCOD with concomitant simple bone cysts.[13] Coleman et al[14] described a case of familial FCOD in a black family in Africa and reviewed the literature on this condition.

2. Clinical and radiologic profile

The clinical features of FCOD are characteristic for the different clinicopathologic variants of the disease, which include solitary, multiple, florid, and periapical according to Ackermann and Altini.[4] The "classic" FCOD is characterized by symmetric bony hard swelling of the jaws, often involving all four quadrants. The masses may become large and cause considerable facial deformity, often the only patient complaint. There may be spacing of the maxillary and mandibular anterior teeth with some degree of displacement. Teeth associated with areas of noninfected FCOD are usually vital. Symptoms such as pain or drainage are mostly associated with exposure of the sclerotic calcified masses in the oral cavity. This may occur as a result of alveolar atrophy under a denture or after extraction of teeth in the area involved. Clinically, purulent discharge or fistula formation may occur as secondary phenomena, and cemento-osteomyelitis with sequestration may occasionally develop. From the differential point of view, chronic diffuse sclerosing osteomyelitis has to be considered in cases of infected lesions. Schneider and Mesa[6] discussed the distinguishing features of both lesions in detail. The blood chemistry of patients with FCODs is essentially normal. In most cases, patients do not have a familial history of the disease. There are, however, reported instances of familial involvement in Italian, French, Scottish, American, Finnish, and black African families.[14] Although in the majority of cases the mode of genetic transmission is unclear, Young et al[15] were able to demonstrate in their study of 55 family members from five generations that FCOD appears to be inherited as an autosomal dominant trait with variable phenotypic expression. The autosomal dominant mode of transmission was also found in the family reported by Coleman et el.[14] Young et al[15] suggested that familial FCOD be regarded as a separate form of the disease, because some differences between the familial and nonfamilial variants were noted. Familial FCOD affects both men and women, some as early as 6 years of age. Except for the family reported by Coleman et al,[14] all cases of familial FCOD were observed in white patients. Lesions were reported to be florid, involving large areas of the jaws. The growth rate in familial FCOD seems to be rapid, affecting the mandibular symphysis. A number of cases were associated with multiple unerupted teeth. Associated SBCs have not been recorded in patients with familial FCOD.[15]

As in FocCOD (see chapter 34), the radiographic appearance depends on the degree of maturation of the lesions. Although proliferative, immature FCOD lesions appear radiolucent, later stages of maturation are characterized by dense radiopaque masses of cemento-osseous material usually located in the tooth-bearing, posterior mandible or maxilla. On panoramic radiographs, FCODs appear as diffuse, lobular, irregularly shaped radiopacities. In some cases, lesions are en-

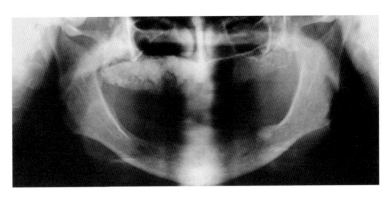

Fig 35-1 Panoramic radiograph of a 72-year-old white woman revealing an extensive radiopaque lesion of the right maxilla. A smaller radiopaque lesion is seen in the left mandible.

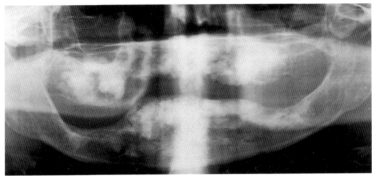

Fig 35-2 Extensive FCOD involving all four quadrants in an elderly black woman. (Courtesy of Professor I. van der Waal, Amsterdam, The Netherlands.)

meshed within poorly defined areas of decreased radiodensity and have a "ground-glass" appearance. The size of FCOD lesions varies between 0.5 and 10 cm[4] (Figs 35-1 and 35-2). If the lesion is infected, a radiolucent border is often discernible. In cases of FCOD associated with SBC, multiple radiolucencies with well-demarcated, scalloped borders and buccal expansion may be observed.[13] Amorphous dense radiopacities may be seen centrally or at the apices of teeth.

The use of computed tomography (CT) and three-dimensional imaging has been described in some cases of FCOD.[5,10,15] Ariji et al[10] found CT to be very useful in the diagnosis of FCOD. The Hounsfield units (HU) of high-density masses were monitored in seven patients with FCODs and ranged from 772 to 1587 HU with a mean of 1337.4 HU. Cyst-like spaces observed in four patients with FCODs revealed a range of 8 to 46 HU, indicating a fluid content. Beylouni et al[5] found axial CT scans to be of use in visualizing the buccolingual aspects of the lesions demonstrating the relationship of FCOD lesions to root apices and cortical plates in the buccolingual dimensions. Vertical and panoramic reconstructions may reveal further details on the relationship of FCOD to the apices of roots and to the canal of the inferior alveolar nerve. Three-dimensional reconstructions enable an anatomic study of the bone surface. Due to high-grade imaging, these authors were able to avoid biopsy of the lesions. They also considered dental imaging helpful in differentiating fibro-osseous lesions from odontomas, in which the HU for enamel is higher than that for cementum. In some cases, scintigraphy with Tc-99m showed increased uptake of the radionuclide in the affected regions of the jaws.

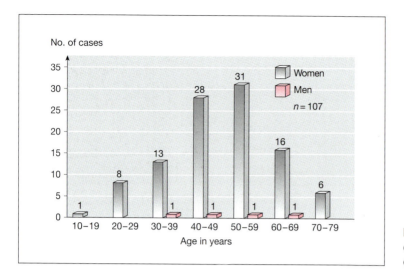

Fig 35-3 Age and gender distribution of 107 cases of FCODs.[4]

The differential diagnoses of FCOD include polyostotic fibrous dysplasia, chronic sclerotic osteomyelitis, Paget disease, Gardner syndrome, and other cemento-osseous dysplasias.

3. Epidemiological data

3.1 Prevalence, incidence, and or relative frequency

Florid cemento-osseous dysplasia has long been considered a rare disease. However, recent studies based on more precise definitions and classifications of cemento-osseous dysplasias[4] have shown this is not the case. The incidence of FCOD is unknown. Shear and Rachanis[16] reported the age-specific morbidity rates for FCOD in the Witwatersrand area of South Africa from 1965 to 1974 as being 0 for white and black men, 0.46 for black women, and 0.21 for white women per million population per year. Since these figures were based on specimens sent to pathology laboratories and many cases remain undiagnosed, the true incidence may be much higher. Only a few cases of FCODs associated with SBC (see chapter 39) have been reported.[8,10,13]

3.2 Age

The age distribution of 107 cases of FCODs[4] is shown in Fig 35-3. The age range of patients was 19 to 76 years. The majority of cases occurred in the 6th and 7th decades. The mean age of 7 Japanese patients with FCODs was 51.3 years (range, 43 to 65 years).[10] The age range at the time of diagnosis for cases of familial FCOD varied considerably among the different families reported.[14]

3.3 Gender

The study by Ackermann and Altini[4] showed that 103 of 107 patients were women with a male:female ratio of 1:26 (see Fig 35-3). Of 7 Japanese patients with FCODs, 6 were women.[10] Of 34 cases of familial FCODs, 20 occurred in women and 14 in men, revealing a different pattern than that of the noninherited variant.

3.4 Location

Florid cemento-osseous dysplasia is only found in the tooth-bearing regions of the jaws and is far more common in the posterior regions. In one study,[4] 78% of the lesions biopsied were located in the mandible. Of the patients studied by Ackermann and Altini,[4] 59% had a single lesion, while the remainder had multiple lesions (29%; two to five lesions in one or more jaw quadrants) or florid lesions (12%; diffuse involvement of periapical and/or alveolar bone in more than one quadrant). Multiple and florid lesions occurred significantly more frequently in black patients and were unusual in patients from other ethnic groups.

3.5 Ethnic distribution

Most reports of FCODs have clearly stated that black women are much more commonly affected than are men or white women. In the study by Ackermann and Altini,[4] 78% of patients were black, 13% were white, 5% were Asians, and 4% were colored. The black:white ratio was 6:1. In contrast, reported cases of familial FCOD have shown that all families except one were white.[14]

4. Pathogenesis

The pathogenesis of FCOD is unknown. However, it has been connected with chronic osteomyelitis and has even been assumed to be inflammatory in origin. Osteomyelitis, however, must be considered only as a complication of FCOD. The periodontal ligament has been considered the tissue of origin of FCOD by most authorities, but some researchers have speculated that FCOD may originate from remnants of cementum left in the bone after extraction.[17]

The etiology of FCOD with SBC differs from that of SBC alone. While SBC, according to some authors, develops after intramedullary hemorrhage following a traumatic injury, Higuchi et al[8] assumed that cystic changes occur after the development of FCOD. Melrose et al[7] suggested that disorderly bone production might result in obstructed drainage of interstitial fluid and thus lead to cyst or cavity formation. This assumption was based on microscopic observations of increased numbers of dilated capillary vessels in FCOD lesions.

5. Pathology

5.1 Macroscopy

Macroscopic descriptions of FCODs have not been published.

5.2 Microscopy

5.2.1 Histologic definition

Both the 1992 WHO classification[2] and the present authors define the FCOD as follows: Lobulated masses of dense, highly mineralized, almost acellular cemento-osseous tissue typically occurring in several parts of the jaws. Black persons are affected more commonly than white persons, and sometimes there is a familial distribution.

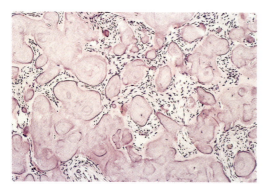

Fig 35-4 Micrograph showing an early FCOD lesion characterized by rounded globules and irregular trabeculae of cementum in a cellular fibroblastic stroma (hematoxylin-eosin [H&E], x120).

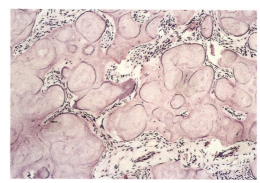

Fig 35-5 Later developmental stage of the FCOD. Globules and trabeculae are now partially fused (H&E, x120).

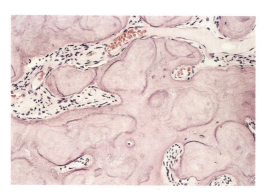

Fig 35-6 Late mature stage of the FCOD. Coalescence and fusion of cemental material is near completion. Note the basophilic resting lines (H&E, x160).

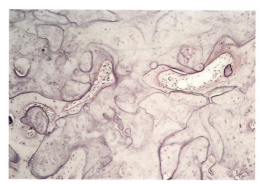

Fig 35-7 Paget disease. Note the similarity between FCOD in Fig 35-6 and the pagetoid globular osteosclerosis here (H&E, x120).

5.2.2 Histopathologic findings

Histopathologically, early-stage lesions are characterized by rounded globules or irregular cementum trabeculae of varying size in a cellular fibroblastic stroma. Some cases may show a proliferative component at the periphery of the lesion. This component consists of cellular fibrous tissue containing rounded globules and/or cementum trabeculae. Ackerman and Altini[4] also observed that the bone around globules of cementum filled in, resulting in fusion of the globules into solid sheets. Fusion of cementum to surrounding bone or inclusion of bone in globules of cementum does not usually occur. The basophilic resting lines may represent the boundaries of the original cementum component.[4] Maturation of the lesions seems to occur at the center with proliferation and an increase in size at the periphery until the lesion "burns itself out." Of the cases studied by Ackermann and Altini,[4] 54% showed signs of infection, resorption, necrosis, and sequestration. These findings were more frequent in cases without a proliferative component (Figs 35-4 to 35-6). The term *pagetoid globular osteosclerosis*,[18] which should not be used to describe FCOD, describes similar histologic features in Paget disease (Fig 35-7).

Cases of familial FCOD reveal a similar histologic appearance as that of the nonhereditary variant. Melrose et al[7] found that most cases exhibited a mixture of cementum-like material and irregular trabeculae of bone, with some trabeculae rimmed by plump osteoblasts and others showing active resorption with apposed multinucleated osteoclasts.

In cases of FCOD with concomitant SBC, the histopathologic features are identical to those of FCOD without SBC. The "cavity wall" consists of a thin, loose fibrous connective tissue layer without epithelial lining as is characteristic for SBC.

Of considerable importance is that in the proliferative phase of FCOD histopathologic features may overlap with those of PCD and cemento-ossifying fibroma.[4] In fact, several biopsies of one lesion may reveal different histologic patterns, some of which may be taken for a cemento-ossifying fibroma. In such instances, differentiation may depend more on clinical and radiographic appearance than on histology.[4]

5.2.3 Histochemical/immunohistochemical findings

Immunohistochemical studies of FCODs and other fibro-osseous lesions of the jaws have rarely been published. Burkhardt[19] studied two "fibro-osteo-cemental" lesions of the jaw using antibodies against vimentin, alpha 1-antichymotrypsin, lysozyme, and S-100 protein. The tumor cells exhibited a positive reaction for the intermediate-size filament vimentin.

5.2.4 Ultrastructural findings

Ultrastructural investigations of FCODs and other non-neoplastic bone lesions of the jaws have not been published to date. Mincer et al[20] published ultrastructural features of sclerotic cemental masses which occurred in the mandible of a 52-year-old black woman. They observed villose cell processes ("cytoplasmic filopodia"), tight junctions, and numerous 7.5 to 10 nm intracytoplasmic filaments occupying a considerable portion of the cell. While the authors interpreted these filaments as contractile elements, Burkhardt[19] argued that it seems unlikely that cells in cemental masses should be equipped for locomotion. He interpreted the vimentin-positive filaments as a cytoskeleton. In recent years, it has been stressed by a number of authorities that more ultrastructural (and immunohistochemical) studies are needed to clarify the nature of immature and mature calcified structures, which have been designated "cementum-like," "osteodentin," and "dysplastic dentin."

6. Notes on treatment and recurrence rate

Usually asymptomatic FCOD lesions do not require any treatment. However, management of FCOD may become a major problem due to the extent and size of the lesions and because they merge with the surrounding bone and cannot be separated easily. In cases of facial deformities, particularly in the familial variant, the jaws can be surgically recontoured; however, cosmetic reshaping of immature lesions has been shown to result in accelerated regrowth (not recurrence).[15] Therefore, the use of surgical recontouring as a treatment option has been questioned by some authors[15] who believe that partial resection of the involved jawbone may be indicated in some cases.

Infection of FCOD may occur after exposure of the avascular sclerotic cemento-osseous masses due to trauma. In such cases, cemento-osteomyelitis with necrosis and sequestration may occur. Sequestrectomy and surgical debridement to remove infected and necrotic tissue is the treatment of choice. Systemic antibiotics should be administered to avoid the spread of infection. However, the avascular nature of FCODs makes the usefulness of antibiotic administration questionable since delivery to the infected site may not be sufficient.

Simple bone cavities associated with FCOD often manifest active enlargement and do not always respond to surgical interventions. In some cases, however, SBCs may "heal" spontaneously. In these cases, the radiographic appearance of the mineralized tissue may be abnormal.[7]

References

1. Pindborg JJ, Kramer IRH. Histologic Typing of Odontogenic Tumours, Jaw Cysts and Allied Lesions. Berlin: Springer-Verlag, 1971.

2. Kramer IRH, Pindborg JJ, Shear M. Histological Typing of Odontogenic Tumours. 2d ed. Berlin: Springer-Verlag, 1992.

3. Waldron CA. Fibro-osseous lesions of the jaws. J Oral Maxillofac Surg 1985;43:249–262.

4. Ackermann GL, Altini M. The cementomas—a clinicopathological reappraisal. J Dent Assoc S Afr 1992;47:187–194.

5. Beylouni I, Farge P, Mazoyer JF, Coudert JL. Florid cemento-osseous dysplasia. Oral Surg Oral Med Oral Pathol Oral Radiol Endod 1998;85: 707–711.

6. Schneider LC, Mesa ML. Differences between florid osseous dysplasia and chronic diffuse sclerosing osteomyelitis. Oral Surg Oral Med Oral Pathol 1990;70:308–312.

7. Melrose RJ, Abrams AM, Mills BG. Florid osseous dysplasia. A clinical-pathologic study of thirty-four cases. Oral Surg Oral Med Oral Pathol 1976;41: 62–82.

8. Higuchi, Y, Nakamura N, Tashiro H. Clinico-pathologic study of cemento-osseous dysplasia producing cysts of the mandible. Oral Surg Oral Med Oral Pathol 1988;65:339–342.

9. Agazzi C, Belloni L. Gli odontomi duri die mascellari. Arch Ital Otol Rinol Laringol 1953;64: 3–102.

10. Ariji Y, Ariji E, Higuchi Y, et al. Florid cemento-osseous dysplasia. Radiographic study with special emphasis on computed tomography. Oral Surg Oral Med Oral Pathol 1994;78:391–396.

11. Ong S-T, Siar CH. Florid cemento-osseous dysplasia in a young Chinese man. Case report. Aust Dent J 1997;42:404–408.

12. Miyake M, Nagahata S. Florid cemento-osseous dysplasia. Report of a case. Int J Oral Maxillofac Surg 1999;28:56–57.

13. Miyauchi M, Ogawa I, Takata T, et al. Florid cemento-osseous dysplasia with concomitant simple bone cysts: A case in a Japanese woman. J Oral Pathol Med 1995;24:285–287.

14. Coleman H, Altini M, Kieser J, Nissenbaum M. Familial florid cemento-osseous dysplasia—a case report and review of the literature. J Dent Assoc S Afr 1996;51:766–770.

15. Young S, Markowitz R, Sullivan S, et al. Familial gigantiform cementoma: Classification and presentation of a large pedigree. Oral Surg Oral Med Oral Pathol 1989;68:740–746.

16, Shear M, Rachanis CC. Epidemiology of odontogenic lesions in South Africa. J Dent Assoc S Afr 1979;34:685–688.

17. Oikarinen K, Altonen M, Happonen R-P. Gigantiform cementoma affecting a Caucasian family. Br J Oral Maxillofac Surg 1991;29:194–197.

18. Musella AE, Slater LJ. Familial florid osseous dysplasia: A case report. J Oral Maxillofac Surg 1989;47:636–640.

19. Burkhardt A. Dentin formation in so-called "fibro-osteo-cemental" lesion of the jaw: Histologic, electron microscopic, and immunohistochemical investigations. Oral Surg Oral Med Oral Pathol 1989;68:729–738.

20. Mincer HH, McGinnis JP, Wyatt JR. Ultrastructure of sclerotic cemental masses. Oral Surg Oral Med Oral Pathol 1977;43:70–81.

Chapter 36

Cherubism

1. Terminology

Cherubism is an uncommon, benign fibro-osseous lesion which causes a progressive, painless, symmetrical expansion of the jaws and is found primarily in the mandible. It was first reported in 1933 by Jones,[1] who described a family in which three of five siblings were affected by bilateral cystic jaw lesions associated with fullness of the cheeks, cervical lymphadenopathy without apparent relationship to the jaw lesions, and an upward cast to the eyes with exposure of the rim of the lower sclera. The "grotesque cherubic appearance" of these children caused Jones to suggest the term *familial multilocular disease of the jaws* for these manifestations. He later coined the term *cherubism* after the cherubs seen in Renaissance art with their "eyes-raised-to-Heaven" look; in cherubism this is caused by enlargement of the lower face with stretching of the skin and consequent retraction of the lower eyelids. A number of other descriptions have also been used; these include *familial fibrous dysplasia of the jaws, hereditary fibrous dysplasia of the jaws, disseminated juvenile fibrous dysplasia, bilateral giant cell tumors of the jaws, fibro-osseous dysplasia of the jaws, familial intra-osseous fibrous swelling of the jaws, familial bilateral giant cell tumor of the jaws, familial multilocular cystic disease of the jaws,* and *familial fibrous swelling of the jaws.*[2]

By 1978, approximately 145 cases of cherubism had been reported, including several families with multiple affected members. Subsequent reports included those by Peters,[3] Zachariades et al,[4] Zohar et al,[5] Kaugars et al,[6] Marck and Kudry,[7] Vaillant et al,[8] Penfold et al,[9] Hitomi et al,[10] Valiathan et al,[11] Southgate et al,[12] von Wowern,[13] and Stiller et al.[14] In 2000, about 280 cases of cherubism had been published, with 80% indicating familial manifestations.[14] Single case reports indicating that cherubism may occur without hereditary origin have been published. A few reports have described cherubism associated with other diseases such as a Noonan-like, multiple giant cell lesion syndrome[15]; Ramon syndrome, comprising short stature, mental retardation, gingival fibromatosis, and epilepsy[16]; as well as fragile X syndrome (mental retardation).[17] Cherubism associated with craniosynostosis has been described also.[14] Intelligence is not usually affected in cherubism.

Although sporadic, non-gender–linked mutations exist, as do unilateral and occasional bilateral cases reported in relatives of known patients, cherubism usually occurs as an autosomal dominant gene with variable expressivity, ranging from 100% penetrance in men to 50% to 75% in women. Mangion et al[18] mapped the gene for cherubism to chromosome region 4p16.3. Critical meiotic recombinants placed the gene in a 3-cM interval between D4S127 and the telomere of 4p. Within this region, a strong candidate is the gene for fibroblast growth factor receptor–3 (FGFR-3). Mutations in this gene have been implicated in a diverse set of bone development disorders.[18] In a recent study of craniosynostosis and cherubism,[14] however, the FGFR-3 gene was excluded as a possible candidate.

2. Clinical and radiologic profile

Cherubism is characterized by bilateral enlargement of the mandible and maxilla with bone loss and replacement with fibro-osseous lesional tissue. In rare instances, ribs or long bones may be affected also. The spectrum of the disease can range from the unilateral subclinical involvement of the jaws to extreme bilateral expansion. The most common site is the mandibular angle. The lesions may spread to involve the retromolar areas and ascending rami. In more severe cases, the coronoid processes may expand so severely as to obliterate the mandibular notch. The condyle is only rarely involved, and most patients can open their mouths adequately.

Maxillary lesions (60%) usually start in the tuberosity and involve the maxillary alveolar processes, resulting in the development of a narrow V-shaped palate. The antral floor may be thickened. In severe cases, the antrum may be completely obliterated. The anterior wall of the maxilla may become enlarged and protrude forward. The lower eyelid is pulled down, producing the characteristic Heavenward "gaze." Orbital compression with impaired vision and proptosis may occur in some cases.

The facial deformities in cherubism are due solely to enlargement and expansion of the underlying fibro-osseous structures. Since these deformities may be of varying severity, a grading system has been proposed[7]:

Grade 1: involvement of both mandibular ascending rami

Grade 2: involvement of both mandibular ascending rami and both maxillary tuberosities

Grade 3: massive involvement of the entire maxilla and mandible except the condylar processes

Grade 4: same as Grade 3 with involvement of the orbits, causing orbital compression.

A number of dental abnormalities have been reported. The fibro-osseous lesions may cause premature loss of deciduous teeth. Agenesis of the second and third molars of the mandible—and the maxilla, when involved—is regularly observed. Displacement of teeth with delayed eruption is also seen. Resorption of roots may occur in severe cases.

Cervical lymph node enlargement may be present in 45% of cases and contributes to the full-faced appearance. Lymph nodes enlarge before the age of 6 years, decrease in size after 8 years, and are rarely enlarged at 12 years. The increase in size is produced by reticuloendothelial hyperplasia with fibrosis. Due to the cumulative enlargement of the submandibular lymph nodes and the expansion of the mandible, the tongue may be displaced, affecting speech, mastication, swallowing, and respiration. Cherubism is not present at birth. Facial swelling first appears between the age of 14 months and 4 years and progresses until the age of 12 to 15 years (Figs 36-1 to 36-3). Typically, the earlier the lesion appears, the more rapidly it progresses. The fastest growth occurs over the first 2 to 3 years with a slowing down after the patient reaches the age of 5 years. Growth of the posterior mandible and maxilla stops first, whereas the anterior mandible

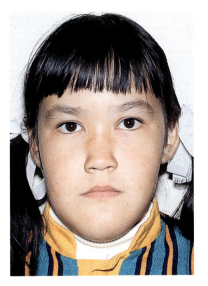

Fig 36-1 Ten-year-old girl with marked mandibular involvement of cherubism.

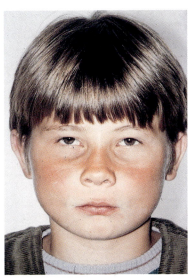

Fig 36-2 Eleven-year-old male patient exhibiting cherubism with bilateral swelling of the cheeks.

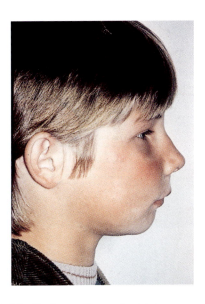

Fig 36-3 Lateral view of the patient shown in Fig 36-2.

may continue to grow for some time. Clinically, cherubism may become quiescent without treatment and may decrease in size at 20 to 30 years, although the jaws may remain somewhat large.

In the vast majority of cases, the characteristic maxillofacial deformities remain within acceptable limits and surgical interventions are unnecessary or limited. Cases of extensive bone destruction resulting in an esthetically monstrous appearance or severe functional disturbances may occasionally be observed. In addition, aggressive forms of cherubism have been described.[19,20]

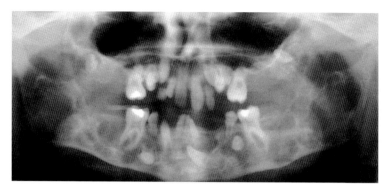

Fig 36-4 Panoramic radiograph of the patient shown in Figs 36-2 and 36-3 at the age of 11 years. Multiple cystic lesions of the mandible are seen with displacement of several permanent teeth. The maxilla is also involved.

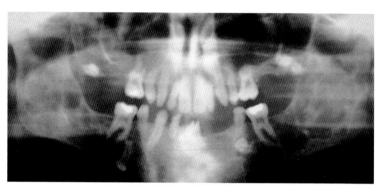

Fig 36-5 Panoramic radiograph of the same patient at the age of 15 years.

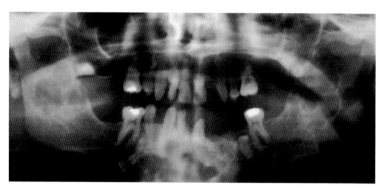

Fig 36-6 Panoramic radiograph of the same patient at the age of 20 years. The mandibular cherubic lesions are still present, but some have become smaller and bone formation has started.

Laboratory findings in cherubism are not diagnostic. Serum calcium, phosphorus, and alkaline phosphatase may be elevated or normal. However, elevated values in children are not unusual and are associated with the physiologic growth of bones. Southgate et al[12] confirmed that the biochemical profile in four children with cherubism was normal (serum calcium, parathyroid hormone, parathyroid-related hormone, calcitonin, alkaline phosphatase); however, urine analysis of pyridinium and desoxypyridinium cross-links, hydroxyproline, and calcium in relation to urine creatinine to assess bone resorption showed values at the upper end of the normal range.

Radiographically, the lesions consist of multilocular radiolucencies with distinct borders divided by bony trabeculae (Figs 36-4 to 36-6). Expansion of the cortical plates associated with marked thinning is also seen. The cortical plates may be perforated. Changes usually begin posteriorly and spread anteriorly. Mandibular lesions may reveal caudal displacement of the inferior alveolar nerve canal, and the lesion may involve the alveolar process, the mandibular angle, and the ascending ramus. Lesions are usually found bilaterally. Teeth may be displaced or unerupted, or they may appear to be floating in the cystlike spaces. Root resorption may be observed as well. Radiographically, maxillary lesions are similar to those of the mandible and are located primarily in the tuberosities. The maxillary sinuses, which are small in children, may be completely obliterated. Occlusal films may reveal a "soap-bubble" appearance.

The bilateral extended osseous destruction changes with age. Whereas trabeculae are sparse during the growth phase, the number and thickness of the septa increase and the lesion becomes more radiopaque when the patient reaches 8 to 12 years of age. During this phase the lesion may take on a ground-glass appearance. By 20 to 30 years of age, the lesion changes to a granular texture. Cystic spaces, however, may still be present at age 70.

Although conventional radiography is helpful in the diagnosis of cherubism, computed tomography (CT) is superior for making the diagnosis and determining the degree of severity. In particular, CT may provide a realistic spatial picture of the lesion, its site, extent, and structure, thus showing some aspects that otherwise would not be demonstrable due to superimposition and the anatomic complexity of the jaws.[10,21]

Three-dimensional reconstructions of the lesions may be helpful in planning surgical interventions in more severe cases of cherubism. Using stereophotographic assessment, the changes of facial swelling may be monitored and compared with the norm. Bone scintigrams have revealed low radioactivity—so-called cold areas—in some cases of cherubism.[10]

3. Epidemiological data

3.1 Prevalence, incidence, and relative frequency

Cherubism is a rare disease. Until 2000, approximately 280 cases had been described.[14] Figures on incidence and prevalence have not been published to date.

3.2 Age

Cherubism manifests in early childhood, usually at 14 months to 5 years,[18] and becomes more marked until puberty. At this time the fibro-osseous lesions begin to regress, but in many cases cherubism may persist throughout life. Data for the creation of a "conventional" age distribution are not available.

3.3 Gender

Men are affected twice as frequently as women, and there is no ethnic dominance.[4]

3.4 Location

While the mandible seems to be involved in all cases, the maxilla is affected in only 60% of cases. Lesions are usually bilateral, although unilateral cases have been reported.[22] Lesions start to develop posteriorly and extend anteriorly during the disease process.

4. Pathogenesis

Jones[1] speculated that cherubism was neoplastic and must be related in some way to the development of the permanent teeth, thus suggesting an odontogenic origin. The odontogenic theory was based on the fact that cherubism is localized in or near the tooth-bearing region. It has also been assumed that cherubism may represent a form of fibrous dysplasia. A perivascular fibrosis that results in reduced oxygenation of bone and an alteration of the mesenchyme during bone development has also been considered in the pathogenesis.[4] Other causation theories include latent hyperparathyroidism; a benign neoplasm with hormonal dependence; trauma (since fibrous dysplasia has been considered a nonspecific, abnormal reaction to trauma); and an aberration of ossification in membranous bone causing fibrous dysplastic lesions of varying manifestations and histopathologic pattern.[2] However, most authors consider cherubism to be of a giant cell nature.

Recent studies have shown that the genetic defect characteristic of cherubism is responsible for a localized increase in osteoclasts which is normalized during puberty with a physiologically increased synthesis of sexual hormones (estradiol and testosterone).[12] In addition, it has been shown that the multinucleate cells in cherubic lesions are osteoclasts; they synthesize tartrate-resistant vitronectin receptor and resorb bone.[12]

5. Pathology

5.1 Macroscopy

Macroscopically, lesional tissue may have a reddish, grayish, yellowish, or bluish color. The consistency may vary from hard to semihard to soft to jellylike. The lesion is not usually encapsulated, and periosteum is not normally found.[4]

5.2 Microscopy

5.2.1 Histologic definition

Both the 1992 World Health Organization (WHO) classification[23] and the present authors define cherubism as follows:
A benign, self-limiting condition in which the lesional tissue consists of vascular fibrous tissue containing varying numbers of multinucleated giant cells arranged diffusely or focally.

5.2.2 Histopathologic findings

The histologic findings vary according to disease stage. Early active lesions are characterized by high cellularity with abundant giant cells and multiple foci of extravasated erythrocytes (Fig 36-7). The highly vascularized fibrous stroma is arranged in whorled patterns and contains numerous fibroblasts. The multinucleated giant cells are of the osteoclast type with prominent nuclei and nucleoli. Blood vessels are well formed, and endothelial cells are large. Perivascular cuffing around small capillaries is observed with use of an acidophilic van Gieson–positive material. This characteristic finding is of unknown significance; however, it has been considered a contributing factor in the development of cherubism since it may support the pathogenetic theory of hypoxemia.[4] In more mature lesions, lesional tissue be-

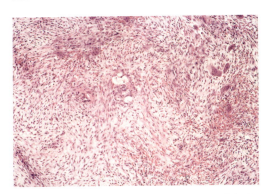

Fig 36-7 Early active lesion with high cellularity and giant cells in a vascular fibrous stroma (hematoxylin-eosin [H&E], x60).

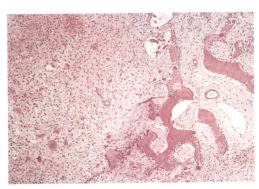

Fig 36-8 A more mature lesion with formation of new bone trabeculae (H&E, x60).

comes more fibrous, and there is a decrease in the number of giant cells; new bone may be formed (Fig 36-8). Remnants of odontogenic epithelium are sometimes scattered throughout. This particular finding has been interpreted as supporting the odontogenic origin of cherubism.[4] The enlarged lymph nodes usually reveal reticuloendothelial hyperplasia, fibrosis, and chronic inflammation.[4]

Morphologically, cherubic lesions are similar to those observed in giant cell lesion, fibrous dysplasia, and hyperparathyroidism. Therefore, the diagnosis of cherubism should never be based on microscopic findings alone but should include anamnestic, clinical, and radiographic findings (eg, early onset of the disease, a positive family history, absence of other bone pathology, histologic picture).

5.2.3 Histochemical/immunohistochemical findings

Cherubic lesions have only rarely been studied systematically by histochemical or immunohistochemical methods. Chomette et al[24] studied three cases of cherubism by histoenzymologic methods. Oxidative enzymes—including acid and alkaline phosphatases, ATPase, and leucine aminopeptidase—were tested. These authors were able to characterize three stages in the morphologic evolution of cherubism. The first (osteolytic) stage is characterized by an osteolytic "granuloma" with numerous giant cells and a high level of acid phosphatase activity. The second stage shows repair with proliferation of highly active fibroblasts and an increase in leucine aminopeptidase activity. The third stage exhibits osteogenesis as a sign of bony restoration with high alkaline phosphatase activity. It was concluded that histologic and histoenzymologic findings may indicate whether involution or progression of the disease should be expected.

Burkhardt and Berthold[25] found histiocytic characteristics in both mononuclear and multinuclear cells by demonstrating alpha-1-trypsin, alpha-1-antitrypsine, and lysozyme. Staining for lysozyme was much more marked in giant cells than in mononuclear cells. The mononuclear cell elements were identified as fibrohistiocytic with marked signs of activity; the multinuclear giant cells were of the osteoclastic type, although it was thought possible that they might assume an intermediate position between mature osteoclasts and histiocytic giant cells (making them preosteoclastic). Since findings in giant cell granulomas are almost identical, the authors suggested a relationship between the two types of lesion.

5.2.4 Ultrastructural findings

Chomette et al[24] and Burkhardt and Berthold[25] studied biopsy specimens of cherubism by transmission electron microscopy. Chomette et al[24] found three types of cells: giant cells, ovoid cells, and fusiform cells. Giant cells had features of osteoclasts and revealed several pale nuclei with marginated heterochromatin. The cytoplasmic membrane showed regular microvillus-like projections and sometimes revealed irregular larger cytoplasmic processes. The cytoplasm contained numerous mitochondria and well-developed cisternae; there were few lysosomes. Ovoid cells were similar to young fibroblasts. Elongated cells were similar to osteoblasts.

Burkhardt and Berthold[25] also revealed a number of different cell types. Mononuclear fibroblastic/fibrocytic spindle-shaped cells and abundant rough endoplasmic reticulum were most common. Other cell types included myxoblast-like cells, myofibroblasts, cells of histiocyte-macrophage differentiation, osteoblasts, and angioblasts. On average, 15 nuclei per giant cell were found.

6. Notes on treatment and recurrence rate

Treatment of cherubism is not uniform or standardized. Cherubism usually is self-limiting and regressive, although aggressive cases have been described.[15] Radiation therapy is absolutely *contraindicated* because of severe sequelae such as osteoradionecrosis and osteosarcomas. Peters[3] reported that of 10 patients with cherubism who had received radiation therapy (25 Gy), a fibrosarcoma developed in 1 patient and 5 others had growth disturbances of the jaws. Because there are few functional disturbances, treatment is usually based on the rate of tumor progression, the extent of involvement, and the psychologic state of the patient. Most authors recommend deferring treatment until after puberty, which makes it difficult to evaluate nontreatment. The general view of the surgical treatment is to follow the patient and perform biopsies, surgical corrections, and removal of ectopically impacted teeth.[13] Early surgical interventions, on the other hand, often result in prompt recurrence and aggravation of the lesions. In 2000, von Wowern[13] showed that surgical treatment did not provoke growth of lesional tissue in any of 22 cases observed over a period of 36 years.

In young patients, the lesions are vascular, and blood loss may be considerable when treated surgically. In one case, [26] vascular transformation occurred after surgery. In cases where treatment is necessary in a young patient, some authorities have proposed radical treatment rather than conservative curettage to avoid multiple recurrences and repeated surgical interventions. Other authors have proposed curettage of the lesions, while still others have suggested unilateral surgery and comparative follow-up. Contouring procedures after age 20 are usually satisfactory in terms of facial esthetics. Calcitonin, which is used as an antiresorptive agent to prevent osteoporosis in postmenopausal women, has recently been discussed as a possible medication for cherubism.[12]

The prognosis for cherubism is generally good, since the disease gradually regresses. The first signs of improvement may be observed in the maxilla; lesions in the mandible may progress until age 20. After 30 years of age, few traces of the disease are still detectable, especially in the mandible.

References

1. Jones WA. Familial multilocular cystic disease of the jaws. Am J Cancer 1933;17:946–950.

2. Riefkohl R, Georgiade GS, Nicholas GG. Cherubism. Ann Plast Surg 1985;14:85–90.

3. Peters WJ. Cherubism: A study of twenty cases from one family. Oral Surg Oral Med Oral Pathol 1979;47:307–311.

4. Zachariades N, Papanicolaou S, Xypolyta A, Constantinidis J. Cherubism. Int J Oral Surg 1985; 14:138–145.

5. Zohar Y, Granskord R, Shabtai F, Talmi Y. Fibrous dysplasia and cherubism as a hereditary familial disease. J Craniomaxillofac Surg 1989;17:340–344.

6. Kaugars GE, Niamtu J III, Svirsky JA. Cherubism: Diagnosis, treatment, and comparison with central giant cell granulomas and giant cell tumors. Oral Surg Oral Med Oral Pathol 1992;73:369–374.

7. Marck PA, Kudryk WH. Cherubism. J Otolaryngol 1992;21:84–87.

8. Vaillant JM, Romain P, Divaris M. Cherubism. Findings in three cases in the same family. J Craniomaxillofac Surg 1989;17:345–349.

9. Penfold CN, McCullagh P, Eveson JW, Ramsay A. Giant cell lesion complicating fibro-osseous conditions of the jaws. Int J Oral Maxillofac Surg 1993;22:158–162.

10. Hitomi G, Nishide N, Mitsu K. Cherubism. Diagnosis imaging and review of the literature in Japan. Oral Surg Oral Med Oral Pathol 1996;81:623–628.

11. Valiathan A, Orth MS, Prashanth VK. Cherubism: Presentation of a case. Angle Orthod 1997;67: 237–238.

12. Southgate J, Sarma U, Townend V, Barron J, Flanagan AM. Study of cell biology and biochemistry of cherubism. J Clin Pathol 1998;51: 831–837.

13. von Wowern N. Cherubism. A 36-year long-term follow-up of 2 generations in different families and review of the literature. Oral Surg Oral Med Oral Pathol Oral Radiol Endod 2000;90:765–772.

14. Stiller M, Urban M, Golder W, et al. Craniosynostosis in cherubism. Am J Med Genetics 2000; 95:325–331.

15. Addante RR, Breen GH. Cherubism in a patient with Noonan's syndrome. J Oral Maxillofac Surg 1996;54:210–213.

16. Pina-Neto JM, Moreno AFC, Silva LR, et al. Cherubism, gingival fibromatosis, epilepsy, and mental deficiency (Ramon syndrome) with juvenile rheumatoid arthritis. Am J Med Genet 1986;25: 433–441.

17. Quan F, Grompe M, Jakobs P, Popvich B. Spontaneous deletion in the FMR1 gene in a patient with fragile X syndrome and cherubism. Hum Molec Genet 1995;4:1681–1684.

18. Mangion J, Rahman N, Edkins S, et al. The gene for cherubism maps to chromosome 4p16.3. Am J Hum Genet 1999;65:151–157.

19. Timosca GC, Galesanu RM, Cotutiu C, Grigoras M. Aggressive form of cherubism: Report of a case. J Oral Maxillofac Surg 2000;58:336–344.

20. Ayoub AF, El-Mofty SS. Cherubism: Report of an aggressive case and review of the literature. J Oral Maxillofac Surg 1993;51:702–705.

21. Bianchi SD, Boccardi A, Mela F, Romagnoli R. The computed tomographic appearances of cherubism. Skeletal Radiol 1987;16:6–10.

22. Reade PC, McKellar GM, Radden BG. Unilateral mandibular cherubism: Brief review and case report. Br J Oral Maxillofac Surg 1984;22:189–194.

23. Kramer IRH, Pindborg JJ, Shear M. Histological Typing of Odontogenic Tumours. 2d ed. Berlin: Springer-Verlag, 1992.

24. Chomette G, Auriol M, Guilbert F, Vaillant JM. Cherubism. Histoenzymological and ultrastructural study. J Oral Maxillofac Surg 1988;17:219–223.

25. Burkhardt A, Berthold H. Cherubism. Klinische and morphologische Beobachtungen. Dtsch Z Mund Kiefer Gesichtschir 1986;10:257–263.

26. Koury ME, Stella JP, Epker BN, Worth F. Vascular transformation in cherubism. Oral Surg Oral Med Oral Pathol 1993;76:20–27.

Chapter 37

Central Giant Cell Lesion (Granuloma)

1. Terminology

Giant cell lesions of the maxillofacial skeleton and other bones are a controversial matter, and uncertainty still exists regarding their basic pathology and biologic behavior. Fifty years ago, giant cell lesions of the jaws were generally diagnosed as giant cell tumors, and these lesions were widely considered to be similar to those that occurred in the extragnathic skeleton.

In 1953, Jaffe[1] proposed the term *giant cell reparative granuloma of the jaws* to distinguish these lesions from the *giant cell tumor* usually found in the epiphyseal regions of long bones. Jaffe believed these jaw lesions were not neoplasms and likely represented a local reparative reaction. This concept was widely accepted, and since then such jaw lesions have generally been designated *giant cell reparative granulomas.* However, because the clinical behavior of many of these lesions is inconsistent with a reparative reaction, the word *reparative* was omitted in more recent classifications. The term *granuloma*—meaning a small, rounded, inflammatory mass of macrophages—may not be appropriate in the light of recent findings[2] showing that the jaw lesions are composed of a relatively small number of macrophages (7%). However, the field seems to be saddled with tradition and the term *giant cell granuloma* persists, although the more general *giant cell lesion* is gaining ground.

Giant cell lesions of the jaws occur in two variants: the *peripheral* and the *central* (endosteal or intrabony) types. The peripheral giant cell lesion is a solitary soft tissue mass located on the gingiva in dentate persons or the alveolar mucosa in edentulous persons. It has been indicated that the ratio between the peripheral and central variants ranges from 3:1 to 4:1. The two variants exhibit identical histologic features. The peripheral variant, which is not likely to give rise to differential diagnostic confusion with odontogenic lesions, is not dealt with in this chapter. Recent studies on the peripheral variant have been reported by Mighell et al,[3] Carvalho et al,[4] and Bodner et al.[5]

Central giant cell lesions (CGCLs) of the jaws and giant cell tumors (GCTs) of the extragnathic skeleton are, according to one theory,[6,7] not distinct and separate entities but rather represent a continuum of a single disease process modified by the age of the patient, tumor location, and other possible factors that are not yet clearly understood. The present authors agree with Whitaker and Waldron[8] that until future research clearly delineates separation of the CGCL from the GCT, this approach seems logical; CGCL is used throughout this chapter for the giant cell lesion.

Chuong et al[9] and Ficarra et al[10] have suggested separating the jaw giant cell lesions into aggressive and nonaggressive types based on clinical and radiologic considera-

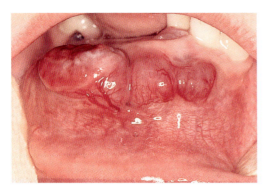

Fig 37-1 Central giant cell lesion which has perforated the labial cortex of the mandible in the incisor region. The clinical appearance mimics that of the peripheral variant.

tions, and Whitaker and Waldron[8] support the view that this distinction may be of aid to the clinician.

2. Clinical and radiologic profile

The CGCL is an intrabony, non-neoplastic, slow-growing lesion affecting women more often than men. The diagnosis is made in most patients (72%) before the age of 30 years. Signs and symptoms vary considerably, but pain is present only rarely. The lesion may occur in either jaw, but it shows a definite predominance in the mandible. Larger lesions may produce localized swelling of the jaws. Sometimes the expansion occurs rapidly. The proliferative periosteal reaction is usually poor. Perforation of the periosteum may result in an overgrowth presenting as a soft tissue mass mimicking the peripheral variant (Fig 37-1). A smaller subset of these lesions, however, are clinically *aggressive* to varying degrees and tend to recur after treatment; they exhibit features more typical of a neoplasm than a reactive process. These lesions are often associated with pain or paresthesia, cortical perforation, and root resorption. The question of whether or not "true" giant cell tumors exist in the jaws has been argued for years and is still unresolved.

Radiographically, there is an area of bone destruction evident with CGCLs. According to Wood and Goaz,[11] the lesion may initially occur as a solitary cystlike radiolucency and as it grows larger, it may develop a soap-bubble type of multilocular radiolucency. Kaffe et al[12] showed that of their 80 analyzed cases, 51% were multilocular, 44% were unilocular, and 5% were "not loculated." The multilocular appearance may bear some similarity to that of an intraosseous, infiltrative ameloblastoma (Fig 37-2). Kaffee et al[12] found that the mean size of multilocular lesions was 7.4 cm, whereas the mean size of the unilocular lesions was only 4.0 cm, a statistically significant difference. The authors also described a not previously reported correlation between root resorption and gender: Root resorption was observed in 24% of male patients and only 6% of female patients (Fig 37-3).

3. Epidemiological data

3.1 Prevalence, incidence, and relative frequency

Central giant cell lesions of the jaw have been described as uncommon,[13] relatively common,[6] and common,[14] the latter authors indicating that the lesion accounts for approximately 7% of all benign jaw tumors. No data on prevalence or incidence of CGCLs are available.

Fig 37-2 A large CGCL in a 15-year-old female patient with multilocular radiolucent destruction of the mandibular right third molar–ascending ramus area. Note the displaced tooth germ of the third molar. The radiologic features resemble those of a solid/multicystic ameloblastoma (SMA).

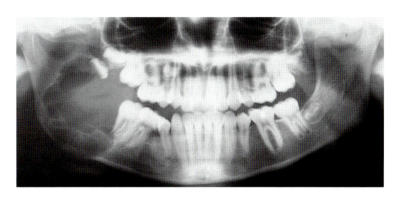

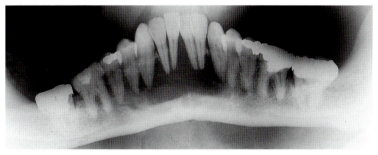

Fig 37-3 Unilocular radiolucent CGCL in a 29-year-old woman. The borders are well defined, and the lesion covers the anterior mandibular area from the left second premolar to the right second premolar. No root resorption is evident.

3.2 Age

Information on age has been collected from reports by Andersen et al[15] (32 cases), Whitaker and Waldron[8] (132 cases), Kaffe et al[12] (18 cases), and Bodner and Bar-Ziv[13] (10 cases). The pooled data from these 192 adequately documented cases show an age range between 2 and 81 years (Fig 37-4). There is a peak in the 2nd decade of life, with 30.7% of patients in this group. Almost three quarters (71.8%) of patients were under the

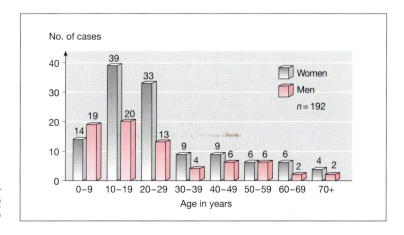

Fig 37-4 Age and gender distribution of 192 cases of CGCLs.[8,12,13,15]

age of 30 at the time of diagnosis. The available data do not allow calculation of the mean age for these patients.

3.3 Gender

There is a female predominance for CGCLs, with 62.5% of all cases occurring in women (see Fig 37-4). The male:female ratio varies, according to age group, from 1:1.5 to 1:3. A female predominance was noted in every decade of life with the exception of the 1st (male:female ratio, 1:0.7).

3.4 Location

Pooled data on tumor location were collected from the same sources as those used for age and gender.[8,12,13,15] The total number of cases for which location was reported was 129. All four studies showed almost identical numbers for the distribution of lesions between the maxilla and mandible. There is a clear mandibular predominance, with between 70% and 75% of the lesions being located there. Kaffe et al[12] pooled data from their own 18 cases with 62 cases collected

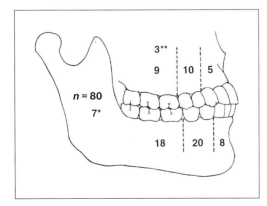

Fig 37-5 Topographic distribution of 80 cases of CGCLs.[12] Single asterisk indicates ramus and condyle; double asterisk indicates maxillary sinus.

from the literature and found that, contrary to what was previously reported, 50% of lesions were located in the posterior areas of the jaws. However, their tabulated data showed that 43% of cases were located in the maxillary and mandibular molar region, mandibular ramus, and condyle area; 54% were located in the anterior (incisor, canine, and premolar) regions (Fig 37-5). Thus, their data actually agree with those of previous authors[7,11,16] that the anterior area of the jaws is most commonly involved.

The frequency of CGCL occurrence in association with the crown of an impacted, unerupted, or developing tooth varies between 10% and 19%.[8,12,13] This probably reflects that the greatest percentage of these lesions occurs in young patients.

4. Pathogenesis

Perhaps the most widely held view is that the initial CGCL is an endosteal hemorrhage. In 1962 (still the "reparative era"), Kramer[17] stated that if the process is concerned with repair following hemorrhage, then the repair follows a peculiar pattern complicated by repeated new hemorrhages. El-Labban,[18] who studied central giant cell lesions ultrastructually 35 years later, demonstrated that Kramer was right in his statement. The majority of vessels showed intravascular fibrin thrombi and endothelial cell damage, with gaps in the cell walls. Plasma, erythrocytes, and fibrin were seen subendothelially. El-Labban and Lee[19] had previously shown evidence of fusion between myofibroblasts and giant cells and postulated that giant cells form and increase in size through this fusion. In El-Labban's 1997 report,[18] she noted that one of the gaps in a vessel had been sealed

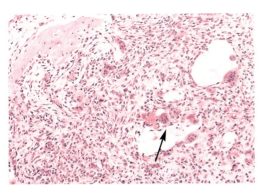

Fig 37-6 Characteristic cellular components of the CGCL: stromal cell population comprising spindle-shaped fibroblast-like cells with oval nuclei and macrophage-like cells containing round, chromatin-dense nuclei. Aggregations of multinuclear giant cells are distributed between the stromal cells and often found near or even situated inside (*arrow*) thin-walled vascular channels. In the upper left corner, an immature osteoid trabeculum can be seen (hematoxylin-eosin [H&E], x80).

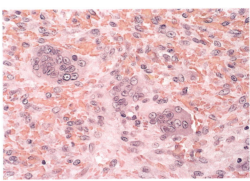

Fig 37-7 Features of metabolically active giant cells in a CGCL with multiple vesicular nuclei, each containing a distinct nucleolus. Note the fresh hemorrhage (H&E, x180).

by a giant cell. The author suggested that the presence of the giant cell closed the gap and stopped hemorrhaging. More information pertaining to the pathogenesis of CGCLs appears later in the chapter.

5. Pathology

5.1 Macroscopy

The surgical specimen consists of a soft, spongy, reddish to brownish friable tissue of varying size. Since the vascular tissue bleeds very easily, the specimen is often coated with fresh or coagulated blood.

5.2 Microscopy

5.2.1 Histologic definitions

According to the 1992 World Health Organization (WHO) classification,[20] the CGCL is "an intraosseous lesion consisting of more or less fibrous tissue containing multiple foci of hemorrhage, aggregations of multinucleated giant cells, and sometimes trabeculae of woven bone forming within the septa of more mature fibrous tissue that may traverse the lesion."

The definition used by the present authors is as follows:

An intraosseous lesion consisting of a stromal cell population admixed with multinucleated giant cells and distributed in a collagenous tissue. The stromal cells may be of at least two types: one resembles (myo)fibroblasts, oval or spindle-shaped with a cigar-shaped nucleus exhibiting sparse chromatin; the other resembles macrophages with smaller round nuclei exhibiting dense chromatin (Fig 37-6). Foci of fresh hemorrhage, hemosiderin granules, and thin-walled vascular spaces are common findings (Figs 37-6 and 37-7). Bone formation with production of immature osteoid trabeculae is found in a high percentage of cases.

5.2.2 Histopathologic findings

The stromal cells project between the giant cells in swirls, with herringbone and storiform focal patterns. The aggregations of giant cells show great variations in size, morphology, and the number of nuclei.

Morphologically, the giant cells are of foreign body type or osteoclast-like. The stainability of the cytoplasm varies from light basophilia to marked eosinophilia; variations may occur within the same giant cell. Some cells contain big ovoid and lightly stained nuclei with prominent nucleoli and sparse chromatin. Other cells contain small, darkly stained nuclei of irregular shape. Cytoplasmic vacuoles of different sizes containing erythrocytes, iron-positive hemosiderin granules, and leukocytes are frequently found. Mitotic figures are rarely present. In many instances, the giant cells show a definite relationship to vascular channels. The function of the multinucleated giant cells that typify these lesions is still controversial, although most investigators believe that the origin of these cells is related to the fusion of stromal cells with either macrophages or (myo)fibroblast-like cells (see the section on ultrastructural findings in this chapter).

The size, number of nuclei, and distribution of the prominent and mysterious multinucleated giant cells has been compared in both jaw lesions and lesions in other bones. Lucas[21] stated that the giant cells in jaw lesions are often smaller than those in giant cell tumors of long bone. Cells in jaw lesions are unevenly distributed throughout, whereas numerous evenly distributed giant cells are present in practically every field of the neoplasm. In a study of 10 cases of each of the two lesions, Abrams and Shear[22] confirmed Lucas' statement but concluded that a few giant cell lesions of long bones had giant cells that were as small as—if not smaller than—those in jaw lesions. In addition, giant cells of the jaw lesions contained significantly fewer nuclei than those of the long bone lesions. The authors further concluded that some giant cell lesions of long bones are morphologically indistinguishable from giant cell lesions of the jaws and vice versa. It is possible, therefore, that some jaw lesions are GCTs and that some giant cell lesions outside the jaws are CGCLs. Lastly, Abrams and Shear[22] suggested that if a giant cell lesion contains giant cells in which the product of length and breadth exceeds 1500 μm^2, the diagnosis of GCT should be considered. Giant cell lesions (granulomas) are likely to have areas of less than 1500 μm^2.

Franklin and colleagues[23] also studied 10 cases of each lesion. Unlike Abrams and Shear,[22] they found that the giant cells in the GCT were smaller than those of the CGCL, but they agreed that there were more nuclei in the cells of the GCT.

Auclair et al,[6] using a semiautomatic image analyzer, studied various parameters for 50 giant cell profiles from each of 42 GCTs and 49 CGCLs. They showed that the mean size (area and volume) of the giant cells in the GCTs was larger than that in CGCLs, but there was a great degree of overlap between the two lesions so this feature should not be used to establish a diagnosis. The authors found, in agreement with Abrams and Shear[22] and Franklin and coworkers,[23] that the number of giant cell nuclei was significantly greater in GCTs than in CGCLs, but overlap among lesions was again marked. The authors concluded that GCTs and CGCLs represent a continuum of a single disease process modified by the age of the patient, the site of occurrence, and possibly other factors.

5.2.3 Histochemical/immunohistochemical findings

Whittaker and Waldron[8] focused on the quantitative AgNOR differences of oral giant cell lesions. The study identified a significantly higher number of AgNORs in the nuclei of both the mononuclear cells and the multinuclear giant cells of recurrent/aggressive lesions as opposed to nonrecurrent/nonagressive lesions. The authors concluded that, with some limitations, AgNOR quantification may correlate with clinical behavior. The histogenesis of the multinucleated giant cells remain controversial, and evidence can be found to support macrophage, osteoclast, and fibroblast origins. Tiffee and Aufdemorte[24] used markers specific for macrophage lineage (1-ACT) and factor XII-la antibodies. For detection of osteoclast characteristics, the authors used an enzyme unique to this cell type—tartrate-resistant acid phosphatase. It was shown that the giant cells were neither macrophages nor osteoclasts, but appeared to represent a precursor cell of the granulocyte/macrophage line that has not been fully characterized and possesses features of both macrophages and osteoclasts.

O'Malley et al[2] found in their study of aggressive versus nonaggressive CGCLs that mononuclear cells, not giant cells, were in cell cycle. The CGCL represented a heterogeneous population of cells in which fibroblasts (some with myofibroblastic differentiation) were the dominant cell type (80% of the mononuclear cells) and probably comprised the proliferative compartment. Macrophages appeared to play a secondary role, similar to that proposed for their role in giant cell tumors of long bone.[25] The authors con-

cluded that it is not yet possible to predict the behavior of CGCLs from known histologic, immunophenotypic, or proliferation parameters.

Lim and Gibbins[26] found no significant difference in staining pattern between CGCLs and giant cell tumors of long bone when using a panel of monoclonal antibodies. According to the authors, the most significant finding was that the blood vessels at the periphery of the CGCLs stained intensely with endothelial cell marker factor VIII—related antigen, *Ulex europaeus 1 lectin*, and Qbend 10 in contrast to the striking lack of reactivity of the blood vessels deeper in the lesion, closer to the multinucleated cell aggregations. The authors interpreted these findings as a result of an absence of a mature functional microvasculature in the deep areas of the CGCLs.

Regezi,[27] in a discussion of the article by Tiffee and Aufdemorte, speculated that fibroblasts are the cells of primary importance in CGCLs, and through their cellular products, they recruit and/or induce mononuclear cells to become multinuclear giant cells. The reactive giant cells seem to be most closely related to osteoclasts. Regezi also believed that CGCLs represent benign neoplasms, or possibly abnormal reparative processes, and proposes that the lesional fibroblasts are dysfunctional and express or overexpress inappropriate cytokines and/or growth factors. Lastly, Regezi suggested that application of modern molecular methods should provide the next level of information on the biology of CGCLs.

5.2.3.1 Giant cell lesions and hyperparathyroidism

Virtually identical lesions to CGCLs have been reported in patients with hyperparathyroidism. The so-called brown tumor is a well-documented feature of this endocrinopathy. This lesion, when occurring in the oral region, can easily be mistaken for a typical CGCL. However, some features like the presence of multiple lesions, multiple recurrences, or loss of the lamina dura around teeth in the involved area would be unusual for a typical CGCL. Should these features be present, additional studies of serum chemistry should be undertaken, including measuring ionized calcium and parathyroid hormone levels measurement of the N-terminal peptide is the recommended method. It should, however, be pointed out that a brown tumor is not a common sequela of hyperparathyroidism. Rosenberg and Guralnick,[28] in a study of 220 patients with this condition, found that only 4.5% had clinically apparent giant cell lesions.

5.2.3.2 Giant cell lesions in vitro and as xenografts

El-Mofty and Osdoby[29] showed in their tissue culture study that the giant cells and macrophage-like cells in CGCLs had a limited life span in culture and survived for up to 2 and 5 weeks, respectively. The spindle-shaped mononuclear cells, however, continued to proliferate and were still actively growing 10 months after isolation. The observation that the giant cells were unable to perpetuate themselves suggested that these cells might represent a fully differentiated end cell. The ability of the spindle-shaped mononuclear cells to undergo active proliferation, as demonstrated by their mitotic activity in vivo and their continuous replication in vitro, is analogous to that of their counterparts in GCTs of long bones.[30] Based on their histochemical and electron microscopic observations, the authors suggested that the spindle-shaped cells were not typical fibroblasts and that they might be myofibroblasts, which is in agreement with ultrastructural findings by El-Laban and Lee.[19]

Further, the mononuclear round cells were interpreted as being macrophages or their derivatives. Finally, positive staining for histiocytic membrane antigens suggested that the giant cells may be derived from stromal macrophages.

Cohen et al[31] transplanted tissue subcutaneously from three CGCLs into nude mice, and the xenografts were harvested at 3, 5, 8, and 13 weeks. One of the most striking features of the harvested xenografts was the early disappearance of giant cells, a finding that agreed with the in vitro study by El-Mofty and Osdoby,[29] suggesting that these cells probably represent an end-stage process in cellular differentiation. Ultrastructural observations showed that these cells could be identified as myofibroblasts both in the original lesional tissue and in the xenografts. The most prominent stromal cells in the graft were those that resembled myofibroblast, and these cells were lying in close apposition to giant cells. The authors suggested that CGCLs of the jaws contain a high proportion of myofibroblast-like cells which fuse to form giant cells.

5.2.3.3 Aggressive and nonaggressive giant cell lesions

In 1986 and 1987, two groups of investigators[9,10] focused on the correlation between the histologic features and clinical behavior of jaw lesions in an attempt to determine whether there are histologic differences between lesions that demonstrate aggressive behavior and those that demonstrate a nonaggressive clinical course. Chuong et al,[9] in their study of 17 cases of giant cell lesions, defined nonaggressive lesions as those characterized by the absence of or minimal symptoms, slow growth, the absence of root resorption or cortical perforation, and a low recurrence rate. The authors noted that giant cells in aggressive lesions showed a higher relative size index than those in nonaggressive lesions and that giant cells in recurrent lesions had a higher size index and higher fractional surface area. It was noted, however, that these histologic differences were not as readily apparent as the differences in biologic behavior.

With the use of computer-aided image analysis, Ficarra et al[10] studied 32 cases of giant cell lesions with the same criteria for clinical behavior as those of Chuong et al.[9] Statistically significant differences in the number and fractional surface area of giant cells were found when comparing aggressive and nonaggressive lesions. The analysis was performed without knowledge of the clinical course and was successful in predicting the clinical course in 70% of the aggressive lesions and 82% of the nonaggressive ones. As mentioned earlier, Auclair et al[6] used similar cytometric methods and were unable to find any significant histologic differences between 5 cases of recurring giant cell lesions and 20 that did not recur.

In 30 CGCLs of the jaw (10 patients with aggressive and 20 patients with nonaggressive lesions), giant cell nuclear DNA was quantified by computer-aided image analysis.[32] DNA content was then used to predict clinical behavior and outcome. The authors concluded that cytometric measurement of giant cell nuclear DNA content is not useful as a predictor of clinical behavior (aggressiveness vs nonaggressiveness) of these lesions. The authors suggested that future investigations might focus on the role of stromal cells in determining the biologic behavior of CGCLs of the jaws.

Whitaker and Waldron[8] used discriminant analysis to study a total of 142 cases of central giant cell lesions of the jaws in an attempt to correlate histologic features with clinical behavior. When comparing aggressive versus nonaggressive lesions, the presence of more irregular-shaped giant cells, as well as a greater proportion of smaller giant cells,

were seen in nonaggressive lesions (60% and 77%, respectively) as compared with aggressive ones (40% and 67%, respectively). Six of the cases behaved in a markedly aggressive manner (presenting with pain or paresthesia, cortical perforation, and root resorption), and the histologic features were those commonly accepted for "true" giant cell tumors of long bones. The authors expressed the opinion that if the slides from these cases were examined by an experienced orthopedic pathologist with the "false" information that the tissue came from a lesion in the epiphysis of a long bone, a diagnosis of GCT would be made. The authors favored the concept that giant cell lesions of the jaws and giant cell tumors of the extragnathic skeleton are not separate entities but represent a continuum or a single disease process.

It seems, however, that a subset of jaw lesions clearly falls within the histologic profile accepted for giant cell tumors, and conversely, some long bone lesions show the histologic features widely accepted for giant cell lesions of the jaws. Giant cell tumors of long bones are considered to be locally aggressive, with recurrence rates of up to 60% after curettage.[33-35]

5.2.3.4 CGCL associated with central and peripheral odontogenic fibroma-like lesions
Recently, two reports[36,37] described a rare, intraosseous, hybrid lesion with the combined histologic features of a giant cell lesion and a central odontogenic fibroma. Histologically, zones of typical giant cell lesions lay in a fibrous stroma containing islands, strands, and clusters of odontogenic epithelium. Osteoid trabeculae were present in 5 of the 10 lesions reported by Odell et al.[37] Although these features cannot be attributed conclusively to a variant of either giant cell lesions of the jaws (or aneurysmal bone cysts) or central odontogenic fibromas, the clinical

features are slightly more suggestive of a giant cell lesion.

Ficarra et al[37] reported an unusual case in which a patient, who 10 years earlier had multiple occurrences of CGCLs of the left maxilla, developed multifocal peripheral odontogenic fibromas (WHO type; see chapter 19), one of which was associated with a giant cell lesion. The authors suggested that this finding was just coincidental or alternatively that the two lesions were somehow related.

5.2.3.5 Noonan-like/multiple giant cell lesion syndrome

Central giant cell lesions of the jaws are usually solitary lesions. The occurrence of synchronous, multiple lesions with the characteristic histology of the CGCL is uncommon. A syndrome has recently been defined in which patients exhibit phenotypical features of Noonan syndrome and multiple giant cell lesions.[39,40] Although this syndrome was first described more than 100 years ago, the first accurate study was not published until 1963.[41] Common oral features of the Noonan syndrome include micrognathia, a highly arched palate, dental malocclusion, delayed tooth eruption, bifid uvula, and (in rare cases) a cleft palate. In addition, patients exhibited multiple giant cell lesions of the jaws. In the case reported by Betts et al,[40] a 14-year-old boy had four separate multilocular lesions of the maxilla and mandible. One and a half years after surgery, the patient returned with a new mandibular lesion as well as an intraosseous, osteolytic process of the middle phalanx of the left index finger. All lesions were giant cell lesions.

Although there are phenotypical similarities between these patients and patients with Turner syndrome, Noonan syndrome does not appear to be the result of a chromosome abnormality as in Turner syndrome.

5.2.3.6 Giant cell lesions of the distal extremities

Giant cell lesions have been described in the small tubular bones of the hands and feet (see Panico et al[42]) with similar, if not identical, clinical behavior and histology to those of CGCLs of the jaws. Initially, this lesion was called a "giant cell reaction." Panico et al[42] described five cases in young and middle-aged adults (range, 16 to 41 years), three in the foot and two in the hand. The correct diagnosis of this lesion is important because a conservative treatment approach is sufficient, even in cases that recur. Compared with the GCT, the CGCL lacks foci of necrosis, has clustered rather than dispersed osteoclast-like giant cells, and exhibits foci in which there is osteoblastic rimming of trabecular osteoid. Immunohistochemically, the authors demonstrated expression of both vimentin and actin in the stromal spindle cells. Panico and coworkers[42] found histologically that the CGCL and the solid and classic aneurysmal bone cyst have many identical features, explaining why the two lesions may be related morphologically with only quantitative histologic differences. A possible relationship between aneurysmal bone cysts and CGCLs of the jaws is discussed in chapter 38.

5.2.4 Ultrastructural findings

Several authors have studied the ultrastructure of the cell populations in CGCLs of the jaws. Andersen et al[15] found two types of giant cells (I and II), of which type II—dominated by an electron-dense cytoplasm and a large number of vacuoles and dilated cisternae—was considered an aging or degenerating cell. Clusters of stromal, fibroblast-like cells were found in close contact with giant cells, the distance between cell membranes being approximately 10 to 20 nm. The presence of lamina densa–like material surrounding these cells suggested that they are pericytes and precursors to the giant cells.

El-Labban and Lee[19] studied CGCL stromal and giant cells and found that the great majority of stromal cell clusters were fibroblast-like cells or myofibroblasts rich in rough endoplasmic reticulum and containing filaments similar to those of smooth muscle cells. Many of these cells were closely apposed to giant cells and often showed evidence of fusion and continuity between their plasma membranes and those of the giant cells. In another study, El-Labban[18] found that approximately 75% of vessels found in CGCLs contained multiple fibrin thrombi or intravascular fibrin deposits. These vessels were lined with damaged endothelial cells with sometimes large gaps between them. The endothelial cells showed an absence of basal lamina, especially in areas where plasma, fibrin, red cells, or giant cells were in close proximity to the outside of their plasma membranes. The gaps between the cells led to extravasation of red cells and leakage of large amounts of plasma, which were altered to fibrin within the tissue.

5.2.4.1 Multifocal central giant cell lesions of the maxillofacial skeleton (craniofacial giant cell dysplasia)

Smith et al[43] presented the case of a 41-year-old woman with a large multilocular radiolucency of the right mandibular angle, ramus, and condylar neck. A biopsy showed central giant cell lesion. Nine years after her initial resection, the patient presented with a large lesion involving the left sinus, left nasal bone, and orbital floor. A second, much smaller lesion was present in the right maxillary sinus. A workup for hyperparathyroidism showed normal values. The lesions proved histologically to be CGCLs. Based on the appearance of new giant cell lesions 9 years after resection of the original lesion, the authors raised the question of possible metastasis via hematogenous seeding. Further, the authors suggested that a new variant of giant cell lesion may exist which demonstrates multifocality; they called this entity "craniofacial giant cell dysplasia."

The occurrence of multiple central giant cell lesions is rare, with only 17 cases having been reported in the literature, according to Miloro and Quinn.[44] In the differential diagnosis, it is essential to rule out other giant cell lesions that present with similar, if not identical, histologic features as the CGCL. These include the brown tumor of hyperparathyroidism, cherubism, and the aneurysmal bone cavity. To document true multifocality, the following factors must be considered. First, involvement of only one bone (eg, bilateral mandible) might suggest that the occurrence of multiple lesions may merely represent contiguous lesions (ie, cherubism) separated by an area of normal bone. Second, the presence of *synchronous* involvement would strongly support the concept of multifocality, whereas reports of *metachronous* occurrence could potentially represent recurrences due to seeding or incomplete surgical excision. Third, many surgeons and pathologists believe that multiple giant cell lesions do not exist in the absence of hyperparathyroidism or a familial history of cherubism. Miloro and Quinn[44] concluded that no previous single case report has proved to be a true synchronous occurrence of multifocal central giant cell lesion. Thus, the authors believed that their report might represent the first documented case in the literature. The 37-year-old woman presented with a large, multilocular, mixed radiolucency/radiopacity of the posterior left maxilla and a smaller multilocular mixed lesion in the anterior mandible.

There are few case reports discussing the association between giant cell lesions and other benign lesions of the jaws such as fibrous dysplasias, ossifying fibromas, Paget disease, and odontogenic fibromas. Ardekian et al[45] added to this list of conditions with their report of a 38-year-old woman with a bilateral, mandibular giant cell granuloma. Her medical history indicated neurofibromatosis and amputation of her right leg due to the disease. Blood tests gave no indication of hyperparathyroidism.

6. Notes on treatment and recurrence rate

The common therapy for CGCLs is curettage or resection, and loss of teeth or (in younger patients) tooth germs is often unavoidable. Several reports have documented the presence of calcitonin receptors in the multinucleated giant cells in lesions of various locations. These cells possess the capacity to resorb bone, adding further support to the speculation that they are related to osteoclasts. Since calcitonin antagonizes osteoclastic bone resorption or may act directly on other cells in the lesion, Harris[46] suggested that the CGCL may respond to systemically applied calcitonin. Two recent reports[47,48] show that calcitonin as a therapy for CGCLs of the jaws is a promising alternative to surgical curettage, particularly for large lesions and in children and young adults (see also chapter 32). The use of intralesional corticosteroid injections is yet another newly introduced management method for central giant cell lesions,[49] but it is too early to judge the benefit of this modality.

Several studies on CGCLs have reported recurrences with rates varying between 11% and 35%. According to Whitaker and Waldron,[8] 57 of their 142 cases of CGCLs were considered to be potentially aggressive lesions. Twelve (46%) of the 26 patients for whom follow-up information was obtained developed one or more recurrences. The age of the patient at the time of initial treatment seems to be a factor in the frequency of recurrence. In Whitaker and Waldron's study, the mean age for patients who demonstrated one or more recurrences was 20 years, whereas the mean age of the 26 patients who were followed and did not show recurrence was 28 years. Although the authors were not able to gather accurate data on lesion size as a factor in recurrence, they had the distinct impression that lesions larger than 3.0 cm at their greatest diameter were more likely to recur than smaller ones.

References

1. Jaffe HL. Giant cell reparative granuloma, traumatic bone cyst, and fibrous (fibro-osseous) dysplasia of the jawbones. Oral Surg Oral Med Oral Pathol 1953;6:159–175.

2. O'Malley M, Pogrel MA, Stewart JC, Silva RG, Regezi JA. Central giant cell granulomas of the jaws: Phenotype and proliferation-associated markers. J Oral Pathol Med 1997;26:159–163.

3. Mighell AJ, Robinson PA, Hume WJ. Peripheral giant cell granuloma: A clinical study of 77 cases from 62 patients, and literature review. Oral Dis 1995;1:12–19.

4. Carvalho YR, Loyola AM, Gomez RS, Araujo VC. Peripheral giant cell granuloma. An immunohistochemical and ultrastructural study. Oral Dis 1995;1:20–25.

5. Bodner L, Peist M, Gatot A, Fliss DM. Growth potential of peripheral giant cell granuloma. Oral Surg Oral Med Oral Pathol Oral Radiol Endod 1997;83:548–551.

6. Auclair PL, Cuenin P, Kratochvil FJ, Slater LJ, Ellis GL. A clinical and histomorphologic comparison of the central giant cell granuloma and the giant cell tumor. Oral Surg Oral Med Oral Pathol 1988;66:197–208.

7. Waldron CA, Shafer WG. The giant cell reparative granuloma of the jaws: An analysis of 38 cases. Am J Clin Pathol 1966;45:437–447.

8. Whitaker SB, Waldron CA. Central giant cell lesions of the jaws. A clinical, radiologic, and histopathologic study. Oral Surg Oral Med Oral Pathol 1993;75:199–208.

9. Chuong R, Kaban LB, Kozakewich H, Perez-Atayde A. Central giant cell lesions of the jaws: A clinicopathologic study. J Oral Maxillofac Surg 1986;44:708–713.

10. Ficarra G, Kaban LB, Hansen LS. Giant cell lesions of the jaws: A clinico-pathologic and cytometric study. Oral Surg Oral Med Oral Pathol 1987;64: 44–49.

11. Wood NK, Goaz PW. Differential diagnosis of oral lesions. 4th ed. St. Louis: Mosby-Year Book, 1991:393–395.

12. Kaffe I, Ardekian L, Taicher S, Littner MM, Buchner A. Radiologic features of central giant cell granuloma of the jaws. Oral Surg Oral Med Oral Pathol Oral Radiol Endod 1996;81:720–726.

13. Bodner L, Bar-Ziv J. Radiographic features of central giant cell granuloma of the jaws in children. Pediatr Radiol 1996;26:148–151.

14. Austin LT, Dahlin CD, Royer QR. Giant cell reparative granuloma and related conditions affecting the jawbones. Oral Surg Oral Med Oral Pathol 1959;12:1285–1295.

15. Andersen L, Fejerskov O, Philipsen HP. Oral giant cell granulomas. A clinical and histological study of 129 new cases. Acta Pathol Microbiol Scand 1973;81:606–616.

16. Cohen MA, Hertzanu Y. Radiologic features, including those seen with computed tomography, of central giant cell granuloma of the jaws. Oral Surg Oral Med Oral Pathol 1988;65:255–261.

17. Kramer IRH. Central giant cell reparative granuloma of the jaws and related lesions. In: Oral Pathology in the Child. New York: International Academy of Oral Pathology, 1963:48–58.

18. El-Labban NG. Intravascular fibrin thrombi and endothelial cell damage in central giant cell granuloma. J Oral Pathol Med 1997;26:1–5.

19. El-Labban NG, Lee KW. Myofibroblasts in central giant-cell granuloma of the jaws: An ultrastructural study. Histopathology 1983;7:907–918.

20. Kramer IRH, Pindborg JJ, Shear M. Histological Typing of Odontogenic Tumours. 2d ed. Berlin: Springer-Verlag, 1992.

21. Lucas RB. Pathology of Tumours of the Oral Tissues. 2d ed. London: Churchill Livingstone, 1972:244.

22. Abrams B, Shear M. A histological comparison of the giant cells in the central giant cell granuloma of the jaws and the giant cell tumor of long bone. J Oral Pathol 1974;3:217–223.

23. Franklin CD, Craig GT, Smith CJ. Quantitative analysis of histological parameters in giant cell lesions of the jaws and long bones. Histopathology 1979;3:511–522.

24. Tiffee JC, Aufdemorte TB. Markers for macrophage and osteoclast lineages in giant cell lesions of the oral cavity. J Oral Maxillofac Surg 1997; 55:1108–1112.

25. Abe Y, Yonemura K, Nishida K, Takagi K. Giant cell tumor of bone: analysis of proliferative cell nuclear antigen antibody and cell culture procedures. Nippon Seikeigaka Gakkai Zasshi 1994;68:407–414.

26. Lim L, Gibbins JR. Immunohistochemical and ultrastructural evidence of a modified microvasculature in the giant cell granuloma of the jaws. Oral Surg Oral Med Oral Pathol Oral Radiol Endod 1995;79:190–198.

27. Regezi JA. Markers for macrophage and osteoclast lineages in giant cell lesions of the oral cavity. J Oral Maxillofac Surg 1997;55:1112–1113.

28. Rosenberg EH, Guralnick WC. Hyperparathyroidism: A review of 220 proved cases with special emphasis on findings in the jaws. Oral Surg Oral Med Oral Pathol 1962;15(suppl 2):84.

29. El-Mofty SK, Osdoby P. Growth behavior and lineage of isolated and cultures cells derived from giant cell granuloma of the mandible. J Oral Pathol 1985;14:539–552.

30. Troise GD, DeLustig ES, Gallardo H. Mitosis in tissue cultures of giant cell tumors of bone. Oncology 1973;28:193.

31. Cohen MA, Grossman ES, Thompson SH. Features of central giant cell granuloma of the jaws xenografted in nude mice. Oral Surg Oral Med Oral Pathol 1988;66:209–217.

32. Eckardt A, Pogrel MA, Kaban LB, Chew K, Mayall BH. Central giant cell granulomas of the jaws. Nuclear DNA analysis using image cytometry. Int J Oral Maxillofac Surg 1989;18:3–6.

33. Schajowicz F. Giant cell tumor of bone (osteoclastoma). J Bone Surg 1961;43A:1–29.

34. McDonald DJ et al. Giant cell tumor of bone. J Bone Joint Surg 1968;68A:235–342.

35. Sanerkin NG. Malignancy, aggressiveness, and recurrence in giant cell tumors of bone. Cancer 1980;46:1641–1649.

36. Allen CM, Hammond HL, Stimson PG. Central odontogenic fibroma, WHO type. A report of three cases with an unusual associated giant cell reaction. Oral Surg Oral Med Oral Pathol 1992;73:62–66.

37. Odell EW, Lombardi T, Barrett AW, Morgan PR, Speight PM. Hybrid central giant cell granuloma and central odontogenic fibroma-like lesions of the jaws. Histopathology 1997;30:165–171.

38. Ficarra G, Sapp JP, Eversole LR. Multiple peripheral odontogenic fibroma, World Health Organization type, and central giant cell granuloma. A case report of an unusual association. J Oral Maxillofac Surg 1993;51:325–328.

39. Cohen MM Jr, Gorlin RJ. Noonan-like/multiple giant cell lesion syndrome. Am J Med Genet 1991;40:159–166.

40. Betts NJ, Stewart JC, Fonseca RJ, Scott RF. Multiple central giant cell lesions with a Noonan-like phenotype. Oral Surg Oral Med Oral Pathol 1993;76:601–607.

41. Noonan JA, Ehmke DA. Associated noncardiac malformation in children with congenital heart disease. J Pediatr 1963;63:468–470.

42. Panico L, Passeretti U, De Rosa N, D'Antonio A, De Rosa G. Giant cell reparative granuloma of the distal skeletal bones. A report of five cases with immunohistochemical findings. Virchows Arch 1994;425:315–329.

43. Smith PG, Marrogi AF, Delfino JJ. Multifocal central giant cell lesions of the maxillofacial skeleton: A case report. J Oral Maxillofac Surg 1990;48:300–305.

44. Miloro M, Quinn PD. Synchronous central giant cell lesions of the jaws: Report of a case and review of the literature. J Oral Maxillofac Surg 1995;53:1350–1355.

45. Ardekian L, Manor R, Peled M, Laufer D. Bilateral central giant cell granulomas in a patient with neurofibromatosis: Report of a case and review of the literature. J Oral Maxillofac Surg 1999;57:869–872.

46. Harris M. Central giant cell granulomas of the jaws regress with calcitonin therapy. Br J Oral Maxillofac Surg 1993;31:89–92.

47. Pogrel MA, Regezi JA, Harris ST, Goldring SR. Calcitonin treatment for central giant cell granulomas of the mandible: Report of two cases. J Oral Maxillofac Surg 1999;57:848–853.

48. de Lange J, Rosenberg AJ, van den Akker HP, Koole R, Wirds JJ, van den Berg H. Treatment of central giant cell granuloma of the jaw with calcitonin. Int J Oral Maxillofac Surg 1999;28:372–376.

49. Kermer C, Millesi W, Watzke IM. Local infection of corticosteroids for central giant cell granuloma: A case report. Int J Oral Maxillofac Surg 1994;23:366–368.

Section Eight

Pseudocysts of the Jaws

Introduction

This section describes four separate lesions or conditions: aneurysmal bone cavity, simple bone cavity, lingual mandibular bone depression, and focal marrow-containing jaw cavity. These lesions have several features in common. They are all largely asymptomatic, have a more or less demarcated radiolucent appearance, are diagnosed incidentally on radiographs, and have an as-yet-unclarified etiology/pathogenesis. As a result, the terminology used for each is cumbersome or chaotic.

The term *cyst* has at one time or another been attached to each of the first three lesions, although *none* of them possesses an epithelialized lining of the bone cavity. So the lesions are, in fact, probably best categorized under a common heading of *pseudocysts*. The focal marrow-containing jaw cavity is often categorized as a "defect," although it does not signal a faulty or imperfect structure but rather is a result of the normal healing process in bone.

The terms preferred and suggested by the present authors for each of the four lesions appear in the chapter titles followed by the nomenclature most often used today.

Only two of the four aforementioned lesions—the aneurysmal bone cyst (cavity) and the simple bone cyst (cavity)—are included in the forthcoming WHO volume *Tumours of the Head and Neck* in chapter 6 under the heading "Neoplasms and Other Lesions Occurring in the Maxillofacial Skeleton."

Chapter 38

Aneurysmal Bone Cavity (Aneurysmal Bone Cyst)

1. Terminology

The aneurysmal bone cavity (ABC), first recognized as a distinct pathologic entity by Jaffe and Lichtenstein in 1942,[1] is an intraosseous, osteolytic lesion which has been reported to affect mainly the metaphysial region of long bones and vertebrae. The distal femur and proximal tibia are the most common sites.

Only 2% of ABC lesions are found in the head and neck region, two thirds of these being located in the jaw, where they appear initially to have been recognized by Bernier and Bhaskar.[2] Despite its recognition, the lesion remains a relatively uncommon finding in the facial bones. ABCs of the jaws are rare; 64 cases (60 cases from the literature and 4 new cases) that fulfilled the clinical and radiologic criteria suggested by White[4] were reported by Kaffe et al.[4] Kalantar Motamedi[5] described the ABC as a giant cell lesion with a fibrous connective tissue stroma, various amounts of bone and osteoid, numerous cavernous channels or blood sinusoids, and no epithelial or endothelial lining. The author claimed to have traced a total of 78 reported cases of maxillofacial ABCs in the international literature up to January 1997.

Prior to 1942, ABCs were reported in the literature as *ossifying hematomas, hemorrhagic osteomyelitis, osteitis fibrosa cystica, expansile hemangioma,* and *aneurysmal giant cell tumors,* to mention but a few descriptions. Currently, a *primary form* of ABC (which may be vascular, solid, or mixed) for which no preexisting lesion is identified is distinguished from a *secondary form* that results from well-recognized predisposing bone lesions such as giant cell lesions, chondroblastomas, osteoblastomas, and fibrous dysplasias. Kershisnik and Batsakis[6] stated that approximately 30% of ABCs are secondary and that these are found most often in long bones and rarely in the jaws. Kramer et al,[7] in the 1992 World Health Organization (WHO) classification of odontogenic tumors, used the term *hybrid lesions* for the secondary form of ABC.

The term most commonly used, *aneurysmal bone cyst,* is unfortunate in that the lesion has nothing to do with vascular aneurysms. It is also not a true (epithelialized) bone cyst but rather a lesion characterized by blood-filled spaces of different sizes separated by connective tissue septa. The bony cavity contains trabeculae of bone or osteoid tissue and osteoclast-like giant cells.

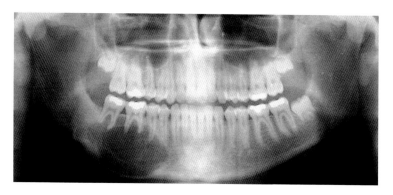

Fig 38-1 Panoramic radiograph of an ABC involving the right mandibular molar region and exhibiting septation. There is some ballooning expansion of the cortex.

2. Clinical and radiologic profile

The clinical signs and symptoms of the ABC are nonspecific and often do not allow a clinical diagnosis. According to patient histories, prior trauma is frequently involved, but its significance in the development of ABC is unclear. As suggested by Eveson and coworkers,[8] the traumatic episode may only serve to initiate an examination, which subsequently reveals the preexisting lesion. Progressive swelling over the area of bone involvement is a common finding in ABCs of the jaws, and it is often insidious at onset. The rate of enlargement, however, is often described as relatively rapid. The lesion generally expands the adjacent bony cortex and may perforate it. Pain or tenderness on palpation may or may not be a concomitant symptom. Fluctuation and crepitus also may be noted. Recent tooth mobility, migration of teeth, or development of a malocclusion have been found, but vitality of the teeth in the involved area is not violated. Aspiration of dark red or brownish hemorrhagic fluid favors a diagnosis of ABC. The aspirate is not arterial, unlike that usually encountered in central hemangioma of bone. Blood chemistry is normal.

The radiographic features of ABCs are not pathognomonic, and there is no consensus in the literature pertaining to these features.[4] The lesion may appear as a unilocular, soap-bubble, honeycomb, multilocular, or moth-eaten radiolucency that causes expansion, perforation, or even destruction of the bony cortices in aggressive cases. There may also be an associated periosteal reaction, with reactive new bone forming a peripheral sclerotic border in some cases (Fig 38-1). Kaffe and associates[4] did a comprehensive study of radiologic and clinical features of 64 cases of ABCs of the jaws and found that 87% of cases (*n* = 53) were radiolucent, 2% were radiopaque, and 11% were mixed. The prevalence of mixed lesions supports the explanation by Farman et al[9] that reactive bone formation within an ABC produces this appearance. Kaffe et al[4] found that 53% were multilocular (and usually large), 43% were unilocular, and 3% showed no loculation. Revel et al[10] found that magnetic resonance imagery (MRI) and computed tomography (CT) were helpful in the differential diagnosis of ABCs because of the additional information that can be obtained on the interface between the tumor and healthy tissue and on tumor contents and composition. Further, MRI is superior to CT scans because it shows the soft tissue and fluid-containing cavities more definitively. There were no fluid levels in CT scans of six maxillary ABCs, a finding that suggests these lesions may be less vascular in this site than elsewhere.[11] As Kaffe and coworkers[4] demonstrated, the expansile character of the lesion and its thin bony walls are better depicted by CT scans.

3. Epidemiological data

3.1 Prevalence, incidence, and relative frequency

In a retrospective study by Leithner et al[12] involving 94 Austrian patients with primary ABCs (specific locations of the lesions were not given), the authors provided population-based analysis of ABC incidence. They found the rate to be 0.14 cases per million individuals. Farole et al[13] indicated that the ABC accounts for roughly 5% of all lesions of the cranial and maxillofacial bones. Additional epidemiological data concerning incidence and prevalence for these lesions are not available.

3.2 Age

Data on age distribution of ABCs of the jaws from the report by Kaffe et al[4] are shown in Fig 38-2. There is a sharp peak in the 2nd decade, 70.3% of the patients being younger than 21 years and 81.3% younger than 31 years. The mean age was 17 years for both men and women, with a range of 4 to 78 years. Two studies specifically dealt with ABCs of the maxilla.[11,14] In his review, Bataineh[14] collected 28 cases from the literature to which he added a new case. Out of the 28 cases, 5 were secondary lesions. If data from the 24 primary cases are analyzed, they reveal that 75% of the patients were younger than 21 and 92% were younger than 31. The mean age was 17.9 years, with a range of 8 to 55 years.

3.3 Gender

A gender distribution based on the data from Kaffe et al[4] (see Fig 38-2) demonstrates that there is an almost equal ratio between men and women (1:0.9). The male:female ratio for maxillary cases alone was 1:1.2.[14] Some authors[6,15] reported a modest female pre-

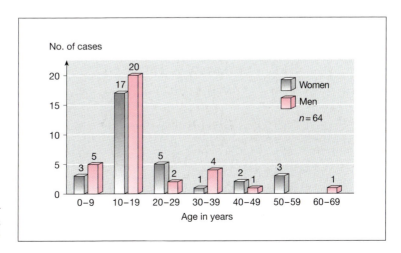

Fig 38-2 Age and gender distribution of ABCs according to Kaffe et al.[4]

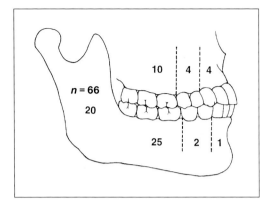

Fig 38-3 Topographic distribution of ABCs according to Kaffe et al.[4]

4. Pathogenesis

The pathogenesis of the ABC is controversial, and a number of theories have been advanced. Although trauma has been postulated, there is little evidence to support this. Some workers have subscribed to the idea that the lesion results from a hemodynamic disturbance or the development of an arteriovenous shunt. Based on angiographic, immunohistochemical, and electron microscopic studies, Szendroi et al[19] found no changes at the arterial site in 16 primary ABCs (long and flat bones) and no signs of an arteriovenous shunt. The authors proposed the hypothesis that the ABC corresponds to a hemodynamic disturbance. Elastic or muscular tissue in the walls of the vascular channels has not been demonstrated, thus casting doubt on the theory that the lesion arises from preexisting engorged vessels. The close connection between ABCs and giant cell lesions (GCLs) (see chapter 37) has been noted by several authors. Yarrington et al[20] believed that histologically the ABC differs from the GCL only in having blood-filled cavernous spaces. Hillerup and Hjørting-Hansen[21] regarded ABCs, GCLs, and simple bone cavities as different expressions of the same disease.

Other authors support the concept that ABCs may develop as a secondary phenomenon in a preexisting bone lesion (secondary ABC). This concept has recently gained considerable support, and there is good evidence to sustain it. A comprehensive discussion of these theories can be found in Shear's monograph *Cysts of the Oral Regions*.[22]

dominance, whereas others[16] reported a higher occurrence in men.

3.4 Location

The distribution of ABCs according to location within the jaw (*n* = 66) is shown in Fig 38-3.[4] The mandible was the location of 48 (72%) of the cases, giving a maxilla:mandible ratio of 1:2.7. With regard to specific locations, 47 (98%) of the mandibular cases were located in the premolar-molar-ramus area, with only 1 lesion located anterior to the premolar region. Of the 18 maxillary lesions, 14 (78%) were found in the premolar-molar regions and the remaining 4 (22%) in the anterior area. Most of the maxillary lesions located in the posterior area projected into the maxillary sinus.

Two cases of ABCs located in the zygomatic bone have been reported.[8,17] A rare case of a secondary ABC was published by Svensson and Isacsson,[18] who described a 14-year-old boy with an ABC associated with a benign osteoblastoma located in the mandibular condyle and ramus.

5. Pathology

5.1 Macroscopy

The operation specimen is brownish to dark blue and soft in consistency. Cross section reveals solid areas interspersed with multiple blood-filled locules. The solid parts may represent areas of repair or remnants of a pre-existing lesion.

5.2. Microscopy

5.2.1 Histologic definitions

The 1992 WHO classification[7] stated the ABC was "a benign intraosseous lesion, characterized by blood-filled spaces of varying size associated with a fibroblastic tissue containing multinucleated giant cells, osteoid, and woven bone."

The definition used by the present authors is as follows:
A benign intraosseous lesion characterized by large and small cavernous channels (Fig 38-4), the walls of which are not muscular or elastic. The stroma has spindle-shaped cells with unevenly distributed osteoclast-like giant cells, many of them arranged around the blood-filled spaces. The loosely textured fibrous tissue contains many dilated capillaries. In more solid areas, the tissue components resemble those seen in central giant cell lesions of the jaw: vascular tissue, large numbers of multinucleated giant cells, fibroblasts, hemorrhage, and hemosiderin deposits (Fig 38-5). Trabecular and lacelike osteoid is a common finding.

5.2.2 Histopathologic findings

The above definition used by the present authors covers a typical primary ABC. In contrast, some solid areas of the secondary form of ABC may have the appearance of fibrous dysplasia, giant cell tumor, cemento-ossifying fibroma, or other benign jaw tumors and conditions. A rarely reported finding in ABC is the occurrence of mitotic figures. De Dios et al[23] found that 82% of cranial and facial ABCs contained 1 to 3 mitotic figures per 10 high-power fields. Atypical mitosis was not seen. The authors stressed, however, that the presence of mitotic figures should not be

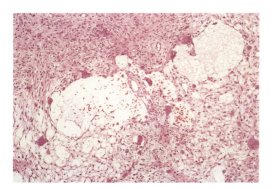

Fig 38-4 The same ABC shown in Fig 38-1 characterized by cavernous channels and loosely textured stroma with osteoclast-like giant cells {hematoxylin-eosin [H&E], x80).

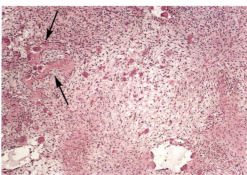

Fig 38-5 ABC with more solid areas of tissue resembling those seen in central giant cell lesions of the jaw. Osteoid trabeculae are indicated by *arrows* (H&E, x80).

considered a worrisome feature in the absence of atypical stromal cells.

5.2.3 Karyotypic changes

Sciot et al[24] studied the cytogenetic-morphologic correlations in ABCs, giant cell tumors of bone, and combined lesions. Three primary ABCs, all extragnathic (two from the tibia, one from the fibula) showed that chromosome segments 16q2 and/or 17p1 are nonrandomly involved. The authors further stated that the consistent chromosome pattern suggests that at least some of these lesions are neoplastic.

6. Notes on treatment and recurrence rate

Treatment of the ABC is generally directed toward complete removal of the lesion. This may prove difficult at times, particularly if the lesion is multilocular and divided by multiple bony septae. A multitude of treatment modalities have been reported (they have included simple curettage, cryotherapy, resection, bone grafting, and no treatment). Block excision or resection is usually reserved for recurrent cases or for secondary forms of ABC, where the associated lesion necessitates such treatment. Evidence from aspiration, CT scans, carotid arteriography, and operative findings confirms that *maxillary ABCs* are relatively avascular, belonging to the "low-pressure" group of lesions. Consequently, they are best treated by conservative surgery, usually using an intraoral approach.[14] Provided that preoperative aspiration and incisional biopsy have been undertaken as precautionary measures, there is no indication for preoperative ligation of major vessels, and

an extraoral approach or blood transfusion is seldom required.

Prognosis is excellent for ABCs. Recurrence of jaw lesions, although uncommon, has been reported, apparently related to inadequate surgical access to the lesion and thus incomplete removal. Recurrence seems to be most frequent within 1 year of initial treatment. Consequently, it is important to follow treated cases and to take periodic radiographs until complete osseous repair and remodeling of the affected area have taken place. Biesecker et al[25] found a 59% recurrence rate following curettage, but only 2 of their 66 cases were in the jaws. Gingell et al[26] reported a 19% recurrence rate of ABCs in the jaws, including three cases with multiple recurrences.

References

1. Jaffe HL, Lichtenstein L. Solitary unicameral bone cyst with emphasis on the roentgen picture, the pathologic appearance and pathogenesis. Arch Surg 1942;44:1004–1025.

2. Bernier JL, Bhaskar SN. Aneurysmal bone cyst of the mandible. Oral Surg Oral Med Oral Pathol 1958;11:1018–1028.

3. White SC. Computer aided differential diagnosis of oral radiographic lesions. Dentomaxillofac Radiol 1989;18:53–59.

4. Kaffe I, Naor H, Calderon S, Buchner A. Radiological and clinical features of aneurysmal bone cyst of the jaws. Dentomaxillofac Radiol 1999;28:167–172.

5. Kalantar Motamedi MH. Aneurysmal bone cysts of the jaws: Clinicopathological features, radiographic evaluation and treatment analysis of 17 cases. J Craniomaxillofac Surg 1998;26:56–62.

6. Kershisnik M, Batsakis JG. Aneurysmal bone cysts of the jaws. Ann Otol Rhinol Laryngol 1994;103:164–165.

7. Kramer IRH, Pindborg JJ, Shear M. Histological Typing of Odontogenic Tumours. 2d ed. Berlin: Springer-Verlag, 1992.

8. Eveson JW, Moos KR, Macdonald DG. Aneurysmal bone cyst of the zygomatic arch. Br J Oral Surg 1978;15:259–264.

9. Farman AG, Nortje CJ, Wood RE. In: Oral and Maxillofacial Diagnostic Imaging. St. Louis: CV Mosby, 1993:228–238.

10. Revel MP, Vanel D, Sigal R, et al. Aneurysmal bone cysts of the jaws: CT and MR findings. J Comput Assist Tomogr 1992;16:84–86.

11. Matt BH. Aneurysmal bone cyst of the maxilla: Case report and review of the literature. Int J Pediatr Otorhinolaryngol 1993;25:217–226.

12. Leithner A, Windhager R, Lang S, et al. Aneurysmal bone cyst. A population based epidemiologic study and literature review. Clin Orthop 1999; 363:176–179.

13. Farole A, Manalo A, Iranpour B. Lesion of the temporomandibular joint. J Oral Maxillofac Surg 1992;50:510–514.

14. Bataineh AB. Aneurysmal bone cysts of the maxilla: A clinicopathologic review. J Oral Maxillofac Surg 1997;55:1212–1216.

15. Waldron CA. Bone pathology. In: Neville, Damm, Allen, Bouquot, eds. Oral and Maxillofacial Pathology. Philadelphia: WB Saunders, 1995;459–461.

16. Pindborg JJ, Hjørting-Hansen E. Atlas of Diseases of the Jaws. Munksgaard, 1974:144–145.

17. Carmichael F, Malcolm AJ, Ord RA. Aneurysmal bone cyst of the zygomatic bone. Oral Surg Oral Med Oral Pathol 1989;68:558–562.

18. Svensson B, Isacsson G. Benign osteoblastoma associated with an aneurysmal bone cyst of the mandibular ramus and condyle. Oral Surg Oral Med Oral Pathol 1993;76:433–436.

19. Szendroi M, Arato G, Ezzati A, et al. Aneurysmal bone cyst: Its pathogenesis based on angiographic, immunohistochemical and electron microscopic studies. Pathol Oncol Res 1998;4: 277–281.

20. Yarrington CT, Abbot J, Raines D. Aneurysmal bone cyst of the maxilla. Association with giant cell reparative granuloma. Arch Otolaryngol 1964;80:313–317.

21. Hillerup S, Hjørting-Hansen E. Aneurysmal bone cyst—simple bone cyst, two aspects of the same pathological entity. Int J Oral Surg 1978;7:16–22.

22. Shear M. Cysts of the Oral Regions. 3d ed. Oxford and Boston: Wright, 1992;179–186.

23. De Dios AMV, Bond JR, Shives TC, et al. Aneurysmal bone cyst. A clinicopathologic study of 238 cases. Cancer 1992;69:2921–2931.

24. Sciot R, Dorfman H, Brys P, et al. Cytogenetic-morphologic correlations in aneurysmal bone cyst, giant cell tumor of bone and combined lesions. A report from the CHAMP study group. Mod Pathol 2000;13:1206–1210.

25. Biesecker JL, Marcowe RC, Huvos AG, Mike V. Aneurysmal bone cysts: A clinicopathologic study of 66 cases. Cancer 1970;26:615–625.

26. Gingell JC, Levy BA, Beckerman T, Tilghaman DM. Aneurysmal bone cyst. J Oral Maxillofac Surg 1984;42:527–534.

Chapter 39

Simple Bone Cavity (Simple Bone Cyst)

1. Terminology

The simple bone cavity (SBC) of the jaw is a unilocular cavity or pseudocyst that occasionally occurs as a bilateral or even multifocal lesion. It closely resembles the *unicameral bone cavity* which is an analog lesion of long bones. Most (75%) cases arise during childhood and adolescence in the metaphyseal region, and the most common sites are the proximal ends of the humerus and femur.[1-3] The unicameral bone cyst, however, is often more aggressive and can frequently undermine the long bone, resulting in pathologic fractures. The SBC is not a common lesion; its behavior and etiology are still far from being established conclusively.

Rushton[4] adopted the following criteria when collecting cases of SBCs: (*1*) the "cyst" should be single, have no epithelial lining, and show no evidence of acute or prolonged infection; (*2*) it should principally contain fluid and not soft tissue; (*3*) its walls should be hard bone which may be thin in parts; and (*4*) the pathologic and chemical findings do not exclude a diagnosis of SBC. In 1875, the German pathologist Rudolf Virchow[5] first drew attention to the lesion ("solitäre Knochenzyste") that is known as SBC today. However, Lucas is often cited as being the first (in more recent years) to have described this lesion. Over the years, the SBC has been known under a variety of names, such as *solitary, traumatic, hemorrhagic, extravasation,* *unicameral, trabecular, idiopathic, progressive,* and *simple bone cyst,* of which traumatic bone cyst and SBC are in common use. The problem with using traumatic bone cyst is that it suggests both that trauma is the cause and that the lesion is in fact a cyst. However, trauma has never satisfactorily been proven to be an important etiologic factor. The other concern is that this lesion is not a true cyst because it lacks an epithelial lining.

The lesion most frequently presents as an empty bone cavity, containing no more than minute quantities of serous or serosanguineous fluid with electrolyte and protein concentrations similar to those of serum. The international histologic classification of odontogenic tumors by the World Health Organization (WHO)[7] uses the term *solitary bone cyst.* However, *simple bone cavity* may be preferable because some lesions show multiple occurrence.[8,9]

2. Clinical and radiologic profile

The SBC is typically a symptom-free, intrabony, cystlike lesion but may occasionally present with pain, swelling,[2,3] paraesthesia,[10] and pathologic fracture.[11] The SBC may occasionally expand the buccal and lin-

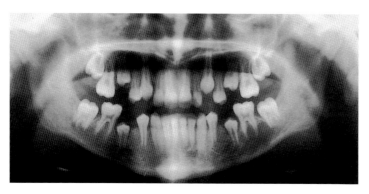

Fig 39-1 Panoramic radiograph showing a simple bone cavity in the left mandible (premolar-molar region) of an 11-year-old girl. Interradicular scalloping is not prominent in this case, and resorption of tooth apices is not present.

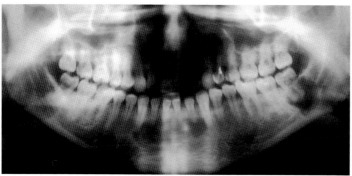

Fig 39-2 Panoramic radiograph of the mandible of a 40-year-old woman exhibiting multiple radiolucent areas (right and left third molars, both canines, and all incisors) representing SBCs.

gual cortical plates,[12] but significant expansion of the jaw is unusual.

The SBC appears radiologically as a well-defined unilocular, roughly oval radiolucency within the alveolar process, and it is frequently a chance radiographic finding (Fig 39-1). It is located above and often in front of the mandibular canal, in contrast to the *lingual mandibular bone depression* (see chapter 40), which is typically situated below and often behind the canal. Bilateral or multiple lesions may occur (Fig 39-2). Based on tracings of the peripheral border of 44 cases of SBCs, Copete et al[3] identified four shapes for this lesion: cone (64%), oval (16%), irregular (16%), and round (4%). The authors found that 22 (50%) had a sclerotic margin; the border scalloped around the roots of adjacent teeth in 68% of cases, a feature that may lead to the lesion being diagnosed on a bitewing radiograph. The characteristic scalloping, a feature first noticed by Waldron,[4] gives the appearance of the root apices "hanging" within the SBC cavity. Root resorption is not a common finding, and the lamina dura is identifiable in most cases. In the past, the scalloped periphery in combination with the occasional occurrence of bony septa has been interpreted as a multilocular, radiolucent lesion, which can lead to an erroneous diagnosis. In the radiographic review of 44 cases of SBCs by Copete et al,[3] the authors searched for the "fallen fragment, or trabecula, sign." This sign, which is seen in unicameral bone cysts of long bones in association with pathologic fractures, represents a fractured cortical fragment that has separated and is suspended in the bone cavity by fluid. The fallen trabecula sign could not be identified in any of the 44 radiographs of

SBCs (of the jaws). Trauma-related radiologic signs were identified in 11 cases (25%), with hairline, nondisplaced fractures being noted in 5 cases.

3. Epidemiological data

3.1 Prevalence, incidence, and relative frequency

The solitary bone cyst is not a common lesion if measured by the number of reported cases in the literature. The estimated number of cases published as of the year 2000 was around 250. No data on prevalence, incidence, or frequency exist. It makes no sense to indicate percentages based on the total number of jaw cysts (as is occasionally done in the literature), since the SBC is a pseudocyst or intrabony, nonepithelialized cavity with no relationship to conventional, odontogenic, or nonodontogenic epithelial jaw cysts.

3.2 Age

Except for classic cases of SBCs diagnosed during the 2nd decade of life, the age of patients ranges from 2[15] to 75 years.[16] Figure 39-3 shows the age distribution in three reported series of SBCs (Hansen et al,[16] Matsumura et al,[17] and Howe[2,3]). All three reports concur in the finding of a major peak in the 2nd decade of life (58.7%,[16] 64.7%,[17] and 75.4%[2,3] of cases). In their 67 reported cases, Kaugars and Cale[8] found a mean age of 24.3 years (range, 9 to 68 years); an even lower mean age, 18.0 years (range, 2.5 to 51 years), was found among 94 cases retrieved from the literature. MacDonald-Jankowski,[9] in his study of 20 SBCs in 14 Hong Kong Chinese patients, found that the mean age for men was 19.8 ± 1.5 years and for women, 40.6 ± 11.7 years. This difference in age between the sexes, which may be difficult to explain, is statistically significant.

3.3 Gender

There is a considerable difference in male:female ratios between series of reported cases. In the review by Kaugars and Cale,[8] there

Fig 39-3 Age and gender distribution of SBCs combined from three studies.[2,3,16,17] The distribution is almost identical in all three studies, with a prominent peak in the 2nd decade of life.

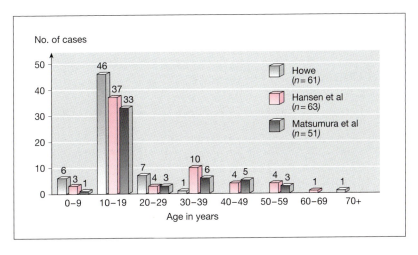

was an equal gender distribution in both their literature survey and their own sample. However, if patients 30 years of age or older (25.4%) were singled out, the male:female ratio was 1:2.4. The male:female ratios in the three studies shown in Fig 39-3 were 1:1 (Hansen et al[16]), 1:1.2 (Matsumura et al[17]), and 1:0.6 (Howe[2,3]).

3.4 Location

The vast majority of SBCs occur in the mandible. In a radiographic survey of 44 cases (Copete et al[13]), 98% occurred in the mandible, predominantly in premolar-molar areas; 13% of the lesions crossed the midline. In the report by Hansen et al,[16] two thirds of cases were located in the mandible. Rare cases have been found in the mandibular condyle[18-20] and zygomatic arch.[21] Bilateral and multiple lesions have been described in 4% to 10% of cases (see review by Shimoyama et al[22]). In MacDonald-Jankowski's series,[9] 14 mandibular lesions were found in 9 women, with no less than 5 SBCs diagnosed in 1 patient. This author also measured the size of the area of the lesions digitally on panoramic radiographs and found that the mean area differs significantly between the sexes (5.2 cm^2 ± 1.4 for men versus 2.5 cm^2 ± 1.1 for women).

4. Pathogenesis

The pathogenesis of the SBC is still unclear. Shear[23] comprehensively surveyed the different theories that have been advanced over the years. In short, the lesion is believed to be of endosteal origin, primarily involving the medullary bone with reactive secondary involvement of the cortical bone. The main theories of orgin are traumatically induced intramedullary hemorrhage with failure of early organization of the hematoma, low-grade infection, cystic degeneration of bone tumors, local alteration of bone metabolism resulting in osteolysis, ischemic marrow necrosis, and failure of differentiation of osteogenic cells. Although trauma has often been suggested as an initiating cause, a history of trauma is either infrequently or not convincingly present.

If one accepts the hypothesis that men experience traumatic injury more frequently than women and combines this with a lack of gender predilection,[8] then the concept of trauma being the sole causative factor is discredited. It is likely that the reason the SBC is so often an incidental finding is the fact that it was detected on a *posttrauma* radiograph. It seems likely that the SBC does not have a single common cause but may be multifactorial in origin.

Melrose et al[24] reported 34 cases of florid cemento-osseous dysplasias with concurrent occurrence of an SBC in 17 cases. Fisher[25] reported cysts in fibro-osseous lesions as "bone cavity in fibro-osseous lesions" and that these cysts could be the result of cystic breakdown of the lesions. Hillerup and Hjørting-Hansen[26] reported a case of aneurysmal bone cyst recurring after surgery on an SBC. They suggested that aneurysmal bone cysts, central giant cell granulomas, and SBCs all arise from some vascular lesion or defect.

5. Pathology

5.1 Macroscopy

When the bone cavity is opened at surgery, it is frequently found to be empty; blood, serous, or serosanguineous fluid may be present. A lining usually is not seen. A thin membrane, granulation tissue, or blood clot has also been described.

5.2 Microscopy

5.2.1 Histologic definitions

According to the 1992 WHO classification,[7] a solitary bone cyst is "an intraosseous cyst having a tenuous lining of connective tissue with no epithelium."

The definition of an SBC used by the present authors is as follows:
An intrabony cacity, the walls of which are lined with a delicate membrane consisting of loose fibrous tissue of variable thickness and/or granulation tissue with hemosiderino-phages and scattered multinucleated osteo-clast-like cells (Fig 39-4). An epithelial lining is not present. If adjacent bone is included in the surgical specimen, the inner surface often shows osteoclastic resorption. The bone may exhibit fibrous or cemento-os-seous dysplasia-like features.

5.2.2 Histopathologic findings

Donker and Punnia-Moorthy[27] suggested a possible subclassification of simple bone cavities based on content: empty cavities would be called idiopathic; those with solid content would be designated according to the histologic appearance of the bulk of the solid (eg, fibrous or granulation tissue); and cavities containing fluid with a biochemical profile similar to that of serum would be called extravasation cysts.

Another approach to the classification of SBCs was proposed by Matsumura et al,[17] who classified 53 cases of SBCs into types A and B based on histology. In type A, the cavity membrane consisted of a thin con-nective tissue lining and in type B, there was a thickened myxofibromatous wall and dys-plastic bone formation usually seen in benign fibro-osseous lesions. The authors found that bone expansion and radiopacity were closely related to histopathologic findings. They concluded that type A and type B bone cysts may have different causes.

5.2.3 Histochemical findings

No histochemical studies are available.

5.2.4 Ultrastructural findings

Using scanning electron microscopy, Schwenzer et al[27] confirmed that epithelium was absent in the cavity lining of SBCs. The lining was composed of a network of colla-gen fibers with embedded erythrocytes.

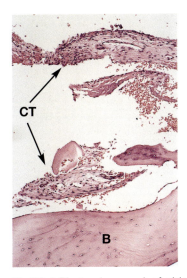

Fig 39-4 Photomicrograph of a biopsy specimen from the edge of the cavity in an SBC. B=bone wall; CT=fragments of the connective tissue wall with a few inflammatory cells (hematoxylin-eosin [H&E], x100).

6. Notes on treatment and recurrence rate

The low prevalence of SBCs in old age and the high prevalence in younger patients suggests that self-healing can occur. Sapp and Stark[29] followed two untreated cases of SBCs, one for 7.5 and the other for almost 3 years. By the time both patients approached age 22, their lesions had resolved, and the trabecular bone pattern had approached a normal radiographic appearance. The treatment used most often for SBCs is curettage. This is usually all that is necessary to institute healing, which takes place within a year.

Some surgeons advocate provoking bleeding by scraping the cavity wall carefully, which should enhance the healing process. However, this procedure may damage the inferior alveolar nerve or the tiny neurovascular bundles to adjacent teeth.

There is too little experience with injection of autogenous blood,[30] insertion of Gelfoam saturated with thrombin and penicillin,[31] bone allografts,[32] or application of methylprednisolone acetate to the cavity to advocate these treatment modalities, although the latter method has been reported to be successful in treating unicameral bone cavities of long bones.[33]

Currently there are no reliable predictors of the behavior of this lesion, although from the few cases of recurrence reported so far, the vast majority of recurrences appear in women.[34-35] An association between multiple SBCs and a tendency toward recurrence finds agreement in some reports[9,30,36] but not in others.[10,37-39] Kaugars and Cale[8] retrieved literature cases of 10 (1 male and 9 female) patients with multiple lesions. A bluish discoloration of the bone or mucosa was seen in 4 patients. A blue appearance of the bone has also been noticed in some cases of unicameral bone cavities and is apparently caused by erosion of the cortical bone, which permits the intrabony fluid to become clinically visible. Shimoyama et al,[22] based on a comprehensive review of 111 published reports, suggested that SBCs have at least two different patterns of clinical behavior: (1) solitary, asymptomatic, self-limiting lesions with a tendency for spontaneous healing, and (2) solitary or multiple progressive lesions with a potential for recurrence. It is important that SBCs be subjected to clinical follow-up, including radiologic examination.

References

1. Jaffe H, Lichtenstein L. Solitary unicameral bone cyst: With emphasis on the roentgen picture, the pathologic appearance and the pathogenesis. Arch Surg 1942;44:1004-1025.

2. Howe GL. "Haemorrhagic cysts" of the mandible. I. Br J Oral Surg 1965;3:55-60.

3. Howe GL. "Haemorrhagic cysts" of the mandible. II. Br J Oral Surg 1965;3:77-91.

4. Rushton MA. Solitary bone cysts in the mandible. Br Dent J 1946;81:37-49.

5. Virchow R. Über die Bildung von Knochenzysten. Sitzung der Akademie der Wissenschaften. Berlin: Abt. F. Math. U. Naturwissenschaften, 1875:760-769.

6. Lucas CD. Do all cysts in the jaws originate from the dental system? J Am Dent Assoc 1929;16:647-661.

7. Kramer IRH, Pindborg JJ, Shear M. Histological Typing of Odontogenic Tumours. 2nd ed. Berlin: Springer-Verlag, 1992.

8. Kaugars GE, Cale AE. Traumatic bone cyst. Oral Surg Oral Med Oral Pathol 1987;63:318-324.

9. MacDonald-Jankowski DS. Traumatic bone cysts in the jaws of a Hong Kong Chinese population. Clin Radiol 1995;50:787-791.

10. De Tomasi D, Hann JR. Traumatic bone cyst: Report of a case. J Am Dent Assoc 1985;111:56-57.

11. Cowan CG. Traumatic bone cysts of the jaws and their presentation. Int J Oral Surg 1980;9:287-291.

12. Harris SJ, Carroll KO, Gordy FM. Idiopathic bone cavity (traumatic bone cyst) with the radiographic appearance of a fibro-osseous lesion. Oral Surg Oral Med Oral Pathol 1992;74:118-123.

13. Copete MA, Kawamata A, Langlais RP. Solitary bone cyst of the jaws. Radiographic review of 44 cases. Oral Surg Oral Med Oral Pathol Oral Radiol Endod 1998;85:221-225.

14. Waldron CA. Solitary (hemorrhagic) cyst of the mandible. Oral Surg Oral Med Oral Pathol 1954; 7:88-95.

15. Robinson RA. Traumatic hemorrhagic cyst of the mandible in an infant. J Am Dent Assoc 1945; 32:774-775.

16. Hansen LS, Sapone J, Sproat RC. Traumatic bone cysts of the jaws. Report of sixty-six cases. Oral Surg Oral Med Oral Pathol 1974;37:899-910.

17. Matsumura S, Murakami S, Kakimoto N, et al. Histopathologic and radiographic findings of the simple bone cyst. Oral Surg Oral Med Oral Pathol Oral Radiol Endod 1998;85:619-625.

18. Gilman RH, Dingman RO. A solitary bone cyst of the mandibular condyle. Plast Reconstr Surg 1982;70:610-614.

19. Persson G. An atypical solitary bone cyst. J Oral Maxillofac Surg 1985;43:905-907.

20. Telfer MR, Jones GM, Pell GM, Eveson JW. Primary bone cyst of the mandibular condyle. Br J Oral Maxillofac Surg 1990;28:340-343.

21. Bradley JC. Solitary bone cyst of the zygomatic bone. Br Dent J 1982;152:203-204.

22. Shimoyama T, Horie N, Nasu D, et al. So-called simple bone cyst of the jaw: A family of pseudocysts of diverse nature and etiology. J Oral Sci 1999;41:93-98.

23. Shear M. Cysts of the Oral Regions. 3d ed. Oxford: Wright, 1992:171-176.

24. Melrose RJ, Abrams AM, Mills BG. Florid osseous dysplasia. A clinical-pathologic study of thirty-four cases. Oral Surg Oral Med Oral Pathol 1976;41: 62-82.

25. Fisher AD. Bone cavities in fibro-osseous lesions. Br J Oral Surg 1976;14:120-127.

26. Hillerup S, Hjørting-Hansen E. Aneurysmal bone cyst-simple bone cyst, two aspects of the same pathologic entity? Int J Oral Surg 1978;7:16-22.

27. Donkor P, Punnia-Moorthy A. Biochemical analysis of simple bone cyst fluid—report of a case. Int J Oral Maxillofac Surg 1994;23:296-297.

28. Schwenzer N, Ehrenfeld M, Roos R. Über die sogenannte solitäre Knochenzyste. Dtsch Zahnärztl Z 1985;40:573-575.

29. Sapp JP, Stark ML. Self-healing traumatic bone cysts. Oral Surg Oral Med Oral Pathol 1990;69: 597-602.

30. Precious DS, McFadden LR. Treatment of traumatic bone cyst of mandible by injection of autogeneic blood. Oral Surg Oral Med Oral Pathol 1984;58:137-140.

31. Thoma KH. The treatment of extravasation cysts with the use of Gelfoam. Oral Surg Oral Med Oral Pathol 1955;8:950-954.

32. Lindsay JS, Martin WR, Green HG. Traumatic bone cyst treated with homogeneous bone graft. Report of a case. Oral Surg Oral Med Oral Pathol 1966;21:536-542.

33. Capanna R, Dal Monte A, Gitelis S, Campanacci M. The natural history of unicameral bone cyst after steroid injection. Clin Orthop 1982;166:204-211.

34. Horner K, Forman GH. Atypical simple bone cyst of the jaws. II. A possible association with benign fibro-osseous (cemental) lesions of the jaws. Clin Radiol 1988;39:59-63.

35. Feinberg SE, Finkelstein MW, Langley Page H, Dembo JB. Recurrent "traumatic" bone cysts of the mandible. Oral Surg Oral Med Oral Pathol 1984;57:418-422.

36. Gardner AF, Stoller SM, Steig JM. A study of the traumatic bone cyst of the jaws. Can Dent Assoc J 1962;28:151-166.

37. Morris CR, Steed DL, Jacoby JJ. Traumatic bone cysts. J Oral Surg 1970;28:188-195.

38. Kuroi M. Simple bone cyst of the jaw: Review of the literature and report of case. J Oral Surg 1980;38:456-459.

39. Raibly SO, Beckett P, Nowakowski A. Multiple traumatic bone cysts of the mandible. J Oral Surg 1979;37:335-337.

Chapter 40

Lingual Mandibular Bone Depression (Stafne's Cavity)

1. Terminology

The lingual mandibular bone depression (LMBD) is yet another bone "defect" or "cyst" that may be classified as a pseudocyst of the jaw. The use of the term *cyst* over the past several years stems from the fact that the bone depression produces a cystic appearance on radiographs. It is occasionally confused with the solitary or simple bone cavity (see chapter 39). A description of 35 cases seen in 34 patients (in one patient, the condition had a bilateral occurrence) was reported by Stafne in 1942[1] under "bone cavities situated near the angle of the mandible." Since then the author's name has been inextricably bound to this bone "defect" through the term *Stafne's cavity* or *cyst*. If knowledge about the etiology/pathogenesis of a particular lesion is restricted or nonexistent, the list of diagnostic terms used often becomes extensive, as in the present case.

The LMBD has been identified as *mandibular embryonic defect, aberrant salivary gland tissue in the mandible, latent hemorrhagic cyst of the mandible, static bone cavity or defect, latent bone cavity, idiopathic bone cavity, ectopic submaxillary gland in the mandible, lingual mandibular salivary gland depression, lingual cortical mandibular defect, lingual mandibular bone concavity, idiopathic lingual mandibular bone "depression,"* and *lingual cavitation defect.*

The present authors suggest that *lingual mandibular bone depression* most appropriately covers the "lesions" in question. Until 1957, the LMBD had been described only as a bone cavity localized in the *posterior* lingual mandible in the area of the angle and characteristically situated below the inferior alveolar canal. In 1957, Richard and Ziskind[2] reported on an *anterior* counterpart (ALMBD) of the posterior LMBD (PLMBD) that was located in the mandibular incisor-canine-premolar region. A recent survey based on 310 cases of LMBDs[3] disclosed 40 ALMBDs and 270 PLMBDs. Data from this report provide the basis for this chapter. A rarely reported or referenced mandibular bone depression localized in the ascending ramus[3-6] and obviously analogous to the LMBD when found elsewhere in the mandible is also presented.

2. Clinical and radiologic profile

Almost all reports on LMBDs agree that these "lesions"—whether anterior, posterior, or ramus-related—are typically asymptomatic with no clinically detectable abnormalities. The bone depressions are almost never disclosed on palpation. The lesions are usually detected incidentally on routine radiographic examination.

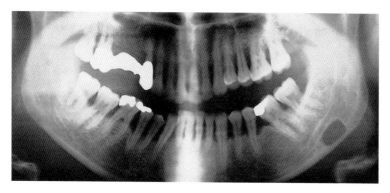

Fig 40-1 Posterior LMBD in a 54-year-old man. The longest diameter of the ovoid depression is parallel to the inferior mandibular border.

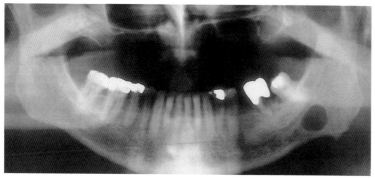

Fig 40-2 Circular PLMBD with a well-defined peripheral border in a 68-year-old man.

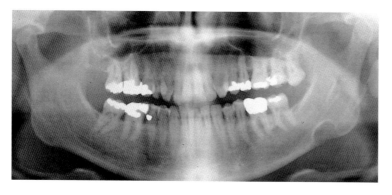

Fig 40-3 PLMBD situated close to the inferior border of the mandible in a 49-year-old man.

On plain radiographs (orthopantomograms), the PLMBD appears as a circular or ovoid (longest diameter parallel to the inferior border of the mandible (Fig 40-1), well-defined radiolucency (Fig 40-2). It classically arises just above or at the inferior border of the mandible (Fig 40-3) from an area of the first molar to the mandibular angle. It is always inferior to the mandibular canal. The border of the depression is often surrounded by an opaque line. On rare occasions the depression may occur bilaterally and, even more rarely, as two adjacent, unilateral depressions.

In recent years, computed tomography (CT) and magnetic resonance imagery (MRI)[7-9] have shown to be valuable and useful as adjuncts to panoramic radiographs.

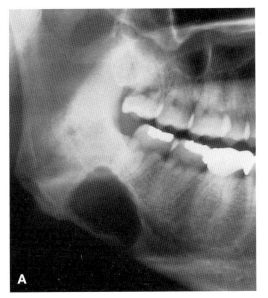

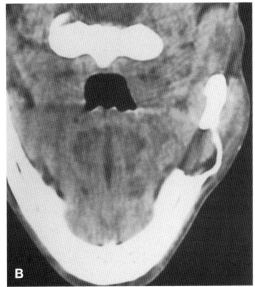

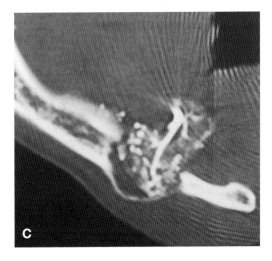

Fig 40-4 A 36-year-old Japanese man with a large PLMBD in the right mandible. A: Panoramic radiograph. B: Axial CT showing extreme lateral extension of the buccal cortical plate. C: Entrapped submandibular gland confirmed by CT sialography. (Courtesy of Dr E. Ariji, Fukuoka, Japan.)

With its enhanced definition of adjacent soft tissue, CT may reveal submandibular salivary gland tissue extending into the lingual bone depressions (Figs 40-4 and 40-5).

The ALMBD may be superimposed on the roots of incisors, canines, and premolars (mimicking a periapical lesion) or may occur in an interradicular location (Fig 40-6). The rare MRBD often appears more circular on radiographs than do the LMBDs and is localized posterior to the mandibular lingual foramen, just below and inferior to the neck of the condyle (Fig 40-7).

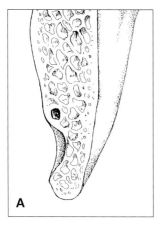
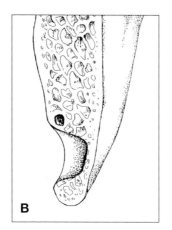
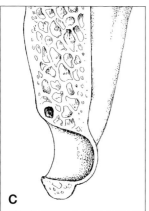
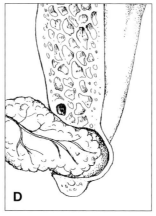
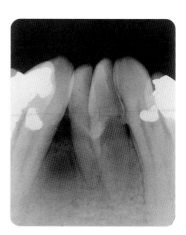

Fig 40-5 Schematic drawing of the development of a PLMBD (modified from Ariji et al[7]). The depression develops from a shallow erosion (A) to a deep cavity (B and C) caused by pressure resorption from a lobe of the submandibular salivary gland (D).

Fig 40-6 Intraoral radiograph showing an ALMBD situated interradicularly between the mandibular right lateral incisor and canine.

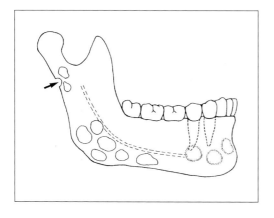

Fig 40-7 Schematic illustration of the location and shape of the PLMBD and ALMBD. Note the depression interrupting the dorsal border of the ramus (MRBD, *arrow*).

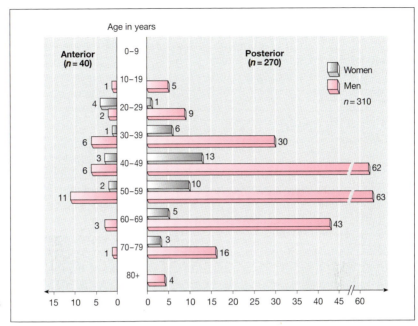

Fig 40-8 Age distribution of ALMBDs (*n*=40) and PLMBDs (*n*=270). Note the peak in the 5th to 6th decades in men.

3. Epidemiological data

3.1 Prevalence, incidence, and relative frequency

According to Samson et al,[10] the prevalence of PLMBDs varies between 0.10% and 0.48% when based on clinical material. Studies involving dry mandibles (archaeological material) give a higher prevalence rate (between 0.66% and 3.84%); this is not surprising since incipient "lesions" that are not evident radiographically are often not detected in clinical materials. From 42,600 orthopantomograms,[3] 65 cases of PLMBDs (prevalence, 0.15%) and 4 ALMBDs (prevalence, 0.009%) were detected. It has been shown that to demonstrate a lesion in bone radiographically, the volume of mineralized matter must be reduced by 12%.[11,12] As pathologic processes are not involved in the pathogenesis of the LMBD, the pressure resorption caused by a salivary gland lobe ad-

jacent to the mandibular bone obviously takes several years to produce a 12% reduction in the volume of mineralized bone mass. However, this fits well with the fact that LMBDs are rarely diagnosed (radiographically) before the age of 40 years.

3.2 Age

Age distribution at the time of diagnosis is shown in Fig 40-8 (range, 11 to 87 years; *n* = 310). There is a significant peak in the 5th to 6th decades for PLMBDs in men. There are still too few cases of the ALMBD to give a trend in age distribution. Of the 13 cases of MRBDs reported so far, 6 were clinical cases[4,5] with a mean age of 48.0 years.

3.3 Gender

The male:female ratio for PLMBD cases (*n*=270) was 6:1, indicating a strong male

355

predominance. The corresponding ratio for ALMBD cases (*n*=40) was 3:1. Presently, there are only 13 reported cases (all of them in men) of the MRBD; 6 were clinical cases as mentioned earlier, and 7 were reported in archaeological material (dried mandibles).[6]

3.4 Location

The PLMBD occurs between the angle of the mandible and the first molar, below the inferior alveolar canal. A detailed analysis of the relationship of PLMBDs to both the inferior alveolar canal and the lower border of the mandible can be found in a report by Chen and Ohba.[13] The ALMBD has appeared in every lingual mandibular location approximated by the sublingual salivary gland, from the central incisor to the second premolar, above the mylohyoid muscle. The ALMBD has well-defined sclerotic borders on plain radiographs less often than do PLMBDs and thus is more difficult to diagnose. The location of the MRBD is shown in Fig 40-7.

4. Pathogenesis

Since the LMBD was first described 60 years ago, there has been a lot of speculation concerning its etiology/pathogenesis. Stafne[1] proposed that the radiolucencies represent areas of Meckel's cartilage that failed to ossify. Peterson,[14] the first to explore such a depression surgically, found that the area was devoid of content, supporting Stafne's concept of a congenital origin. However, the congenital theory is unlikely since no such occurrence has been documented in children under the age of 11 years. In fact, Stafne abandoned the congenital hypothesis and proposed that the lesion was developmental

in origin when he and Tolman[15] reported two cases in which the radiolucencies developed after middle age.

Fordyce[16] was the first author to describe the presence of salivary gland tissue in the radiolucencies of PLMBDs after doing biopsies on two cases; he suggested that the cause is inclusion of salivary gland tissue within the mandible during ossification. He further suggested the use of sialography in investigating such lesions. Kay,[17] in reviewing dry skull specimens, proposed that the depression was caused by abnormal vascular pressure in the facial artery as it pursues its course over the inferior border of the mandible, thereby producing necrosis and resorption of bone similar to that of an aortic aneurysm causing resorption of the ribs. Lello and Makek[18] argued that the defect was a result of ischemia due to the combined effect of unfavorable hemodynamics of the facial artery and the degenerative arterial change in middle age. These ideas have not yet been substantiated.

Surgical exploration and biopsy results from various authors have yielded equivocal results. The majority of reports described salivary gland tissue with a few yielding lymphatic tissue, muscle, and blood vessels; some were devoid of contents. Simpson[19] reported on a PLMBD containing a pleomorphic adenoma, but the only documentation presented—an out-of-focus photomicrograph—is not convincing. The diverse results of surgery and biopsy may be explained by the fact that surgeons have simply displaced the contents of the defect and have taken biopsies from tissues adjacent to the bone depression.

The present theory is that the LMBD in its various subtypes is caused by a hyperplastic (or hypertrophic) lobe or an aberrant lobe of the sublingual (ALMBD), submandibular (PLMBD), or parotid salivary glands (MRBD), leading to focal atrophy or resorption in response to pressure. As pointed out by Sandy and Williams,[20] "when the mobility of the floor of the mouth is considered, it is perhaps surprising that the gland remains in close proximity to the mandible for sufficiently long periods to cause resorption." It is, however, well known that with increasing age, the major salivary glands are the sites of nonspecific (lymphocytic) inflammatory infiltrations with resulting fibrosis, hypertrophy, and hyperplasia of varying intensity. These processes gradually change the consistency of the glands from a soft to a fibrous, and sometimes quite hard, tissue mass. In youth and middle age, pressure exerted by a fibrous gland on the mandibular bone may be sufficiently intense over time to produce focal bone resorption. However, it should be added that there is a lack of substantiation evidence for this phenomenon.

Support of an explanation involving local resorption of an earlier intact inner cortical plate was supplied by Harvey and Noble.[21] These authors made a histologic examination of PLMBDs diagnosed in dry mandibles and found that the surface of the depressions showed an osteoclastic resorption in all six cases examined. They also presented evidence in two cases for active resorption of bone with nearby regions of bone deposition, the typical response of bone to an expanding lesion. These observations strongly favor the conclusion that the depressions develop after initial ossification of the mandible.

Individuals with LMBDs who have been followed with periodical radiographic examination for some years have shown no change in the size or shape of the mandibular depressions. However, Oikarinen and Julku,[22] who studied 10 cases of PLMBDs, found that the largest depressions were seen in the oldest of the series. It seems the focal bone resorption that eventually produced the depressions diagnosed radiologically in clinical material (in the majority of cases from dry mandible material) is clearly visible around the age of 35 to 40 years. Obviously, it takes another 10 years before the reduction in mineralized bone volume reaches a stage where the depressions become evident radiographically—that is, when they are quite advanced. (For a more detailed account of the etiology/pathogenesis of LMBDs, see the review by Philipsen et al.[3])

5. Pathology

5.1 Macroscopy

The LMBD varies in size from a few millimeters across to 35 x 20 mm or (occasionally) more.

5.2 Microscopy

5.2.1 Histologic definition

The LMBD and MRBD are not included in any of the World Health Organization (WHO) classifications. The present authors define these defects as follows:
Bone depressions with various locations in the mandible; as such, they are not characterized by histologic features apart from the fact that the surface of the depressions show osteoclastic activity. If meticulous surgical interventions and biopsy procedures can be performed, the depressions are seen to "contain" normal, hyperplastic, or hypertrophic salivary gland tissue from the sublingual, submandibular, or parotid glands, respectively.

6. Notes on treatment and recurrence rate

Since LMBDs have been shown to be anatomic rather than pathologic in origin, the present authors support the conservative use of knowledge-based radiologic diagnosis with appropriate clinical follow-up rather than surgical biopsy. With the aid of CT, CT sialography, and MRI, surgery can be avoided. The clinical significance of these bony depressions is that they must be differentiated from other lesions that may require treatment.

It seems irrelevant to discuss recurrence rate when dealing with LMBDs.

References

1. Stafne EC. Bone cavities situated near the angle of the mandible. J Am Dent Assoc 1942;29:1969–1972.

2. Richard EL, Ziskind J. Aberrant salivary gland tissue in mandible. Oral Surg Oral Med Oral Pathol 1957;10:1086–190.

3. Philipsen HP, Takata T, Reichart PA, Sato S, Suei Y. The lingual and buccal mandibular bone depression: A review based on 583 cases from a world-wide literature survey, including 69 new cases from Japan. Dentomaxillofac Radiol 2002;31:281–290.

4. Wolf J. Bone defects in mandibular ramus resembling developmental bone cavity (Stafne). Proc Finn Dent Soc 1985;81:215–221.

5. Barker GR. A radiolucency of the ascending ramus of the mandible associated with invested parotid salivary gland material and analogous with a Stafne bone cavity. Br J Oral Maxillofac Surg 1988;26:81–84.

6. Mann RW, Shields ED. Cavitation defects on the lingual ramus: A further expression of Stafne's defect. J Craniofac Genet Dev Biol 1992;12:167–173.

7. Ariji E, Fujiwara N, Tabata O, et al. Stafne's bone cavity. Classification based on outline and content determined by computed tomography. Oral Surg Oral Med Oral Pathol 1993;76:375–380.

8. Slasky BS, Bar-Ziv J. Lingual mandibular bone defects: CT in the buccolingual plane. J Comput Assist Tomogr 1996;20:439–443.

9. Graham RM, Duncan KA, Needham G. The appearance of Stafne's idiopathic bone cavity on magnetic resonance imaging. Dentomaxillofac Radiol 1997;26:74–75.

10. Samson J, Carlino P, di Felice R, Fiore-Donno G. Inclusioni intramandibolari di tessuto ghiandolare salivare. Minerva Stomatol 1990;39:573–585.

11. Bender IB. Factors influencing radiographic appearance of bony lesions. J Endod 1982;8:161–170.

12. Leff GS, Schwartz SF, del Rio CE. Xeroradiographic interpretation of experimental lesions. J Endod 1984;10:188–198.

13. Chen CY, Ohba T. An analysis of radiological findings of Stafne's idiopathic bone cavity. Dentomaxillofac Radiol 1981;10:18–23.

14. Peterson LW. Cystic cavity in the mandible: Report of a case. J Oral Surg 1944;2:182–187.

15. Tolman DE, Stafne EC. Developmental bone defects of the mandible. Oral Surg Oral Med Oral Pathol 1967;24:488–490.

16. Fordyce GL. The probable nature of so-called latent haemorrhagic cysts of the mandible. Br Dent J 1956;101:40–42.

17. Kay LW. Some anthropologic investigations of interest to oral surgeons. Int J Oral Surg 1974;3:363–379.

18. Lello GE, Makek M. Stafne's mandibular lingual cortical defect. J Maxillofac Surg 1985;13:172–176.

19. Simpson W. A Stafne's mandibular defect containing a pleomorphic adenoma. J Oral Surg 1965;23:553–556.

20. Sandy JR, Williams DM. Anterior salivary gland inclusion in the mandible: Pathological entity or anatomical variant? Br J Oral Surg 1981;19:223–229.

21. Harvey W, Noble HW. Defects on the lingual surface of the mandible near the angle. Br J Oral Surg 1968;6:75–83.

22. Oikarinen VJ, Julku M. An orthopantomographic study of developmental mandibular bone defects (Stafne's idiopathic bone cavities). Int J Oral Surg 1974;3:71–76.

Chapter 41

Focal Marrow-containing Jaw Cavity (Focal Osteoporotic Bone Marrow Defect)

1. Terminology

The focal osteoporotic bone marrow defect, first described by Cahn in 1954,[1] is an uncommon and entirely innocuous jaw condition or cavity. It represents a focal radiolucent process accompanied by proliferation of red or fatty bone marrow. The terminology has varied over the years and has included *osteoporotic marrow defect of the jaw,*[2] *hematopoietic defect of the jaw,*[3] and *focal osteoporotic bone marrow defect of the jaw*[4]—the latter term is the most commonly used. Hematopoietic bone marrow in adults is normally found in the region of the mandibular angle, the maxillary tuberosity, and the condylar process. The bone marrow may be stimulated in response to unusual demands for increased blood cell production, and in such instances, the hyperplastic marrow may extend between adjacent trabeculae, producing "osteoporosis" and even a thinning of the cortex.

The bone resorption associated with red marrow hyperplasia was first demonstrated by Box[5,6] in the early 1930s in human jaw material and in the mandibles of rabbits that had been made anemic by repeated bleedings. In 1993, Reichart et al[7] performed a literature review of 278 cases and added 27 cases of their own, bringing the total number at the time to 305 cases. The authors suggested what they considered a more appropriate term: *focal marrow-containing jaw cavity* (FMJC). The clinical importance of FMJCs is that, in dental radiographs, they closely simulate other lesions which may require urgent therapy. This is the reason the FMJC should be included in the diagnostic armamentarium of all clinicians interpreting dental radiographs and also why an exact diagnosis should be established by histologic means.

2. Clinical and radiologic profile

The FMJC is generally asymptomatic and usually occurs in edentulous mandibular molar regions where extractions or surgical interventions have been performed. Lipani et al[3] and Schneider et al[8] reported that 87.5% and 80%, respectively, of their cases occurred in edentulous areas. The condition is found in middle-aged patients and appears to have a strong female predominance. It is often diagnosed by chance, almost always from radiographic findings.

Radiographically, the FMJC presents as an irregular round or oval radiolucency, varying in size from 8 to 40 mm horizontally and from 6 to 20 mm vertically (Figs 41-1 and 41-2). According to Makek and Lello,[9] the anterior border is usually well delineated and may even appear sclerotic, while the posterior border is usually poorly delineated. How-

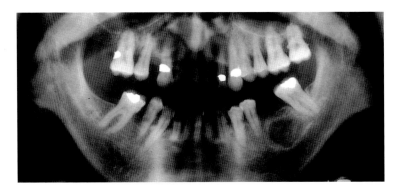

Fig 41-1 Orthopantomogram of a 49-year-old woman with an FMJC in the edentulous mandibular left first molar area. The first molar was extracted 7 years previously. The cavity is well delineated.

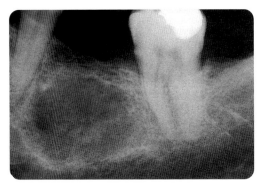

Fig 41-2 Intraoral radiograph of the FMJC shown in Fig 41-1. Note that the delineation of the cavity is not as evident as in the orthopantomogram.

ever, most authors agree that the radiologic features vary considerably, and the radiographic appearance of the FMJC is not sufficiently characteristic to permit an unequivocal diagnosis to be established. The bone cavity may be structureless, or definite intralumenal trabeculations may be present. All mandibular cases have been found above the inferior alveolar canal.

3. Epidemiological data

3.1 Prevalence, incidence, and relative frequency

No data are available for FMJCs.

3.2 Age

Based on the pooled data from six series of FMJCs[2-4,7,9,10] age at the time of diagnosis for 277 cases is shown in Fig 41-3. There is a marked female peak in the 4th and 5th decades. The mean ages given in four of the six studies differed only slightly and were as follows: 42 years (men and women)[4]; 41.3 years (women) and 45.5 years (men)[2]; 42 years (men and women)[10]; and 43 years (men and women).[3] The mean age for 42 cases of FMJCs retrieved from individual data in reports by Lipani et al[3] and unpublished data from Reichart et al[7] was 40.2 years (range, 25 to 71 years). The fact that most cases are diagnosed by chance and are asymptomatic makes it likely that age at the time of diagnosis is probably not indicative of age at onset.

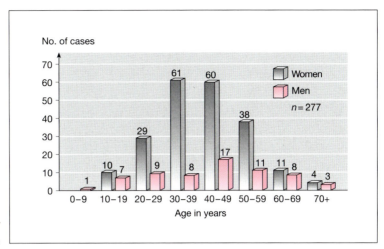

No. of cases

Fig 41-3 Age and gender distribution of 277 FMJCs.

3.3 Gender

The male:female ratio of 277 cases[2-4,7,9,10] (see Fig 41-3) was 1:3.3, confirming a clear female predominance (76.9%).

3.4 Location

The distribution of FMJCs according to location within the jaw (Fig 41-4) is compiled from data retrived from the same six publications mentioned earlier.[2-4,7,9,10] Figure 41-4 shows the greatest occurrence of this condition in the molar and ramus regions of the mandible (79.6%), followed by the premolar region of the mandible (8.5%) and the maxillary tuberosity (6.1%). The maxilla:mandible ratio was 1:9.5.

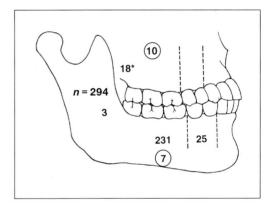

Fig 41-4 Topographic distribution of 294 FMJCs. Circled numbers indicate unspecified sites within the maxilla and mandible. Asterisk indicates maxillary tuberosity.

4. Pathogenesis

Several theories have been advanced concerning the pathogenesis of this lesion.[7,10] The theory proposing an aberrant form of bone healing with the focal formation of hematopoietic bone marrow seems the most plausible, because the FMJC occurs most often in regions where previous extractions or surgical interventions have been performed 1 year (or more) prior to diagnosis of the cavity.

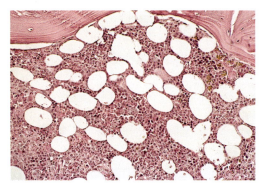

Fig 41-5 Tissue excised from the FMJC shown in Figs 41-1 and 41-2. Normal cellular hematopoietic marrow with scattered fat cell spaces is evident (hematoxylin-eosin [H&E], x160).

5. Pathology

5.1 Microscopy

5.1.1 Histologic definition

The FMJC is *not* included in any of the World Health Organization (WHO) classifications of odontogenic tumors. The definition used by the present authors is as follows:
An intraosseous jaw cavity containing normal erythroid, myeloid, and megakaryocytic bone marrow elements. Scattered fat cells or fat vacuoles may be present.

5.1.2 Histopathologic findings

Standish and Shafer[4] noted that many of their hematopoietic cavities were in premenopausal woman (younger than 50 years) and that the cavities in older women were mainly fatty (Fig 41-5). A large lymphatic follicle containing an active germinal center was an unusual finding in the marrow specimen taken by Syrjänen et al.[11] The authors explained the presence of the germinal center was caused by a coexisting inflammatory process in an adjoining tooth.

6. Notes on treatment and recurrence rate

Therapeutically, no treatment is necessary for FMJCs, provided that the diagnosis is satisfactorily established and routine follow-up care is proposed (no recurrence has been described). The presence of a radiolucency of the nature described here for FMJCs usually leads to an explorative procedure followed by curettage (biopsy) in order to make a definitive diagnosis. In establishing a diagnosis, Syrjänen et al[11] pointed out that the application of fine-needle aspiration cytology should be considered because it is a reliable and technically simple procedure that causes minimal harm to the patient. The irregularity in the trabecular pattern often persists after curettage. In addition, the odontogenic keratocyst, residual cyst, and even ameloblastoma are lesions that have been brought forward in a differential diagnostic context.[7] Most essential for differential diagnosis of "osteoporotic" defects or cavities is a thorough and comprehensive medical history. It is particularly important in women 40 years or older—in whom metastatic lesions of the breast, lung, and parathyroid are not uncommon—and in posthysterectomy patients, whose jaws frequently have an osteoporotic appearance.[3]

Lastly, it should be pointed out that the FMJC has been described as a feature of some patients with sickle cell anemia.[12] It is therefore recommended that patients with diagnosed or suspected FMJCs receive a hematologic examination.

References

1. Cahn LR. Comment on hematopoietic marrow in the jaws. Oral Surg 1954;7:790.

2. Crawford BE, Weathers DR. Osteoporotic marrow defects of the jaws. J Oral Surg 1970;28:600–603.

3. Lipani CS, Natiella JR, Greene GW. The hematopoietic defect of the jaws: A report of sixteen cases. J Oral Pathol 1982;11:411–416.

4. Standish SM, Shafer WG. Focal osteoporotic bone marrow defects of the jaws. J Oral Surg 1962;20:123–128.

5. Box HK. Red bone marrow in human jaws. Can Dent Res Found Bull 1933;20:3–31.

6. Box HK. Bone resorption in red marrow hyperplasia in human jaws. Can Dent Res Found Bull 1936;21:3–27.

7. Reichart PA, Hjørting-Hansen E, Philipsen HP, Martinez MG. Fokale Knochenmarkskavität der Kiefer. Mund Kiefer Gesichtschir 1993;17:310–312.

8. Schneider LC, Mesa ML, Fraenkel D. Osteoporotic bone marrow defect: Radiographic features and pathogenic factors. Oral Surg Oral Med Oral Pathol 1988;65:127–129.

9. Makek M, Lello GE. Focal osteoporotic bone marrow defects of the jaws. J Oral Maxillofac Surg 1986;44:268–273.

10. Barker BF, Jensen JL, Howell FV. Focal osteoporotic bone marrow defects of the jaws. An analysis of 197 new cases. Oral Surg Oral Med Oral Pathol 1974;38:404–413.

11. Syrjänen SM, Syrjänen KJ, Lamberg MA, Saino P. Focal osteoporotic bone marrow defects of the jaws. Report of a case and survey of the literature. Proc Finn Dent Soc 1980;76:219–224.

12. Sanner JR, Ramin JE. Osteoporotic, haematopoietic mandibular marrow defects: An osseous manifestation of sickle cell anaemia. J Oral Surg 1977;35:986–988.

Section Nine

Nonodontogenic Jaw Tumor of Neurocrest Origin

Introduction

This section comprises only one chapter describing a fairly rare, benign tumor, the melanotic neuroectodermal tumor of infancy (MNTI). Although it is considered nonodontogenic, this tumor was included in the 1992 WHO classification of odontogenic tumors. Recent ultrastructural and histochemical studies indicate a neural crest origin. It should be noted that in the forthcoming WHO volume *Tumours of the Head and Neck*, MNTI is excluded from chapter 6 (Odontogenic Tumors) but is described in chapter 1 (Nasal Cavity, authored by S. B. Kapadia). The MNTIs are included in the present book mainly for differential diagnostic purposes.

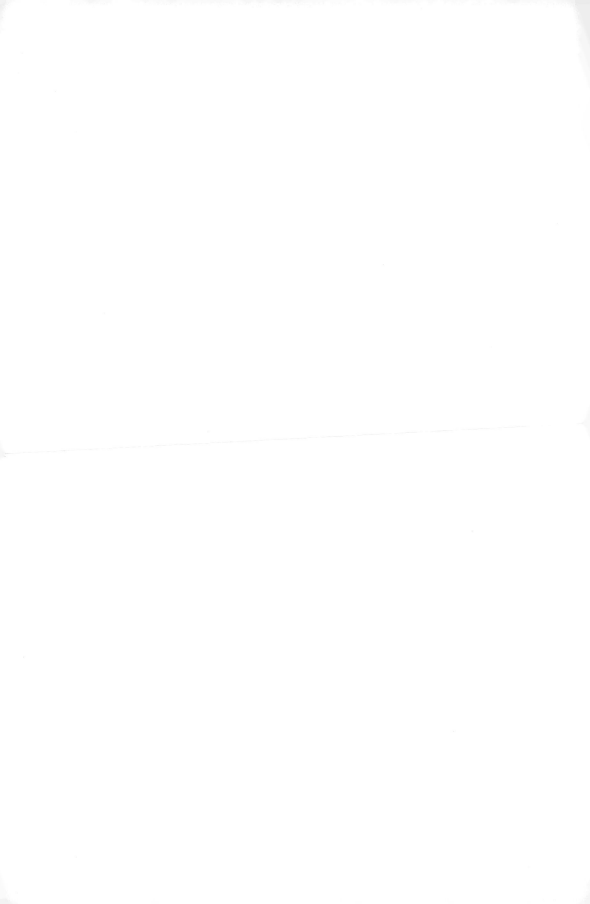

Chapter 42

Melanotic Neuroectodermal Tumor of Infancy

1. Terminology

The melanotic neuroectodermal tumor of infancy (MNTI) is a fairly rare, benign, pigmented lesion that commonly occurs in the anterior maxilla of infants younger than 1 year and mainly in the first 6 months of life. The tumor was first described by Krompecher in 1918[1] as a *congenital melanocarcinoma.* The multiplicity of terms that have been used throughout the years mirrors the confusing and conflicting pathogenetic theories that have been advocated for this lesion: *melanotic epithelial odontome, melanotic progonoma, pigmented adamantinoma, melanotic ameloblastoma, congenital pigmented epulis, retinal anlage tumor, melanocytoma,* and *pigmented neuroectodermal tumor of infancy.* A complete list of synonyms can be found in a report by Nozicka and Spacek.[2] The current consensus favors the use of the term *melanotic neuroectodermal tumor of infancy*, a designation accepted by and used in the 1992 World Health Organization (WHO) classification of odontogenic tumors.[3] As the end of 2000, an estimated 250 cases of MNTIs have been published in the literature.

2. Clinical and radiologic profile

The MNTI usually presents as a rapidly enlarging exophytic mass most often localized in the anterior alveolar ridge of the maxilla of an infant. Lesions are occasionally described in the mandible (Fig 42-1) and in extragnathic sites such as brain, epididymis, uterus, ovary, and mediastinum. The MNTI usually presents as a single lesion, but multiple lesions have been reported.[4,5] The lesion often appears to have irregular pigmentation, although this pigmentation is not always clinically evident. The nontender growth is of a rubbery consistency, may con-

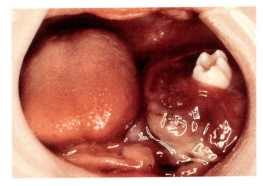

Fig 42-1 Intraoral appearance of an MNTI in a 5-month-old girl. The presence of the tumor has resulted in premature eruption of the mandibular left second deciduous molar. Note the brownish-blue pigmentation of the tumor surface. (Courtesy of Prof A. Eckardt, Hannover, Germany.)

367

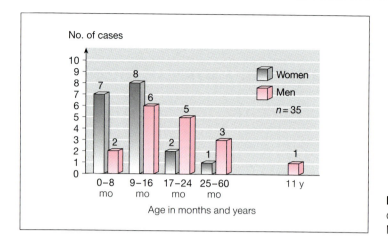

No. of cases

Women
Men
$n = 35$

Age in months and years

Fig 42-2 Age and gender distribution of 35 cases of MNTI.

tain prematurely erupted or displaced primary teeth and may have an ulcerated surface. Most tumors measure from 1 to 4 cm at their greatest diameter. The case of a gigantiform MNTI occurring in a 7-month-old girl and measuring 18 cm in greatest diameter was recently published by Bouckaert and Raubenheimer.[6]

The typical radiographic appearance of the MNTI is that of an intrabony radiolucent lesion with poorly demarcated borders, presumably caused by rapid growth and a tendency to locally invade bone. The area of bone destruction may be traversed by bone septa. Teeth involved in the lesion may appear to be floating within the radiolucent area of the tumor because they are displaced from their normal development sites. This radiographic appearance can understandably mislead a clinician into making a provisional diagnosis of malignancy. Another potentially misleading feature is a common osteogenic reaction that exhibits a "sunray" radiographic pattern which may be mistaken for an osteosarcoma. Computed tomography and magnetic resonance imagery[7,8] are able to define the extent of the lesion precisely, localize possible multiple sites, and

thus greatly assist in surgical planning. These radiographic methods subject very young patients to significant radiation exposure, but they can provide important information and are diagnostically superior to other routine imaging methods.

3. Epidemiological data

3.1 Prevalence, incidence, and relative frequency

No data are available.

3.2 Age

Figure 42-2 shows the age distribution of 35 MNTI cases. The data are retrieved from a review of cases published between 1980 and 1992.[8] The lesion was usually not present at birth, and 85.7% of the cases occurred before the age of 24 weeks (6 months).

3.3 Gender

Male and female infants are almost equally affected (see Fig 42-2).

3.4 Location

According to pooled data from two literature surveys[8,9] comprising 237 cases of MNTIs from all sites published between 1918 and 1997, 61% of cases were located in the maxilla; 13% were located in the skull (particularly in the anterior fontanelle); and only 6% were found in the mandible. The remaining cases (20%) were found in other extragnathic sites. The reason for the maxillary predominance is unknown.

4. Pathogenesis

Five principal theories regarding the origin of MNTIs have arisen from the cases reported in the literature. They may be described as (1) malignant transformation of odontogenic epithelium,[1] (2) ameloblastoma variant,[10] (3) origin from Jacobson's vomeronasal organ,[11] (4) origin from retinal anlage (progonoma),[12] and (5) origin from neuroectodermal rests.[13] Little if any evidence exists to support the first four theories, whereas the fifth has considerable merit. Evidence for this derivation stems from tissue culture and immunohistochemical and ultrastructural studies,[13] and the neural crest is currently the most commonly accepted tissue of origin for MNTIs.

5. Pathology

5.1 Macroscopy

The consistency of the surgical specimen is fibrous or rubbery and has a dark blue or brownish color on the cut surface.

5.2 Microscopy

5.2.1 Histologic definitions

According to the 1992 WHO classification, an MNTI is a tumor that "consists of varying proportions of two cell types—epithelium-like cells, often arranged in strands, and small darkly staining lymphocyte-like cells—in a cellular, fibrous stroma. Melanin is found within the epithelium-like cells and to a lesser extent within the lymphocyte-like cells."

The definition used by the present authors is as follows:
A tumor, which is usually unencapsulated or partially encapsulated, demonstrates a characteristic biphasic cell pattern composed of irregular nests of cells separated by a dense fibrous stroma (Fig 42-3). One consists of

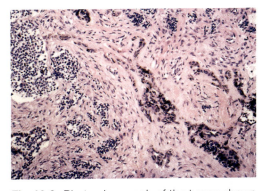

Fig 42-3 Photomicrograph of the tumor shown in Fig 42-1 showing the biphasic cell pattern of pigmented epithelium-like cells and clusters of smaller, nonpigmented neuroblast-like cells (hematoxylin-eosin [H&E], x100). (Courtesy of Prof A. Eckardt, Hannover, Germany.)

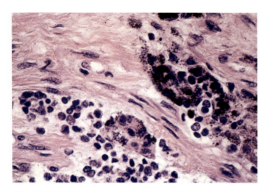

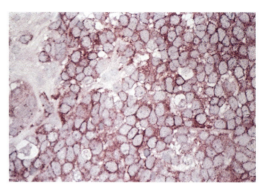

Fig 42-4 Higher magnification of the same tumor showing the pigmented cells and scattered smaller neuroblast- or lymphocyte-like cells (H&E, x250). (Courtesy of Prof A. Eckardt, Hannover, Germany.)

Fig 42-5 A cluster of neuroblast-like cells showing strong positivity for neuron-specific enolase (NSE, x400). (Courtesy of Prof A. Eckardt, Hannover, Germany.)

loose groups of large and epithelium-like cells usually exhibiting abundant brown pigment that is positive for melanin. The second cell type consists of clusters of poorly cohesive nests of smaller, non-melanin-containing ovoid cells with minimal cytoplasm and a hyperchromatic nucleus, resembling neuroblast- or lymphocyte-like cells are present in the alveolar spaces or as isolated nests in the stroma (Fig 42-4). Nuclear atypia and mitotic figures are noticeably absent. Invasion of tumor cells into possibly existing tooth germs may occur.

5.2.2 Histochemical/immunohistochemical findings

Immunohistochemically, the large melanin-containing epithelium-like cells react with a monoclonal antibody directed against anti-human melanoma HMB-45.[9] The same authors also found that the small lymphocyte-like cells were positive for neuron-specific enolase (NSE) (Fig 42-5). Antibodies directed against S-100 protein did not label the tumor cells. Bouckaert and Raubenheimer[6] confirmed these findings and also found that

vimentin was focally expressed in the pigmented cells. De Souza et al[14] studied the immunohistochemical expression of several cell cycle proteins (p53, MDM-2, cyclin D1, cyclin A, and proliferating cell nuclear antigen [PCNA]) in three cases of MNTI. A diffuse immunoreactivity of the melanin-containing cells for MDM-2 and a complete absence of p53 expression were found. These findings suggest that the large epithelium-like cells are the proliferative element of the tumor and that MDM-2 protein may be important for MNTI development.

Khoddami et al[15] performed an immunohistochemical, molecular genetic, and fluorescence in situ hybridization (FISH) study with the purpose of elucidating a possible relationship between MNTIs and other pediatric small cell tumors with neuroectodermal features (such as neuroblastomas, Ewing sarcomas/peripheral primitive neuroectodermal tumors, and desmoplastic small round cell tumors). The melanin-containing large cells showed strong reactivity for low-molecular keratin, epithelial membrane antigen, and HMB-45 and weak positivity for NSE. The smaller neuroblastic cells were strongly positive for NSE. Neither cell type manifested S-100 protein reactivity. According to the authors, the molecular genetics and FISH tests showed that there is no basis to link MNTIs with any of the other small cell tumors with neuroectodermal features.

5.2.3 Ultrastructural findings

Several reports give details about the ultrastructure of the *benign* melanotic neuroectodermal tumor of infancy, as well as the *malignant* variant.[22,23] All except Palacios[22] describe three basic cellular constituents: a pigmented cell, a small immature neuroblast-like cell, and fibroblasts. Cutler et al[16] detailed the intercellular junctions between tumor cells, the occurrence of cilia and melanocyte filaments, and patterns of melanin granule formation—all findings that are compatible with cells of neural crest origin.

5.2.4 Tissue culture findings

The predominance of melanin-containing dendritic cells in culture from MNTIs was reported by Claman et al,[18] who found that this was the only cell type present after prolonged passage in vitro. In their study on a case of malignant MNTI, Dehner et al[23] placed samples of the original maxillary tumor in tissue culture, but a fibroblast growth was the only result. In contrast, tissue explants from the two recurrences yielded three cell types in vitro after 14 days' growth: pigment-producing cells, small round cells with processes consistent with neuritis, and bipolar fibroblasts.

5.2.5 Biochemical findings

Borello and Gorlin[13] reported high urinary vanillyl mandelic acid (VMA) levels in a patient with an MNTI. The VMA levels returned to normal after excision of the tumor. In pa-

tients with MNTIs, VMA is believed to be strongly circumstantial evidence of a neuroectodermal origin. However, most patients with MNTIs show normal levels of VMA.[8,24-27] The fact that Dehner at al[23] reported elevated VMA levels in a malignant transformed MNTI, whereas other malignant cases were not associated with its elevation,[24,26] seems to indicate that VMA levels have no relation to biologic behavior.

6. Notes on treatment and recurrence rate

Although the MNTI displays a disturbingly rapid growth and invasive radiographic appearance, it has a benign course in most cases. There is a 15% propensity for local recurrence and a malignancy rate of about 7%.[21] The few available studies using flow cytometry analysis[21,28] suggest that tumors with aneuploid cells may recur more often than those without. The need for aggressive surgery is usually not advocated for MNTIs. The recommended treatment involves conservative excision, enucleation, and curettage. Conservative local excision of recurrent tumors is almost invariably curative. However, some recurrent cases, particularly multifocal MNTIs, may require a wider excision. The apparent success of a conservative approach to surgical removal does not reduce the need for regular follow-up examinations, because the potential for recurrence still remains.[29]

References

1. Krompecher E. Zur Histogenese and Morphologie der Adamantinome und sonstiger Kiefergeschwülste. Beitr Pathol Anat 1918;64:165–197.

2. Nozicka Z, Spacek J. Melanotic neuroectodermal tumor of infancy with highly differentiated neural component: Light and electron microscopic study. Acta Neuropathol (Berl) 1978;44:229–233.

3. Kramer IRH, Pindborg JJ, Shear M. Histological Typing of Odontogenic Tumours. 2d ed. Berlin: Springer-Verlag, 1992.

4. Steinberg B, Shuler C, Wilson S. Melanotic neuroectodermal tumor of infancy: Evidence for multicentricity. Oral Surg Oral Med Oral Pathol 1988;66:666–669.

5. Pontius EC, Dziabis MD, Foster JA. Multicentric melanoameloblastoma of the maxilla. Cancer 1965;18:381–387.

6. Bouckaert MMR, Raubenheimer EJ. Gigantiform melanotic neuroectodermal tumor of infancy. Oral Surg Oral Med Oral Pathol Oral Radiol Endod 1998;86:569–572.

7. Atkinson GO, Davis PC, Patrick LE, et al. Melanotic neuroectodermal tumor of infancy. MR findings and a review of the literature. Pediatr Radiol 1989;20:20–22.

8. Mosby EL, Lowe MW, Cobb CM, Ennis RL. Melanotic neuroectodermal tumor of infancy: Review of the literature and report of a case. J Oral Maxillofac Surg 1992;50:886–894.

9. Hoshina Y, Hamamoto Y, Suzuki I, et al. Melanotic neuroectodermal tumor of infancy in the mandible. Report of a case. Oral Surg Oral Med Oral Pathol Oral Radiol Endod 2000;89:594–599.

10. Kerr DA, Pullon PA. A study of the pigmented tumours of jaws of infants. Oral Surg 1964;18:759–772.

11. Stownes D. A pigmented tumor of infancy: The melanotic progonoma. J Pathol Bacteriol 1957;73:43–51.

12. Halpert B, Patzer R. Maxillary tumor of retinal anlage. Surgery 1947;22:837–841.

13. Borello ED, Gorlin RJ. Melanotic neuroectodermal tumor of infancy—a neoplasm of neural crest origin. Report of a case associated with high urinary excretion of vanilmandelic acid. Cancer 1966;19:196–206.

14. de Souza PEA, Merly F, Maia DMF, et al. Cell cycle-associated proteins in melanotic neuroectodermal tumor of infancy. Oral Surg Oral Med Oral Pathol Oral Radiol Endod 1999;88:466–468.

15. Khoddami M, Squire J, Zielenska M, Thorner P. Melanotic neuroectodermal tumor of infancy: A molecular genetic study. Pediatr Dev Pathol 1998;1:295–299.

16. Cutler LS, Chaudhry AP, Topazian R. Melanotic neuroectodermal tumor of infancy: An ultrastructural study, literature review, and reevaluation. Cancer 1981;48:257–270.

17. Nikai H, Ijuhin N, Yamasaki A, et al. Ultrastructural evidence for neural crest origin of the melanotic neuroectodermal tumor of infancy. J Oral Pathol 1977;6:221–232.

18. Claman LJ, Stetson D, Steinberg B, Shuler CF. Ultrastructural characteristics of a cell line derived from a melanotic neuroectodermal tumor of infancy. J Oral Pathol 1991;20:245–249.

19. Nelson ZL, Newman L, Loukota DM. Melanotic neuroectodermal tumour of infancy: An immunohistochemical and ultrastructural study. Br J Oral Maxillofac Surg 1995;33:375–380.

20. Sousa SOM, Arauno NS, Sesso A, Araujo VC. Immunohistochemical, ultrastructural, and histogenic considerations in a patient with melanotic neuroectodermal tumor of infancy. J Oral Maxillofac Surg 1992;50:186–189.

21. Pettinato G, Manivel JC, d'Amore ES, et al. Melanotic neuroectodermal tumour of infancy: A re-examination of a histogenetic problem based on immunohistochemical, flow cytometric, and ultrastructural study of 10 cases. Am J Surg Pathol 1991;15:233–245.

22. Palacios JJN. Malignant melanotic neuroectodermal tumor. Light and electron microscopic study. Cancer 1980;46:529–536.

23. Dehner LP, Sibley RK, Sauk JJ, et al. Malignant melanotic neuroectodermal tumor of infancy. A clinical, pathologic, ultrastructural and tissue culture study. Cancer 1979;43:1389–1410.

24. Ogata A, Fujioka Y, Nagashima K, et al. Malignant melanotic neuroectodermal tumor of infancy arising from the pineal body. Acta Neuropathol (Berl) 1989;77:654–658.

25. Hupp JR, Topazian RG, Krutchkoff DJ. The melanotic neuroectodermal tumor of infancy. Report of two cases and review of the literature. Int J Oral Surg 1981;10:432–436.

26. Johnson RE, Scheihauer BW, Dahlin DC. Melanotic neuroectodermal tumor of infancy. A review of seven cases. Cancer 1983;52:661–666.

27. Nagase M, Ueda K, Fukushima M, Nakajima T. Recurrent neuroectodermal tumor of infancy: Case report and survey of 16 cases. J Maxillofac Surg 1983;11:131–136.

28. Kapadia S, Frisman D, Hitchcock C, et al. Melanotic neuroectoderrmal tumor of infancy (MNTI), immunohistochemical and flow cytometric study. Mod Pathol 1992;5:71A. Abstract.

29. Demas PN, Braun TW, Nazif MM. Melanotic neuroectodermal tumor of infancy: A report of two cases. J Oral Maxillofac Surg 1992;50:894–898.

Index

375